THE ESSENTIAL BOOK OF TRADITIONAL CHINESE MEDICINE
VOLUME 2: CLINICAL PRACTICE

THE ESSENTIAL BOOK
OF
TRADITIONAL CHINESE
MEDICINE

VOLUME 2: CLINICAL PRACTICE

LIU YANCHI

Translated by

FANG TINGYU *and* CHEN LAIDI

Editorial Consultant: BARBARA GASTEL

New York
COLUMBIA UNIVERSITY PRESS
1988

The illustrations on the jacket and within the text were specially commissioned for this volume and drawn by Cheng Duoduo.

Columbia University Press
New York   Guildford, Surrey

Copyright © 1988 Columbia University Press and
The People's Medical Publishing House

Library of Congress Cataloging-in-Publication Data

Liu, Yen-ch'ih (Liu Yanchi)
The essential book of traditional Chinese medicine.

Includes bibliographies and index.
Contents: v. 1. Theory.   1. Theory—v. 2. Clinical practice.
1. Medicine, Peter.   III. Title. [DNLM: 1. Medicine,
Oriental Traditional—China. WB 50 Chinese.   I. Vian, Kathleen.
II. Eckman, Peter.   III. Title.   [DNLM: 1. Medicine,
Oriental Traditional—China.   WB 50 JC6 L85e]
R601.I713   1987   610   87-10349
ISBN 0-231-06520-5 (set)
ISBN 0-231-06196-X (v. 1)
ISBN 0-231-06518-3 (v.2)

This book is a joint effort of
The People's Medical Publishing House
(Beijing)
and
The United States–China Educational Institute
(San Francisco)

Supported by
The Educational Foundation of America
(Westport, Connecticut)

CONTENTS

FOREWORD

　　中國傳統醫學是中國人民長期與疾病做鬥爭的智慧結晶，內容豐富，源遠流長。它具有獨特的理論體系和豐富的臨床實踐經驗，千百年來爲中華民族的繁衍昌盛做出了貢獻。西方醫藥界不少人士對中國傳統醫學具有濃厚興趣，美中敎育學院、人民衞生出版社、哥倫比亞大學出版社組織了有關專家，合作出版了這本《中醫入門》。這本書肯定會增進西方對中國傳統醫學的瞭解。我祝願通過這樣的橋樑，中美醫學交流將取得巨大成功。

崔月犁
中國衞生部部長

FOREWORD

Traditional Chinese medicine is the crystal of wisdom of the Chinese people in their long period of struggle against diseases. Its content is substantial and it is of long standing and well established. It has its own theoretical system and rich clinical experience, having made contributions to the prosperous growth of the Chinese nation in the past thousands of years. Many of the figures in the Western medical world have found traditional Chinese medicine interesting. The United States–China Educational Institute, the People's Medical Publishing House, and Columbia University Press have solicited a group of experts to publish cooperatively this *Essential Book of Traditional Chinese Medicine*. It is expected that this book will enhance the understanding of traditional Chinese medicine in the Western world. It is hoped that the exchange in medical science between the United States and China will result in great successes through such a bridge.

Cui Yueli
Minister of Public Health,
People's Republic of China

ACKNOWLEDGMENTS

The writing and production of *The Essential Book of Traditional Chinese Medicine* began over six years ago with a decision between the People's Medical Publishing House and the United States–China Educational Institute to cooperate together on this project. But the credit for these two volumes really should be given to all the traditional Chinese medical scholars who have contributed to this extraordinary body of knowledge for over 4,000 years. The Ministry of Public Health of the People's Republic of China should also be acknowledged for their foresight in organizing a system of institutions for the understanding and the development of traditional Chinese medicine.

For over four thousand years, scholars and medical practitioners have documented the ways of maintaining health and treating illness through the use of herbs, acupuncture, and intelligent life-style practices. As early as 4000 B.C., there were legends about Shen Nong, who tasted hundreds of herbs before they were used medicinally. During the third century B.C., the *Classic of Internal Medicine,* an eighteen-volume document, laid the theoretical foundation for traditional Chinese medicine and it is considered to be one of the greatest medical classics in China. Hua Tuo, a renowned surgeon in the third century A.D., was the first practitioner in China to perform operations under local anesthesia. Yang Jizhou, a prominent acupuncturist during the Ming dynasty, compiled the *Compendium of Acupuncture and Moxibustion,* a work that is still revered by modern acupuncturists.

The human body is a fascinating and intricate system and Chinese scholars have long been studying the ways of conceptualizing the body, with its abundance of energy and physiological activities, and of promoting its health. The gathering of information about the functions of the human body and how to treat illnesses for many thousands of years is an impressive accomplishment and it has resulted in traditional Chinese medicine permeating into the consciousness of the Chinese people. It has become a cornerstone in the foundation of Chinese culture. Today, people think about their health as a balance of the person and the environment, the active and the receptive.

In 1954, the Chinese Ministry of Public Health decided to undertake a major effort to systematically organize this body of knowledge and it has resulted in some impressive achievements. Its policy was to combine the resources and experiences of traditional Chinese doctors with those of Chinese scientists and physicians who are trained in Western medicine, and to channel this intellectual energy into developing traditional Chinese medicine. The Chinese Ministry of Public Health broadened its base of information by organizing scholars to research historical documents. Two-year postgraduate training programs in traditional Chinese medicine were designed for Chinese physicians trained in Western medicine. Research scientists were encouraged to investigate specific research agendas related to traditional Chinese medicine and its integration with Western medicine. Finally, the Ministry of Public Health developed a policy to protect and improve the resources of Chinese medicinal herbs.

To implement these policies, the Ministry established a Bureau of Traditional Medicine within its organization and departments of traditional Chinese medicine in every province and autonomous region in China. In the late 1950s, the Academy of Traditional Chinese Medicine was set up in Beijing, and colleges of traditional Chinese medicine and research institutes were organized in most provinces and autonomous regions. Currently, China has 300,000 doctors and paraprofessionals of traditional Chinese medicine. There are more than 1,100 hospitals of traditional Chinese medicine and some 9,000 general hospitals nationwide which have departments of traditional Chinese medicine. Most recently, the Ministry of Public Health announced plans to step up the training of doctors of traditional medicine so that by 1990 there will be three such doctors for every ten thousand people as compared to only one per ten thousand at the moment.

This enormous undertaking by the Ministry of Public Health to develop traditional Chinese medicine is leading to improved health care practices, new scientific breakthroughs, and a greater understanding and interest in this field among people all over the world. To provide Western health practitioners and scientists with updated information about traditional Chinese medicine and to stimulate the integration of traditional Chinese medicine with Western medicine, the People's Medical Publishing House of the Ministry of Public Health and the United States–China Educational Institute decided to cooperate on the production of *The Essential Book of Traditional Chinese Medicine,* volumes 1 and 2.

This project was made possible by a grant from the Educational Foundation of America, and we are deeply appreciative of its support. Producing *The Essential Book of Traditional Chinese Medicine,* volumes 1 and 2, was a major undertaking that could not have been realized without the full support and confidence given to us by Richard and Sharon Ettinger, Cyrus and Elaine Hapood, Barbara Ettinger, Robert Kalinonski, Edward Anderson, Richard Hansen, and the other members of the Board of Trustees of the Educational Foundation of America.

The People's Medical Publishing House was responsible for determining the author to write about the theory and the clinical practice of traditional Chinese medicine. It was also responsible for identifying the experts to do the translation work. The United States–China Educational Institute would edit and, in some cases, would add to, the manuscript in a way that would preserve the intentions of the author while making changes that would help Westerners understand what the author intended. The editing would also preserve the integrity of the Chinese culture represented in the writing and develop a style that is familiar to the Western mind. These were the principles used by the staff of the Institute.

We thought that if information about the theoretical and the practical components of traditional Chinese medicine were presented in a manner that was readily understood in the West, it might enhance the practice of traditional Chinese medicine in the West and foster more interest in the West in cooperative research activities with Chinese scientists. There would also be an opportunity to synthesize the knowledge and experiences of both Chinese and Western medicine, and we were very much interested in encouraging this kind of synthesis.

Over the last five years, the Chinese portion of this project has been administered by Vice-President Wang Shuqi of the People's

Medical Publishing House. After he transferred to the Peking Union Medical College, the project was led by Vice-President Dong Mianguo. Their dedication and untiring energy in solving inevitable problems which arose during our cooperation have impressed the staff of the United States–China Educational Institute. Dr. Liu Yanchi has a distinguished career as associate professor at the Beijing College of Traditional Chinese Medicine. He is currently head of the Teaching Section of Basic Theory of Traditional Chinese Medicine and is on the editing commissions of the *Chinese Medical Encyclopedia* and the *Digest of Traditional Chinese Medicine.* Mr. Fang Tingyu and Ms. Chen Laidi, chosen as the translators, have much experience in translation work. Mr. Xu Wei and Ms. Chang Zexun, editors at the People's Medical Publishing House, provided valuable assistance and carried out their responsibilities remarkably well. Dr. Ou Mujie and Ms. Nissi Wang reviewed the manuscripts and meticulously and conscientiously ensured that the thinking and the clinical practices were written, translated, and edited with accuracy and integrity. Nissi Wang, a Chinese-American at the People's Medical Publishing House in Beijing, has played an invaluable role in the development of these two volumes. In fact, all these scholars at the People's Medical Publishing House and the Beijing College of Traditional Chinese Medicine played a vital role in transmitting the knowledge and experiences of traditional Chinese medicine to the West.

The main task of the Institute was to communicate effectively in English the concepts and the treatment modalities of traditional Chinese medicine. This was an extremely complicated process and required agile and creative minds with sensitivity to both cultures. Our editors and collaborators needed to understand the Chinese way of thinking and to communicate these concepts in a format that was easily understood in the West. We were fortunate to have Kathleen Vian, Ph.D., and Dr. Peter Eckman, who collaborated with Dr. Liu Yanchi in the writing and editing of the first volume, on the theoretical aspects of traditional Chinese medicine. Dr. Vian applied her unique sensitivity to and understanding of traditional Chinese medicine and Chinese culture, and she effectively communicated these concepts in the English language. Dr. Peter Eckman, a graduate of New York University, where he received both an M.D. and a Ph.D. in physiology, has devoted over ten years to the study, practice, and teaching of traditional Chinese medicine, which is now the focus of his professional life. The editorial consultant for Dr. Liu's volume on clinical practice was Barbara Gastel, M.D., M.P.H. Dr. Gastel has distinguished herself as a scientific writer who spent two years in Beijing as a Fellow of the United States–China Educational Institute teaching scientific writing and communication to medical scholars at Beijing Medical University and at the *Chinese Medical Journal.* Prior to her work in Beijing, she was an assistant professor in the Writing Program of the Massachusetts Institute of Technology. While Dr. Gastel was in Beijing, she worked with Ms. Nissi Wang and the staff of the People's Medical Publishing House in editing volume 2 of *The Essential Book of Traditional Chinese Medicine.* Drs. Vian and Gastel are some of the most intellectually talented writers that we have had the privilege to know, and they have an abundance of respect for traditional Chinese medicine and culture. They spent many hours writing and rewriting this manuscript. To them, we express our indebtedness and our appreciation.

Early in our discussions with the administrators of the People's Medical Publishing House, we realized the importance of communicating the concepts of traditional Chinese medicine through visual means. The Institute sought the assistance of Mr. Cheng Duoduo, who is a talented painter from Shanghai. We also sought out the assistance of Mrs. Sally Yu Leung, a sensitive and thoughtful Chinese-American, who provided unending assistance in the development of the illustrations. Mr. Cheng and Mrs. Yu Leung were attracted to the issue of how to communicate traditional Chinese concepts to Westerners and they accepted this assignment with a great deal of interest. All the illustrations were painted with a Chinese brush technique called *bai miao* or Chinese brush-line drawing. As you will see, the beginning of each chapter has Mr. Cheng's illustrations which summarize the concept of each chapter. He paints with unusual sensitivity and imagination, two qualities which are so essential to promoting communication and understanding about traditional Chinese medicine.

Many of us who have worked on this project were inspired to initiate the production of *The Essential Book of Traditional Chinese Medicine* by our association with Jennifer Mei, Dr. Sadja Greenwood, and Dr. Ho Wingtong at the Min An Health Center. Min An is a community health facility located in San Francisco's Chinatown. At Min An, Western and traditional Chinese practitioners work side by side. Together they provide a variety of health services, including women's health, family practice medicine, pediatrics, internal medicine, herbal medicine, acupuncture, general dentistry and nutrition, and exercise counseling. The patients who visit Min An have the opportunity to view their health and illness from both these perspectives. They may choose their therapies from either or both traditions.

In addition to the fellows of the Institute, there were members of the Institute's Board of Directors, Board of Advisers, and members of our network who played an important part in this project. Their assistance enhanced the quality of our work and they are: Jane Lurie, Charlotte Calhoun, Professor James Cahill, Dr. Stella Ling, Dr. Jerome Steiner, Dr. May Tung, Dr. Thomas Killip, and many other health professionals at major medical centers in the United States. While most of the final copies of the manuscripts were typed in China, there were many drafts that were prepared here at the Institute. We are deeply appreciative of the assistance of Dr. Wayne Payne, Judith Peck, and Faith Tan.

It was a great experience for us to work with Susan Koscielniak, Executive Editor, Columbia University Press. Ms. Koscielniak understood the vision that we had for this book. She was willing to undertake this innovative project and help us in every step of the way. We are very impressed with her insight and her publishing skills.

These bright and talented scholars in China and the United States have used their sophisticated skills and creative powers to communicate the concepts and practices of traditional Chinese medicine to the West. The effort took over six years and involved the cooperation of over twenty-four scholars to realize *The Essential Book of Traditional Chinese Medicine.*

Hanmin Liu   Dong Mianguo
President   President
United States–China   People's Medical Publishing House
  Educational Institute   December 1986
December 1986

As described in volume 1, traditional Chinese medicine is based on several related theories. On the basis of these theories and the findings derived through various diagnostic methods, the physician categorizes the patient's current signs and symptoms as a specific symptom-complex. Then the physician prescribes treatment accordingly.

The current volume deals with treatment in traditional Chinese medicine. The early chapters address such aspects as principles, widely used methods, important herbs, and common prescriptions. The rest of the book describes how various disorders are treated according to the differentiation of symptom-complexes.

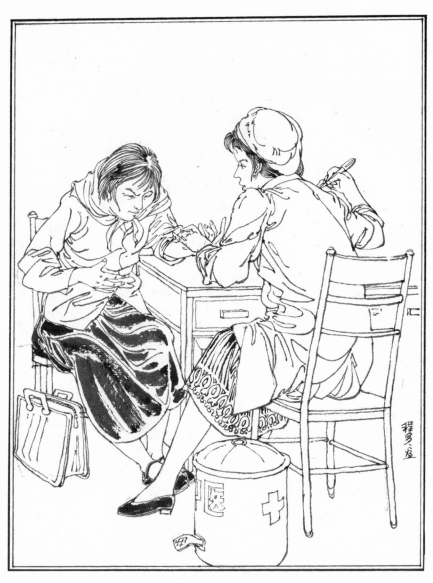

A patient describing her symptoms to her doctor.

CHAPTER ONE

Treatment:
Principles and Basic Methods

PRINCIPLES OF TREATMENT

IN TRADITIONAL CHINESE MEDICINE, practice is based on theory. Thus, general principles derived from the theories described in volume 1 guide the choice of treatment. Discussed below are the basic principles of treatment: integrity and the correct handling of relationships between part and whole, emphasizing the internal cause and correctly handling the relationship between the pathogenic factor and antipathogenic factor, distinguishing the disease's essence from its appearance and treating the root cause, and making a concrete analysis of concrete conditions (analyzing each case individually). Then methods of treatment are described.

Integrity and the Correct Handling of Relationships Between Part and Whole

In traditional Chinese medicine, treatment is based on the concept that the human body is a unified organic entity (i.e., the concept of integrity). Every disease or local condition, without exception, is related to the whole, for there are integral relationships between the parts of the body and between the part and the whole. Thus, one should not merely notice the local condition and treat only the head when the head aches, or only the foot when the foot hurts; one should also notice the whole. Nor should one perceive the whole but not the part and apply a general treatment instead of treating the diseased part. One can affect the whole by treating the part and vice versa.

The commonly applied principles of treatment based on the concept of integrity and the close relationships of the *zang-fu* organs are the following: the reconciliation of *yin* and *yang,* indirect reinforcing and reducing, removing disturbance from an organ by treating the organ exterior-interiorly related to it, and treating the five *zang* organs to relieve disturbances from the five sense organs as well as selecting acupoints. Each of these principles is discussed below.

RECONCILIATION OF *YIN* AND *YANG*

On the most fundamental level, disease results from a breakdown in the equilibrium of *yin* (vital essence) and *yang* (vital function) in the body. In disease, the normal interconsuming-supporting relationship of *yin* and *yang* is replaced by an abnormal condition: either a preponderance or a deficiency of *yin* or *yang.* Thus a cardinal principle of treatment is to reconcile the two and restore them to a relative balance. In practice, the principles most directly related to readjusting this balance are "reducing the redundancy" and "reinforcing the deficiency."

When there is only a preponderance of either *yin* or *yang, the principle of reducing the redundancy* (i.e., counteracting the preponderance) is applied. This approach is used chiefly in conditions resulting from an excess of either *yin* or *yang* due to the invasion of the body by pathogenic factors. As discussed in volume 1, *yang* in excess injures *yin;* for example, exogenous or endogenous heat (a *yang* factor) injures vital essence and body fluid (*yin* factors). And *yin* in excess injures *yang;* for example, when exogenous or endogenous cold (a *yin* factor) prevails, vital function of the internal organs (a *yang* factor) is impaired. Therefore, the principle of reducing the redundancy is applied to restore the balance of *yin* and *yang.*

This concept may be further explained in terms of treatment. For instance, as will be discussed in subsequent chapters, in heat-excess symptom-complexes caused by exogenous-heat pathogenic factors, drugs cold in nature should be given to dispel heat and correct the preponderance of *yang*. And in cold-excess symptom-complexes due to invasion of the body by exogenous-cold pathogenic factors, drugs pungent in flavor or hot in nature should be given to dispel cold and reduce *yin* to normal. *The principle of reinforcing the deficiency* (i.e., correcting the insufficiency) is applicable mainly in conditions marked by symptom-complexes of deficient *yin* or *yang*. The simplest resolution to this imbalance is reinforcing *yang* in patients with a deficiency of *yang,* and invigorating *yin* in patients with a deficiency in *yin*. However, this approach is often not suitable in actual cases because of the interrestraining relationship of *yin* and *yang*. This may be explained as follows.

If *yin* is deficient, it often fails to check or restrain *yang;* thus a deficiency-heat symptom-complex or exuberance of *yang* due to deficiency of *yin* can occur. Likewise if *yang* is deficient it often fails to check *yin,* and a deficiency-cold symptom-complex or preponderance of *yin* develops. Therefore, the *yin* aspect is treated in diseases of *yang* nature and the *yang* aspect is treated in diseases of *yin* nature.

More explicitly, exuberance of heat due to deficiency of *yin* must be considered not as an actual excess of *yang* but as insufficiency of *yin*. Thus, drugs cold in nature are contraindicated for dealing immediately with the heat. The correct approach is to nourish *yin*. This is also known as "replenishing vital essence to check exuberance of vital function in order to restrain *yang*." For example, if deficiency of *yin* (vital essence) of the kidney and intense fire of the vital gate are present, a deficiency-heat symptom-complex due to preponderance of *yang* occurs. In this condition, special attention must be devoted to replenishing *yin* of the kidney. Abundant kidney *yin* may relieve hyperactivity of fire of the liver or kidney.

An analogous condition is preponderance of cold caused by deficiency of *yang* or lowered vital function rather than by an actual excess of *yin*. The cold, therefore, cannot be dispelled by drugs pungent in flavor and warm in nature. Instead, it is essential to invigorate *yang* and check *yin,* i.e., "to reinforce the fire of the vital gate to treat debility caused by cold symptoms." For instance, deficiency of *yang* (vital function) of the kidney due to hypofunction gives rise to a cold symptom-complex manifested by the collection of water-dampness. In this condition, invigorating the vital function of the kidney with drugs warm in nature is the approach often used. When the kidney function returns to normal and the water-dampness is relieved, the preponderance of cold also subsides.

In patients with deficiencies of both *yin* and *yang,* the two should be reinforced simultaneously. Furthermore, when treating cases due to deficiency of *yin,* it sometimes is advisable to activate *yang* when *yin* is replenished—and vice versa. The basis for doing so is the theory of the interdependence of *yin* and *yang* (i.e., that each of the two aspects is the condition for the other's existence and neither can exist in isolation). Thus, when *yin* is to be replenished, appropriate drugs to invigorate *yang* sometimes are given, and vice versa. it should be noted, however, that in practice one must differentiate the primary cause from the secondary and not equate invigoration of *yang* with replenishment of *yin,* and vice versa.

INDIRECT REINFORCING AND INDIRECT REDUCING

As described in volume 1, the five *zang* organs are interrelated in a manner analogous to the five elements. Thus, each organ has a "mother" organ and a "son" organ. These relationships give rise to two important approaches to therapy. The first is that if insufficiency is found in an organ, not only should the weakened organ be invigorated but also its generating or "mother" organ should be reinforced. For example, to cure chronic consumptive diseases of the lung, the lung is strengthened by reinforcing its "mother" organ, the spleen. The second is that if excess is found in an organ, its "son" should be treated with dispelling measures. For instance, in the flaring up of excessive heat in the liver, removal of intense heat from the heart by purgation is more effective than quenching fire in the liver. These two approaches are known as indirect reinforcing and indirect reducing, respectively.

REMOVING DISTURBANCE FROM AN ORGAN BY TREATING THE ORGAN EXTERIOR-INTERIORLY RELATED TO IT

We know that the *zang-fu* organs are exterior-interiorly related. Thus one organ in a pair may be treated when the other organ is affected. For example, because the lung and large intestine are exterior-interiorly related, asthma can be caused by constipation; in this instance, purgation can be an effective treatment for asthma. Or consider another example. Pathogenic heat of the heart may be transmitted to the small intestine and lead to oral ulceration, concentrated urine, and painful urination. This condition can be relieved by removing intense heat from the heart to expel excessive heat from the small intestine, as the two organs are exterior-interiorly related.

TREATING THE FIVE *ZANG* ORGANS TO RELIEVE DISTURBANCES IN THE FIVE SENSE ORGANS

This approach is effective because the five *zang* organs and the five sense organs are related. For example, the liver has its specific opening in the eye. Thus, eye troubles due to fire are treated by quenching fire in the liver, and those due to deficiency are treated by nourishing and soothing the liver with blood tonics.

SELECTION OF POINTS FOR ACUPUNCTURE AND MOXIBUSTION

Selection of points for acupuncture and moxibustion is also based on the concept that the body is an organic whole. Points on the lower portion of body may be selected to treat disorders of the upper portion. (For example, Yongquan [K 1] or Taichong [Liv 3] is often selected to treat hypertension due to exuberance of *yang* of the liver.)[1] Similarly, points on the upper portion of the body may be selected to treat disorders of the lower portion. (For example, Baihiu [Du 20] is often selected in moxibustion treatment for prolapse of the rectum.) Also, points on the left side may be selected to treat disorders on the right side and vice versa. (For example, points on the healthy side are selected to treat hemiplegia.) All the principles of point selection aim at restoring harmony of *yin* and *yang*.

1. See volume 1, chapter 4 for more detail on the points used in acupuncture. The nomenclature is based on *The Essentials of Chinese Acupuncture* (Beijing: Foreign Languages Press, 1980).

Emphasizing the Internal Cause and Correctly Handling the Relationship Between the Pathogenic Factors and the Antipathogenic Factors

The course of a disease always represents a contest between the pathogenic factor and the antipathogenic factor. In other words, it is a manifestation of the conflict between the body resistance (the internal cause) and the pathogenic factor (the external cause). It is said that "excess symptom-complexes occur when pathogenic factors are in abundance, and deficiency symptom-complexes occur when the patient's vital essence and energy are severely damaged." In other words, whether a disease is of excess or of deficiency nature depends on the relative levels of the pathogenic and antipathogenic factors. When the antipathogenic factor is in abudance, the human body adapts well to the environment, and its resistance to disease and ability to repair itself are strong. Thus, the pathogenic factor either cannot invade or is expelled. Chinese medicine therefore devotes particular attention to the internal cause.

A cardinal principle of treatment in Chinese medicine is to dispel pathogenic factors and to restore the normal functioning of the human body in order to change their relative strengths and cure the disease. On the basis of this principle, various prescriptions and other treatments have been developed.

And since the relationship between the antipathogenic factor and the pathogenic factor varies during the course of a disease, the following approaches to treatment take into consideration this fluctuating relationship.

The category *strengthening resistance in order to dispel the invading pathogenic factors* includes several measures (e.g., medication, dietary regimens, exercise therapy) to strengthen the body's resistance, build up a good physique, and increase restorative ability, so that the body can remove pathogenic factors and return to health. This is applicable mainly when the body's resistance to exogenous pathogenic factors is lowered. Then, according to the root cause, different therapeutic methods may be adopted (e.g., reinforcing vital function, replenishing vital essence, tonifying vital energy, blood, and body fluid—the material base maintaining normal functional activities of the *zang-fu* organs and channels).

Dispelling pathogenic factors to restore the normal functioning of the body can be accomplished through various measures such as medication, surgery, acupuncture and moxibustion, and cupping therapy. This approach is applicable chiefly when the pathogenic factor and anti-pathogenic factor are both abundant or when there is insufficiency of the antipathogenic factor and preponderance of the pathogenic factor. It has been proved empirically that when the two factors are undergoing a sharp conflict, it is essential to launch a vigorous attack against the pathogenic factor to eradicate it. Furthermore, clinical observation shows that any disease caused by exogenous pathogenic factors is of excess symptom-complex; therefore removal of the pathogenic factors is most important. Different drugs are given to eliminate different pathogenic factors. Methods used include dispelling pathogenic factors from the exterior of the body by diaphoresis, removing toxic heat with febrifugal and detoxicant drugs, purging, dispelling phlegm, resolving dampness, promoting diuresis, eradicating blood stasis, dispersing blood stasis, dispelling masses, expelling parasites, and destroying intestinal parasites.

First administering medicines to drive out the pathogenic agents and then giving tonics for recuperation is applicable to cases in which strong path-ogenic agents must be removed urgently and the antipathogenic fac-tor will not be further impaired by drastic remedies. It is especially suitable in cases in which the attack by pathogenic factors has weak-ened resistance. For instance, in a febrile disease due to exogenous pathogenic factors and accumulation of heat in the intestines and stomach, common manifestations are distending abdominal pain and constipation, a reddened tongue with a dry dark-red coating, absence of saliva, thirst, dry throat, and delirium (due to internal collection of heat, which impairs vital essense and consumes body fluid). The urgent need is to remove excess heat in order to prevent further loss of fluid; this is done by administering drastic purgatives. Then drugs are given to replenish vital essence and body fluid so that the normal functioning of the body is guaranteed.

First administering tonics to improve the patient's general condition and then giving drastic drugs to drive out the pathogens is applicable mainly in conditions characterized by preponderance of the pathogenic factor and extreme weakness of the antipathogenic factor, so that vital func-tion is diminished and vital essence is exhausted. In this case, one should first give tonics to improve the patient's general condition and then give drastic drugs to drive out the pathogenic factors. If the order were reversed, the patient would be harmed.

Simultaneously administering medicines to drive out invading pathogens and tonics to reinforce body resistance is applicable chiefly when vital function is weakened and pathogenic factors prevail. When this approach is used, the pathogenic factors can be driven out without injuring the antipathogenic factor. But when using this common approach, it is important to determine which is the key problem: lowered body resistance or strong pathogens. If pathogenic factors prevail, one should give many drugs to dispel them and only a few drugs to strengthen body resistance. However, in chronic diseases in which the antipathogenic factor has suffered considerable stress, treatment should concentrate on reinforcing body resistance, and only a few drugs should be given to drive out the pathogens.

Dispelling the pathogenic factor and reinforcing the antipathogenic factor are two distinct but complementary principles of treatment. When the body's resistance is strengthened, the patient is better able to fight pathogenic factors, and when the pathogenic factor is eradicated, body resistance is restored.

Distinguishing the Disease's Essence from Its Appearance and Treating the Root Cause

Another important principle is to distinguish a disease's essence from its appearance and to treat its root cause. Disease is an intricate process characterized by an ongoing confrontation between the antipathogenic factor and pathogenic factor. This process has various manifestations, some of which (e.g., cold symptom-complex, heat symptom-complex, deficiency symptom-complex, and excess symptom-complex) are true indications of the disease state but others of which (e.g., pseudo-heat or pseudo-cold symptoms, and false insufficiency or excessiveness symptoms) are misleading. Only by seeing through the appearance of the disease to its essence and distinguishing the primary from the secondary aspect can one select an appropriate treatment. This principle is the basis for such concepts as "differentiation of the fundamental from the incidental aspect" and "treatment of a disease in a routine way or by reverse process."

DIFFERENTIATION OF THE FUNDAMENTAL FROM THE INCIDENTAL ASPECT

There is a saying, "Before treating a disease, one must determine the fundamental aspect." A disease's nature is considered more basic than its symptom-complexes, body resistance more basic than pathogenic factors, the disease itself more basic than its symptoms, and the primary effects of the disease more basic than complications. In general, fundamental rather than incidental aspects should be treated. However, this principle should not be regarded as absolute. Sometimes in emergency cases, it is necessary to treat the manifestations first. Also, in chronic diseases, treating symptoms sometimes may contribute to alleviation of the fundamental cause. The following three principles—treatment of the fundamental aspect, treatment of acute symptoms first in emergency cases, and treatment of both the fundamental aspect and the incidental aspect—exemplify the above concepts.

TREATMENT OF THE FUNDAMENTAL ASPECT. When a disease is being treated, its nature and cause must be understood and eliminated. For instance, in consumptive disease caused by a deficiency of vital essence of the lung and kidney, such signs and symptoms as cough, mild fever, dry mouth and throat, feverish sensation in the palms, soles, and chest, night sweats, and flushed cheeks may be present. Treatment should be aimed at replenishing vital essence and moistening the lung to remove the deficiency symptom-complex rather than, for example, relieving cough and inducing expectoration of sputum.

TREATMENT OF THE ACUTE MANIFESTATIONS FIRST IN EMERGENCY CASES. Usually, treating the fundamental aspect of a disease is the cardinal principle. But in some emergency cases, one must relieve the acute condition first and then eliminate the cause of the disease. Otherwise, the unrelieved acute condition may endanger the patient's life or impede treatment. For instance, in massive hemorrhage, emergency measures must be taken to stop bleeding first; only then can one try to remove the cause. Another example is the occurrence of ascites in liver disease. Ascites is a manifestation; the liver disease is the cause and generally would be treated first. But if ascites leads to acute problems such as shortness of breath, difficulty in breathing when lying flat, constipation, and anuria, it is urgent to expel the retained water with purgatives in order to alleviate the symptoms; only then should the liver trouble be treated with means to soothe or nourish the liver. In some chronic diseases complicated by new acute affections, it is necessary to cure the new affection first, and the chronic disease second. Thus, in emergencies, it sometimes is necessary to treat the incidental aspect first, even though the final goal is to eradicate the disease cause. Sometimes, alleviation of the incidental aspect creates favorable conditions for the treatment of the fundamental aspect.

TREATMENT OF BOTH THE FUNDAMENTAL ASPECT AND THE IN-CIDENTAL ASPECT. This approach is applied to severe cases with marked symptoms. For example, in dysentery, downward drive of dampness and heat into the lower portion of the body is considered the cause of the disease; abdominal pain, tenesmus, frequent stools containing blood and mucus, slimy yellow tongue coating, and slippery, rapid pulse are considered manifestations. In this condition, treatment is aimed at both eliminating damp-heat in order to clear heat from the intestines and regulating the flow of vital energy to relieve abdominal pain and tenesmus. As another example, febrile diseases due to exogenous pathogenic factors often consume vital essence and result in fullness and pain in the abdomen, constipation, feverish sensation of the body, dry mouth and lips, and a dry tongue coating. All these suggest a severe illness with marked manifestations. Here purgation and the nourishment of vital essence are adopted simultaneously to treat both the cause and the manifestations; if the former method is used alone, body fluid may be further injured, and if the latter is used alone, internal heat may not be dispelled thoroughly. When the two methods are applied together, excessive heat is expelled and vital essence maintained; when vital essence is replenished and dryness is removed, constipation is also relieved.

It should be noted that the relationship between the fundamental and incidental aspects is not absolute and immutable. One type of aspect can be transformed into the other under certain conditions. Therefore, one should know the laws of transformation well, grasp the principal contradiction, and determine the cause of the disease.

TREATMENT OF A DISEASE IN A ROUTINE WAY OR BY REVERSE PROCESS

When the manifestations correlate with the nature of the disease, one should use drugs that oppose the manifestations. This commonly used principle is known as "treatment of a disease in a routine way." For example, cold symptom-complexes should be treated with drugs warm or hot in property, and heat symptom-complexes should be treated with drugs cold in property. Likewise, deficiency symptom-complexes should be treated with reinforcing or replenishing methods, and excess symptom-complexes should be treated with purgation and reduction methods.

Sometimes a pseudo-symptom-complex—i.e., manifestations opposite to the nature of the disease—occurs. Then treatment should be according to the nature of the disease, not that of the symptom-complex. In other words, the disease is "treated by reverse process." For instance, in a case of true heat showing pseudo-cold symptoms (e.g., one in which the limbs are cold because intense internal heat has accumulated and failed to dissipate), drugs cool or cold in property should be used; in a case of true cold showing pseudo-heat symptoms (e.g., preponderance of internal cold that hinders heat outside), one should use drugs warm or hot in nature.

Another approach is called "treating the disease in a routine and regular way together with corrigents." As the name implies, this approach consists of treating a disease in a routine way but adding measures to counteract side-effects of the therapy. This approach is often applied to cases of excessive endogenous cold with pseudo-febrile symptoms or of high fever with pseudo-cold symptoms. Applying routine treatment in these cases may sometimes cause a further schism between the pseudo symptoms and the true disease. Vomiting may then result, so that the drugs are not retained. In order to prevent the vomiting, one should prescribe a few additional drugs with properties opposite to those of the principal ingredients.

Making a Concrete Analysis of Concrete Conditions (Analyzing Each Case Individually)

Appropriate treatment is determined through concrete analysis of each individual and disease so as to suit the remedy to the case.

Diagnosis and treatment based on the differentiation of symptom-complexes should never be handled rigidly. Factors to be considered include the climate and the season, the geographic locality, and the patient's constitution and other characteristics.

Seasonal differences in weather affect physiology and pathology, and treatment must be adjusted accordingly. For example, the texture and interstices of muscles (i.e., the superficial layers of the body) are loose in summer and tight in winter. Thus, in summer it is inadvisable to use drugs pungent in flavor and warm in property for the common cold, for they may cause profuse sweating and impairment of body fluid. But in winter it is advisable to give such drugs to dispel pathogenic factors from the exterior of the body through sweating. Drugs cold or cool in property should be used with great care in autumn and winter unless the symptom-complex is of intense heat.

The characteristics of the *geographic locality* should also be considered. For instance, the northwestern highland areas of China are cold and dry. Diseases of cold and dry nature often occur there, and so it is advisable to use drugs pungent in flavor. However, the southeastern lowlands are hot and wet, and diseases caused by damp-heat often occur there; in treatment it is advisable to remove heat and dampness. Even when the same disease occurs in different areas, one must consider geographic factors. For instance, diaphoretics pungent in flavor and warm in property are administered for affections from exogenous wind-cold. But in the southeast a lower dosage of the drug should be used than in the northwest, or milder drugs for the treatment of exterior symptom-complexes should be given. Furthermore, geographic factors should be kept in mind when treating epidemic diseases.

Treatment should also be in keeping with the patient's *sex, age, constitution, customs,* and *habits.* Physiology differs between males and females; care must be taken because women experience menstruation, pregnancy, and delivery. People of different ages show different physiology and pathology. If old people, who want of blood and vital energy and whose body functions are declining, fall ill, lowered body resistance and abundant pathogenic factors are common. Thus, reinforcing methods should be applied. Also, when using drastic drugs to eliminate pathogenic factors in old patients, great care should be taken not to injure vital energy. In infants, who do not have enough vital energy and blood and are susceptible to illness due to improper diet or climatic changes, drastic drugs are contraindicated.

While dosage also depends on age, it must be noted that too low a dosage of medicine may not be effective against disease, and too high a dosage may harm vital energy. Furthermore, different medications are used in individuals who have different constitutions because of inborn and acquired vital energy. Constitutions can be strong or weak, hot or cold. Therefore, different medications are often used in different people with the same kinds of disease. For example, drugs warm in property are seldom given to patients with hot constitutions, and drugs cool in property are rarely given to those with cold constitutions. Other factors, such as occupation and working conditions, are also related to the occurrence of certain diseases and should be taken into account.

As noted above, correct treatment is based on concrete analysis of each individual and disease. It is therefore imperative to remember that different symptom-complexes can occur in the same disease, and different diseases sometimes produce the same symptom-complexes. Thus, two important concepts are *applying different methods of treatment to the same kind of disease* and *treating different diseases by the same method.*

Different methods of treatment are often applied to the same kind of disease, with the same cause and pathogenesis, if the clinical manifestations differ. Take asthma as an example. There are four types of asthma: deficiency, excess, cold, and hot. The deficiency type may be relieved by reinforcing lung and kidney function, the excess type by ventilating and soothing a troubled lung or by quenching fire in the lung, the cold type by administering drugs warm or hot in property, and the hot type by giving drugs cool or cold in property.

Different diseases are often treated by the same method if they are associated with similar symptom-complexes. For example, Chinese medicine contends that gastroptosis, hysteroptosis, nephroptosis, and prolapse of the rectum are all due to sinking of vital energy of the spleen. Therefore, in all these conditions, it is considered advisable to invigorate the function of the spleen in sending vital energy and nutrients upward. Similarly, hiccups, vomiting, cough, and asthma are all considered to be caused by adverse upward flow of vital energy, the treatment for which is to keep vital energy going down.

In short, for a patient to be treated appropriately, it is necessary to obtain a comprehensive understanding of the disease and the patient's condition through a concrete analysis; then suitable therapy can be applied.

COMMON METHODS OF TREATMENT

In traditional Chinese medicine, methods of treatment are classified as *therapeutic methods* and *concrete methods*. The former, also known as basic therapies, are broad, general approaches to treatment (e.g., purgation, heat reduction, and tonification). The latter are treatments for specific diseases.

Therapeutic methods are the link between, on the one hand, the basic theory of Chinese medicine, and, on the other hand, drugs and prescriptions. The methods are based on the theories of the *zang-fu* organs, channels and collaterals, etiology, and pathogenesis; they also are derived from diagnosis according to the differentiation of symptom-complexes and from the general principles of treatment. Only when the appropriate methods of treatment are determined can correct prescriptions be made.

Traditionally, in Chinese medicine there are eight commonly used therapeutic methods: diaphoresis, emesis, purgation, regulation, invigoration, heat reduction, tonification, and elimination. However, additional methods have now been developed. The rest of this chapter introduces fourteen therapeutic methods, as well as concrete methods. Subsequent chapters provide further detail.

Diaphoresis

Diaphoresis consists in dispelling pathogenic factors from the exterior of the body with diaphoretics. It causes the texture and interstices of muscles to open in order to regulate the function of the *ying* (nutrient) system and *wei* (superficial defensive) system. Chinese medicine contends that pathogenic factors first attack the external part of the body and then the interior. Thus it is important to eradicate pathogenic factors before the interior is invaded.

Diaphoretic methods are good for treating exterior symptom-complexes; relieving fever, rheumatism, cough, and asthma; promoting eruption in measles; and causing detumescence.

INDICATIONS

- Affections due to exogenous pathogenic factors, including various infectious diseases such as influenza in their early and second stages, incipient pneumonia, eruption in incipient measles.
- Rheumatic or rheumatoid arthritis.
- Incipient suppurative infections on the body surface, deep-rooted boils, incipient edema.

METHODS COMMONLY USED

Exterior symptom-complexes are of various types, and so their manifestations differ. Thus, various diaphoretic methods are used.

Dispelling pathogenic factors from the exterior of the body with sudorifics pungent in flavor and warm in property is indicated for:

- Exterior cold symptom-complexes marked by aversion to cold, mild fever, headache, generalized aching, thin moist white tongue coating, floating and tight pulse.
- Incipient edema characterized by marked swelling on the upper portion of the body and accompanied by aversion to wind and by fever.
- Rheumatism, especially if associated with pains in the exterior of the body.

Dispelling pathogenic factors from the exterior of the body with drugs pungent in flavor and cooling in property is indicated for:

- Exterior heat symptom-complexes marked by high fever, slight intolerance of cold, thirst, reddened and painful throat, reddened tongue with thin white or yellow coating, floating and rapid pulse.
- Promoting the development of eruption in incipient measles.
- Suppurative infection on the body surface, deep-rooted boils complicated by fever and intolerance of cold.

The above two methods differ in that they employ drugs with different flavors and properties. The first method removes cold and promotes vigorous sweating, but the second is used chiefly to relieve heat by mild perspiration. Experience indicates that in the early stage of febrile disease due to exogenous pathogenic factors, simultaneous administration of drastic diaphoretics and antipyretics is often useful.

Strengthening vital energy and resolving exterior symptom-complexes is used mainly in patients deficient in vital energy who are suffering from secondary affection by exogenous pathogenic factors or from repeated common colds and excessive sweating. Patients deficient in vital energy are susceptible to exogenous pathogenic factors because of lowered superficial resistance. In addition, the invading pathogenic factors are hard to dispel because deficiency of vital energy and profuse sweating exist. Thus, to eradicate the pathogenic factors, it is necessary to add drugs to reinforce vital energy and superficial resistance.

Nourishing vital essence and resolving exterior symptom-complexes is used to expel exogenous pathogenic factors attacking the external parts of the body of a patient deficient in vital essence. We know that sweat is formed from body fluid and blood. Consumption of vital essence invariably leads to deficiency of sweat and so to absence of sweating. Thus, the pathogenic factors cannot be brought out with perspiration. Therefore, drugs to replenish vital essence must be given along with diaphoretics. Clinically, drugs pungent in flavor and cool in property for dispelling pathogenic factors from the exterior of the body are used together with drugs for replenishing vital essence and body fluid.

CAUTIONS

These methods are effective only for exterior symptom-complexes, not for the interior symptom-complexes that ensue when a disease is transmitted from the exterior to the interior of the body. Use of the methods should be discontinued once intolerance of cold and fever subside, which shows that the pathogenic factors have been expelled by sweating. Profuse perspiration should be avoided because excessive sweating may injure vital essence and result in collapse, as sweat is derived from body fluid. After perspiration, the pores of the body are loose, and so one must avoid wind and cold so as not to catch cold again.

Futhermore, the methods should be used with care in patients of weak constitution or with severe vomiting and massive bleeding. Their use is inadvisable when boils or furuncles have festered or the eruption of measles has already been fully brought forth. In summer, extensive use of diaphoresis is not allowed because the body perspires easily on hot days.

Emesis

Emesis consists of using emetics or mechanical stimulation to induce vomiting and thus to expel noxious substances. It is an emergency measure used to restore normal flow of vital energy and expel pathogenic factors in patients with collections of noxious substances in the stomach. The goal is to prevent pathogenic factors from entering the intestines and worsening the condition.

INDICATIONS

- Poison ingestion or food poisoning (when the toxin has not yet been absorbed).
- Retention of undigested food in the stomach, causing pain and a sensation of fullness.
- Obstruction of the stomach by retention of phlegm, so that respiration is impeded.

METHODS COMMONLY USED

Emesis is induced by medicine, salt solution, or mechanical stimulation (e.g., with the fingers or a chicken feather).

CAUTIONS

Induction of emesis is an emergency measure. If it is properly used, results are favorable. However, it may injure vital energy and vital essence of the stomach.

It is enough to induce vomiting once. Repetition does no good.

Emesis is contraindicated in patients with chronic diseases (e.g., deficiency of vital energy, asthma) or with weak constitutions (e.g., in senile debility, in pregnancy, post partum, after loss of blood), for it can injure vital energy and worsen the condition.

Purgation

Purgation is used to relieve constipation, to clear stagnation of food or blood, and to expel internal heat and excessive fluid. Experience indicates that it is very useful. Any interior excess symptom-complex due to accumulation of pathogenic factors in the interior may be removed by purgation. However, the body's resistance and the pathogenic factors should be known before purgation is used.

Purgation methods are used extensively to treat acute abdominal conditions such as intestinal obstruction, acute cholecystitis, and acute pancreatitis.

INDICATIONS

- Interior excess symptom-complexes marked by constipation and dry yellow tongue coating and due to collection of pathogenic heat in the stomach and intestines.
- Retention of undigested food, intestinal parasitosis, stagnated blood in an organ, retention of phlegm and fluid.
- Food or drug poisoning.
- Hemorrhage due to excessive internal heat.
- Incipient dysentery marked by abdominal pain, tenesmus, and discharge of red and white mucus and due to accumulation of damp-heat in the intestines.

METHODS COMMONLY USED

Purgation with drugs cold in nature is indicated for:

- Excess symptom-complexes manifested by hectic fever, abdominal fullness, abdominal pain aggravated by pressure, constipation, flatulence, deep yellow or dark tongue coating, prickly tongue, and deep and slippery pulse; and, in severe cases, by delirium and mania due to fecal impaction in the intestines, or by passing of yellowish, foul, and watery stool, due to the downward drive of dampness and heat into the urinary bladder and intestines; or by dysentery with discharge of red and white mucus.
- Febrile diseases due to exogenous pathogenic heat and marked by restlessness, delirium, and convulsions; macula due to invasion of

the blood system by pathogenic heat causing the escape of blood from vessels (in these conditions many febrifugal and detoxicant drugs are administered simultaneously).

- Sore throat, ulcers of the mouth and tongue, swollen and painful gums, epistaxis, constipation, and halitosis caused by retention of heat in the lung and stomach (in this condition, drugs to remove heat from the lung and stomach are added).

- Headache, flushed face, yellow tongue coating, constipation, tinnitus, deafness, restlessness, and irritability due to flaring up of excessive heat in the liver (in this condition extra drugs are given to eliminate liver heat).

Purgation with drugs warm in nature consists of administering purgatives together with drugs pungent in flavor and warm in nature to remove stagnated pathogenic cold. It is good for interior cold symptom-complexes manifested by distending pain in the abdomen, thick white and slimy tongue coating, constipation, absence of thirst or preference for hot drinks, intolerance of cold, and cold limbs. At present, the method is used for the following conditions: retention of undigested food associated with affection by exogenous pathogenic factors, chronic bacillary dysentery, chronic nephritis, uremia.

Mild purgation consists of administering mild laxatives along with drugs to replenish vital essence and body fluid so as to relieve acute or chronic constipation. It is used in elderly and debilitated patients, patients with consumption of vital essence due to protracted illness, and puerpera with deficiency of blood and fluid.

Expelling retained water with drastic purgatives is effective in water retention (e.g., hydrothorax, ascites accompanied by constipation and ischuria) resulting in dyspnea and a forceful pulse. In cases in which the pathogenic factors are strong but the body resistance is not impeded, drastic purgatives can be administered. The method is especially applicable to ascites due to cirrhosis. It should be noted that this method is radical in action and tends to injure body resistance; thus the tonifying method is often used along with it. Sometimes tonification immediately follows purgation or vice versa; sometimes the two are used at the same time.

The attacking-phlegm method is used for treating psychotic depression, epilepsy, schizophrenia, infantile convulsions, wheezing and convulsions due to accumulation of persistent phlegm.

The attacking-blood-stasis method, in which drugs for eradicating blood stasis and softening hard lumps are added, is used to remove stagnated blood that has accumulated in a channel or an organ. The indications are as follows:

- Distending pain or lumps in the lower abdomen, dark stools, scanty menstruation with discharge of dark blood, mania, constipation caused by stagnation of blood in organs.
- Absence of menstruation, scanty menses with discharge of dark blood, menstrual disorders due to blood stasis.
- Lumps in the uterus and foul vaginal discharge.
- Extra-uterine pregnancy.

In the *parasite-expelling method,* anthelmintics are administered along with purgatives to expel parasites. This method is especially effective in ascariasis and cestodiasis.

CAUTIONS

It is inadvisable to use these methods when an exterior symptom-complex is not yet relieved or the affection is located between the exterior and interior and is accompanied by vomiting. Furthermore, the methods are contraindicated in old, weak patients, in patients with chronic disease (in whom it may injure body fluid), and in pregnant and postpartum women (in whom it may harm body resistance).

Overdosage is forbidden. When the condition is alleviated, purgatives should be discontinued. It is inadvisable to use the drugs continuously. Greasy and indigestible foods should be avoided after taking purgatives.

Regulating (Mediation) Methods

These methods consist in using drugs with regulatory action to restore normal coordination among the internal organs, the channels and collaterals, the nutrient and defensive systems, and the vital energy and blood systems.

INDICATIONS

- Disorders of the Shaoyang Channel, which runs between the exterior and interior of the body.
- Disharmony of the liver and spleen and of the liver and stomach.
- Derangement of vital energy, blood, nutrient, and superficial defensive systems.
- Stagnancy of vital energy of the liver.

METHODS COMMONLY USED

Interior-exterior mediation is used to treat febrile diseases marked by alternating spells of fever and chills, bitter taste in the mouth, dry throat, restlessness, nausea, a sensation of fullness in the chest and hypochondria region, anorexia, and taut pulse. It is used when the pathogenic factors are located between the exterior and the interior of the body.

Coordination of the nutrient and superficial defensive systems is often used to treat disharmony of the nutrient and superficial defensive systems that results from invasion of the exterior of the body by exogenous pathogenic factors and is manifested by aversion to cold and wind, mild fever, headache, and perspiration. Drugs pungent in flavor and warm in nature should be simultaneously administered with drugs that consolidate vital essence by arresting profuse sweating.

Regulating the flow of vital energy and blood is applicable chiefly to stagnancy of vital energy in the liver and disorders of the blood system, both marked by depression, irritability, pain in the hypochondria, a distended feeling in the thoracic region and breast, irregular menstruation, and dysmenorrhea. Drugs to restore the normal functioning of a depressed liver and to regulate the flow of vital energy, as well as blood tonics, are given. If there is marked pain or blood stasis, drugs to activate blood circulation and eliminate blood stasis are also administered.

Coordination of the functioning of the liver and spleen is good for stagnancy in the liver leading to diminished function of the spleen and for disharmony of the liver and spleen due to rage, irregular food

intake, overexertion, or lack of exercise. Common manifestations include distending pain in the chest and hypochondria, depression,
abdominal distension, sticky loose stools, anorexia, constipation,
borborygmi, and diarrhea. The onset of the disease is due to intense
emotion or a drastic change in emotion. Therefore, drugs to restore
the normal functioning of a depressed liver and spleen are often administered.

Soothing the liver and regulating the functioning of the stomach is used
chiefly to relieve depression, stagnancy of vital energy in the liver,
and adverse flow of exuberant vital energy of the liver leading to
dysfunction of the stomach. These are all manifested by distending
pain in the chest, hypochondria, and stomach, fullness of the stomach, belching, acid regurgitation, irritability or depression, thin yellow tongue coating, and taut pulse. Drugs to soothe the liver and to
nourish the vital essence of the stomach so as to normalize the stomach's functioning are often administered.

CAUTIONS

It is inadvisable to use the method when the pathogenic factors
are located on the exterior or in the interior of the body.

Mild drugs are gentle and should only be used for regulating;
continued use may prolong the course of disease.

Invigoration (Warming) Methods

These methods consist of treating interior cold symptom-complexes with drugs warm in property to activate vital function and
dispel pathogenic cold.

INDICATIONS

• Deficiency cold symptom-complexes of the spleen and stomach
  due to invasion of the interior of the body by pathogenic cold,
  leading to lowered vital function and manifested by cold feeling
  and pain in the stomach, belching, diarrhea, cold limbs, and intolerance of cold.

- Collapse due to lowered vital function of the kidney and internal growth of cold; marked by profuse sweating, intolerance of cold, cold limbs, and exceedingly feeble pulse.
- Edema due to insufficient vital function of the spleen and kidney.
- Arthralgia due to invasion of the channels and collaterals by pathogenic factors, stagnation of vital energy, and stasis of blood; manifested by pain in the bones and muscles that is aggravated by cold and manifested by contraction of the limbs, motion impairment, or painful hernia due to accumulation of cold in the Liver Channel.

METHODS COMMONLY USED

Warming the spleen and stomach and dispelling cold from them is applicable to hypofunction of and presence of cold in the spleen and stomach due to continuous lowered vital function of the internal organs. It also is applicable to impairment of vital function of the spleen caused by transmission of cold from the exterior to the interior. Hypofunction of the spleen and stomach are manifested by signs and symptoms such as listlessness, pale tongue with moist white coating, deep slow pulse or soft slow pulse; or cold limbs, diarrhea, abdominal pain relieved by pressure and heat, constipation, deep and taut pulse, stomachache, and vomiting of clear fluid. Drugs to warm the spleen and stomach and reinforce their function are administered. If marked cold symptoms are present, drugs to activate vital function are added.

Restoring yang *(vital function) from collapse* is usually effective in collapse due to preponderance of cold and severe impairment of vital function. This condition is marked by intolerance of cold, lying with the body curled up, cold limbs, abdominal pain, vomiting, diarrhea, cold sweats, decrease in blood pressure and body temperature, pale complexion, and a thready and feeble or a rapid and weak pulse. Drugs to restore vital function and reinforce vital energy are administered. In cases of impairment of vital essence and body fluid due to profuse sweating, drugs to replenish and preserve vital essence are added.

Invigoration and promotion of vital function to induce diuresis is applicable chiefly to systemic or local edema due to insufficient function of the spleen and kidney and manifested by cold limbs, intolerance of cold, pale tongue, thready pulse, and ascites. Drugs to strengthen vital function of the kidney and diuretics are given.

Warming the channels and dispelling cold from them is effective in rheumatic and rheumatoid arthritis due to affection by wind, dampness, and especially cold. These conditions are marked by pain in the joints and by restriction of joint motion, and they are exacerbated by cold and relieved by heat. The method is also effective in painful hernia and gastrointestinal neurosis caused by an upward drive of pathogenic cold. The goal of treatment is to warm the channels to remove obstruction. In protracted rheumatism, drugs to activate blood circulation and strengthen the tendons and bones are administered. For patients with weak constitutions, blood tonics and drugs for reinforcing vital energy are added. If there is a painful hernia, drugs to soothe a depressed liver are used. For gastrointestinal neurosis, drugs to regulate the flow of vital energy are given.

CAUTIONS

Because the drugs used are dry and warm in property, it is inadvisable to use these methods in patients with a weak constitution, reddened tongue, or dry throat. It is also inadvisable to use them in patients with hemoptysis, hematuria, or bleeding per rectum and in pregnant women. Overdosage is prohibited as it may impair vital essence and consume body fluid.

When use of these methods is being considered, it is essential to distinguish true from pseudo cold symptom-complexes, for these methods should not be used in cases of heat showing pseudo-cold symptoms.

Heat Reduction (Febrifugal) Methods

In these methods, medicines cold in property are used to treat acute febrile diseases and other diseases characterized by internal heat. The methods remove toxic heat, preserve body fluid, cool blood, dispel summer heat, relieve thirst and convulsions, and subdue endogenous wind.

INDICATIONS

- Various interior heat symptom-complexes, such as intense heat in the superficial defensive, nutrient, and blood systems, and damp-heat symptom-complexes (generally, the method is applicable throughout the course of a febrile disease).
- Suppurative infections on the body surface leading to toxemia.
- Deficiency heat symptom-complexes marked by insufficient vital essence and abundant vital function (in which case measures to replenish vital essence are also administered).

METHODS COMMONLY USED

Heat symptom-complexes are of both deficiency and excess types. Furthermore, pathogenic heat may reside in the superficial defensive, the nutrient, or the blood system. Sometimes it is accompanied by dampness. Hence, different febrifugal methods are used according to the site and nature of the disease.

Reducing intense internal heat is a method in which drugs bitter in taste and cold in property are used to treat intense heat retained in the lung, heart, stomach, and liver. Common manifestations of conditions treated by this method are high fever, delirium, unconsciousness, cough, asthma, chest pain, dizziness, bloodshot eyes, and constipation.

Dispelling pathogenic heat from the blood is effective in the advanced stages of febrile infectious diseases, when the nutrient system is attacked by pathogenic heat and manifestations such as delirium, deep-red tongue, hemoptysis, epistaxis, and rash are present. It should be noted that some diseases marked by intense heat in the blood are complicated and cannot be relieved by this method alone; drugs for removing pathogenic heat to effect resuscitation, as well as anticonvulsives, are also given.

In the *removing toxic-heat* method, febrifugal and detoxicant drugs bitter in taste and cold in nature are used to treat febrile diseases and pyogenic inflammations (such as epidemic infectious diseases, ulcers, erysipelas, pulmonary and intestinal abscesses, dysentery, painful urination, scanty red urine) that are marked by fever, painful swelling, suppuration, and necrosis. Some febrifugal and detoxicant drugs possess curative effects for specific diseases. They should be administered as indicated.

Removing pathogenic heat and resolving dampness is a method to treat damp-heat symptom-complexes due to exogenous affection by pathogenic heat. Manifestations of this condition are protracted intermittent fever, suffocating feeling in the chest, nausea, anorexia, scanty red urine, sticky loose stools, slimy yellow tongue coating, or dysentery, urination disturbance, eczema, furuncles, and jaundice.

The above four different kinds of drugs are given in different types of cases. For example, when there is excessive damp-heat or damp-heat that turns into fire, it is advisable to use drugs bitter in flavor and cold in property, which can not only eliminate damp-heat but also dispel noxious heat. For cases with major dampness and minor heat in the spleen and stomach—manifested by distension of the stomach and abdomen, nausea, anorexia, loose stools, and intermittent fever—drugs bitter in flavor and warm in property are used to expel dampness. And for cases with minor dampness and major heat, fragrant drugs for resolving dampness, as well as febrifuges bitter in flavor and cold in property, are used. Also, in this method, diuretics are often administered to dispel dampness. For some damp-heat symptom-complexes found in skin disorders, drugs for eliminating heat and dampness by drying are administered.

Replenishing vital essence and removing intense internal heat is used to treat deficiency heat symptom-complexes caused by impairment of vital essence or by deficiency of vital essence accompanied by flaring up of pathogenic heat. These symptom-complexes are found in the advanced stages of febrile disease due to exogenous pathogenic factors or in chronic diseases such as tuberculosis. The aim of treatment is to nourish vital essence, reduce fever, and relieve dryness.

CAUTIONS

Many of the drugs used in these methods are of cold or cool property and thus can hurt the spleen and stomach. Therefore, it is inadvisable to administer them to patients with lowered vital function of the spleen and stomach, reduced digestive function, and loose stools. For fear of injuring the spleen and stomach, the drugs are not given to patients who have just recovered from a severe illness or to postpartum women.

Also, the method is contraindicated in patients with weak constitutions and decreased vital function of the *zang-fu* organs.

True and pseudo heat should be clearly distinguished. The method is forbidden in cases of cold showing pseudo-heat symptoms.

Drugs for eliminating intense heat are given in cases with abundant pathogenic heat. If vomiting occurs after the medicine is taken, it is necessary to add some fresh ginger juice or to administer drugs cold in nature in hot decoction form.

Tonifying Methods

This category includes methods of treating various deficiency symptom-complexes to enhance vital energy, blood condition, vital essence, and vital function so as to strengthen the antipathogenic factor and eliminate pathogenic factors.

INDICATIONS

Any illness caused by deficiency of vital energy, blood, vital essence, or vital function and marked by decreased functioning of the *zang-fu* organs.

METHODS COMMONLY USED

Reinforcement of vital energy consists in using tonics to correct deficiencies of vital energy in the spleen and lung. Manifestations of deficiency of the spleen are listlessness, anorexia, loose stools, and prolapse of the rectum or uterus; those of deficiency of the lung are shortness of breath, weakness, sighing, and spontaneous sweating due to lowered superficial resistance. In addition, pallor, listlessness, asthma precipitated by exercise, and spontaneous sweating often occur in deficiency of vital energy. The method also involves tonifying the lung to invigorate the functioning of the spleen, reinforcing the spleen and stomach, replenishing vital energy, and activating the function of the spleen in sending vital energy upward. Generally, these actions are accomplished by adding drugs benefiting the spleen, blood condition, and so forth, in addition to using large doses of vital energy tonics. In patients with massive hemorrhage due to extreme deficiency of vital energy, it is most important to replenish vital energy first by administering large amounts of vital energy tonics, for vital energy can generate growth of blood and stop hemorrhage.

Tonifying the blood is a method used chiefly to treat blood deficiency caused by acute or chronic hemorrhage, chronic consumptive disease, or delivery. Such deficiency is manifested by pallor, pale tongue and lips, dizziness, palpitation, tinnitus, deafness, insomnia, dream-disturbed sleep, scanty menstruation, and thready pulse. Not only blood tonics but also vital energy tonics are given because the latter may generate the growth of blood. In addition, drugs for activating blood circulation, hemostatics, and sedatives are administered.

Reinforcing vital function is a general method in which tonics are used to correct insufficient vital function of the spleen and especially of the kidney, common manifestations of which include intolerance of cold, cold limbs, soreness of the lower back, retrograde ejaculation, frequent urination, polyuria, edema, pale tongue, and thready pulse. The method promotes vital function, especially virility. When marked deficiency and cold symptom-complexes are present, it is advisable to give vital energy tonics to reinforce the function of the spleen and tonics good for vital essence and blood.

Replenishing vital essence is a general method in which tonics are used to correct deficiency of vital essence in the spleen, liver, and kidney. Common manifestations of such deficiency include emaciation, mild fever, soreness of the lower back, tinnitus, spermatorrhea, hectic sweating, feverish sensation in the palms, soles, and heart area, insomnia, dry mouth and throat, hemoptysis, reddened tongue with little coating or shedding of the tongue coating, and thready and rapid pulse. With these manifestations the methods for replenishing vital essence and body fluid are applied. If deficiency of vital essence and preponderance or exuberance of vital function of the liver are present (marked by dizziness, tinnitus, and headache), drugs for subduing hyperactivity of the liver, putting down upward adverse flow of vital energy, and controlling fever are added.

RELATIONSHIPS AMONG THE ABOVE FOUR METHODS. In clinical practice, the above methods are usually applied in combination rather than singly. For example, both vital energy and blood are replenished or both vital function and vital essence are reinforced. In addition, when deficiencies of both vital energy and vital essence occur in convalescence from febrile disease due to exogenous pathogenic factors or in pulmonary tuberculosis, vital energy and vital essence should be replenished simultaneously. Because vital energy and blood have a common source and *yin* and *yang* are interdependent, it is necessary to replenish vital energy in patients with loss of blood. For deficiency of vital function, drugs for nourishing vital essence should be given in addition to vital function tonics, and vice versa.

When both vital function and vital essence are deficient, they should be replenished together. But it should be noted which of these two aspects is the more deficient: if it is vital essence, then treatment should be directed at reinforcing it, while vital function is given secondary priority; and if it is vital function, then the opposite action is taken.

In patients with deficiency of vital function and abundant heat (usually found in neurasthenia, chronic nephritis, and climacteric hypertension, and marked by intolerance of cold, cold limbs, soreness of the lower back, listlessness, weakness of the legs, restlessness, insomnia, and spermatorrhea), drugs to nourish vital essence and eliminate intense heat are given in addition to invigorating the function of the kidney.

Drugs sweet or pungent in flavor and warm in property are administered for deficiency of vital energy and vital function. For deficiency of vital essence and vital function of the kidney, medicines made from animals are given in addition to vital essence tonics.

CAUTIONS

In chronic illnesses causing debility, nutrition and physical exercises are necessary in addition to tonics.

In extreme debility that may lead to collapse, drastic tonics often are ineffective. In this condition functioning should first be improved with general tonics. When vital energy is insufficient and pathogenic factors are abundant, drugs to drive out invading pathogenic agents and tonics to reinforce the body resistance should be administered at the same time; during convalescence, a long course of tonics is pre-scribed.

It is important to consider the condition of the spleen and stomach when toncis are administered. If these organs are malfunctioning, drugs for nourishing vital essence and blood may be ineffective. Therefore it is advisable to give some fragrant drugs to regulate vital function and activate the function of the spleen. Thus, stagnancy of the spleen and stomach is avoided. Because drugs for replenishing vital energy or vital function are of dry property, it is advisable to add drugs that replenish and preserve vital essence so that it is not impaired.

In patients with dyspepsia due to deficiency of vital energy in the spleen, one should be cautious when using blood tonics good for vital essence. In those with insufficient vital essence associated with inter-nal heat, one should be cautious in using drugs for reinforcing vital energy and vital function.

It is essential to know the nature of a case. In excess symptom-complexes mimicking insufficiency, tonifying methods are contrain-dicated.

It is unwise to misuse tonics, for although they are good for health, they may prevent the destruction of pathogenic factors.

Elimination Methods

These methods include removing stagnated food, dispelling harm-ful masses formed through stagnation of vital energy and blood, dis-solving calculi, and resolving phlegm. The purgation method and the elimination method differ as follows. The former removes dry stools, stagnant blood, collected phlegm, and retained fluid with drastic purgatives. The latter removes long-standing masses in the abdomen by a slow process.

INDICATIONS

• Stagnation of vital energy, disturbance in upward and downward functional activities, dysfunction of the stomach, dyspepsia.

- Masses in the abdomen due to blood stasis, stagnancy of vital energy, and obstruction of the vessels.
- Internal obstruction by phlegm, coagulation of excessive phlegm.
- Edema caused by retained fluid.

METHODS COMMONLY USED

Removing food stagnancy is a method in which stomachics and laxatives are used to cure dyspepsia. Among the common manifestations of the condition are a distended feeling in the stomach and fullness in the abdomen, anorexia, belching, acid regurgitation, nausea, abdominal pain, and constipation or sticky loose stools. Stomachics and drugs for regulating vital energy to strengthen the function of the spleen are used together because stagnation of food is often accompanied by accumulation of phlegm-dampness and stagnancy of vital energy. In severe dyspepsia, small amounts of laxatives are also given.

Dispelling masses is a method for treating masses caused by stagnancy of vital energy, blood, and phlegm and by blood stasis. It is applicable to conditions such as tuberculous cervical lymphadenitis (including lymphadenovarix), goiter (thyroid enlargement), calculi (including urinary and biliary calculi), and masses (such as enlargement of the liver and spleen, tumors, and other masses in the abdomen). According to the type of mass, different drugs are used. For instance, drugs for replenishing vital essence and dispelling toxic heat are given for tuberculous cervical lymphadenitis, diuretics and drugs for alleviating urinary disorders are given for urinary calculi, and drugs for soothing the liver and gallbladder are administered for biliary calculi. Different methods and drugs are used to dispel abdominal masses caused by different conditions (stagnancy of vital energy, coagulation of phlegm, stasis of blood). In addition, drugs for replenishing blood and vital energy are given at the same time to enhance body resistance. Masses are commonly treated by frequent administration of pills containing small amounts of drugs.

Resolving phlegm is a group of measures to dispel phlegm, usually by administering expectorants. If phlegm remains in the lung, antitussives and expectorants are used. If the Heart Channel is obstructed by phlegm (as a pathogenic factor), it is necessary to resolve phlegm and induce resuscitation. Dispelling wind and resolving phlegm are employed in cases with obstruction of the Heart Channel by phlegm, marked by facial paralysis, rigidity of the tongue, and infantile convulsions. In patients with retention of phlegm in the stomach (manifested by vomiting, nausea, etc.), it is advisable to normalize the functioning of the stomach and resolve phlegm. For cases with coagulated phlegm causing goiter, the method of disintegrating the goiter and resolving phlegm is used.

Two other frequently used methods are the following:

Resolving phlegm and stopping cough is a method to cure cough and produce expectoration of sputum. Mild expectorants are effective in symptom-complexes of cold phlegm, damp phlegm, hot phlegm, and dry phlegm. Expectorants warm in property are applicable to cold and damp phlegm, expectorants cool in property to hot and dry phlegm.

Dispelling wind and resolving phlegm is a method to disperse stirring-up of wind due to overabundance of phlegm. Common manifestations of this condition include dizziness and vertigo, wheezing due to excessive phlegm, coma, facial paralysis, rigidity of the tongue, and hemiplegia. Drugs for dispelling wind, clearing obstructed channels, and removing phlegm are used. These drugs also reduce heat and induce resuscitation.

Diuresis is a measure to cure edema. *Dispelling dampness through diuresis by using mild-flavored drugs* is used to treat edema due to retention of dampness and to treat oliguria. Drugs for removing obstruction of vital energy, invigorating the function of the spleen, and resolving dampness are employed. *Diuresis and removal of urinary troubles* is used to treat urodynia, urinary frequency, urgency, and scanty red urine caused by downward drive of damp-heat into the urinary bladder. If severe hematuria is present, hemostatics and drugs for cooling the blood are administered.

CAUTIONS

These methods are only for physical accumulations of matter in the body. Otherwise they are contraindicated.

If used over a long period, these methods may injure vital energy. Therefore, it is advisable to combine them with tonifying methods. Also, the drugs used are drastic. Thus one should be cautious when administering them to patients with insufficient vital energy and blood or lowered functioning of the spleen and kidney.

Scanty urination and retention of urine are often due to hypofunction of the spleen and kidney and to disturbance in water metabolism, and they cannot be cured by diuresis alone. One must also invigorate the functioning of the kidney, or enhance the functioning of the spleen to resolve dampness. In scanty urination caused by want of body fluid, diuresis in contraindicated.

Regulating the Flow of Vital Energy

These methods are used to treat any disorder in the flow of vital energy.

INDICATIONS

- Stagnation of vital energy.
- Adverse flow of vital energy due to stagnancy of vital energy and disturbance in upward and downward functional activities.

METHODS COMMONLY USED

Restoring the normal functioning of a depressed liver to promote the flow of vital energy is used to restore the normal function of a liver that is depressed because of emotional disturbance. In such depression, vital energy can stagnate in the chest and hypochondria (causing distending pain in that area), in the stomach (causing a sensation of fullness there), or in the abdomen (causing distending pain there). For stagnancy of vital energy, drugs for soothing a depressed liver and promoting the normal flow of vital energy are used together. The latter drugs vary in their sites of action; some relieve stagnancy of vital energy in the chest and hypochondria, some do so in the stomach, and some do so in the abdomen. In cases with stagnancy of vital energy and accumulation of phlegm, expectorants are administered along with the drugs for promoting the normal flow of vital energy. For stagnancy of vital energy accompanied by either cold or heat, drugs hot or cold in property are added. If there is blood stasis, it is advisable to remove it in addition to promoting the normal flow of vital energy.

Regulating vital function of the stomach and maintaining the downward flow of vital energy is used to correct stagnancy of vital energy due to retention of phlegm and fluid or to adverse upward flow of stomach *qi* (marked by belching, hiccups, nausea, and vomiting).

Relieving asthma by sending qi *downward* is applicable to adverse upward flow of *qi* caused by exogenous pathogenic factors and to collection of phlegm manifested by cough and asthma. Drugs for ventilating and soothing the lung and dispelling phlegm are used along with drugs for sending down *qi*. It should be noted that different cases must be treated in different ways. For example, when adverse flow of *qi* is accompanied by deficiency of vital energy, drugs for the latter problem are added.

CAUTIONS

Although stagnancy of vital energy and adverse flow of gas are associated with excess symptom-complexes, the condition of vital energy should be considered. Drugs for regulating the normal flow of vital energy are administered with care or discontinued if shortness of breath and listlessness occur. In pregnant and postpartum women and the elderly, the method should be used with care for fear of injuring vital energy.

Regulating Blood Conditions

In general, disorders of the blood system are divided into four classes: deficiency of blood, intense heat in the blood, blood stasis, and hemorrhage. Deficiency of blood is treated by the tonifying method; intense heat in the blood is corrected by the febrifugal method. Blood stasis and hemorrhage are treated mainly by the methods described below.

INDICATIONS

- Stagnancy of vital energy and stasis of blood (e.g., dysmenorrhea, absence of menstruation).

- Persistent rheumatism.
- Trauma causing local swelling, pain, bruising, and blood stasis.
- Incipient carbuncle, suppurative infection on the body surface without ulceration.
- Hemorrhage (e.g., uterine bleeding, hematuria, hematemesis, epistaxis).

METHODS COMMONLY USED

Activating blood circulation to eliminate blood stasis. Before applying this method, one must determine the site and complications of the blood stasis and choose drugs accordingly. For instance, in patients with blood stasis in the Heart Channel, drugs for removing stagnancy of vital energy from the chest and unblocking the channel are often administered. Drugs for dispelling masses are often given to patients with abdominal masses caused by blood stasis. If blood stasis is associated with stagnancy of vital energy and collection of phlegm, drugs for regulating flow of vital energy and resolving phlegm should be added. If there is marked pain, drugs for regulating flow of vital energy and analgesics are added. Early carbuncles are generally treated by giving febrifugal and detoxicant drugs in addition to drugs for invigorating blood circulation and eliminating blood stasis. Furthermore, different drugs are given in cases of different severity. For example, mild drugs are administered in mild cases and drastic drugs in severe cases (e.g., masses in the abdomen).

Hemostasis by dispelling pathogenic heat from the blood is used to cure hemorrhage due to failure of the spleen to keep the blood circulating within the vessels. This condition is marked by a feverish sensation, flushed face, dry mouth and throat, hematemesis, epistaxis, hematuria, rash, and slippery and rapid pulse.

Replenishing vital energy to stop chronic hemorrhage is also known as strengthening the function of the spleen, since this organ is responsible for keeping blood in the vessels. This method is used to stop hemorrhage (e.g., bleeding per rectum, minute bleeding in the skin, profuse menstrual bleeding, other uterine bleeding) associated with deficiency of vital function of the spleen. It should be noted that drugs for invigorating blood circulation should be added if blood stasis is present.

CAUTIONS

Drugs for invigorating blood circulation to eliminate blood stasis are contraindicated in patients with profuse menstrual bleeding who do not show prominent signs of blood stasis. They are also contraindicated in pregnant women, because they may induce abortion.

When the method of activating blood circulation to eliminate blood stasis is used, blood tonics are added so that blood is not impaired and consumed when blood stasis is corrected. Also, hemostatics are often given with drugs for eliminating blood stasis.

Methods for Relieving Rheumatic Conditions

These methods are used to treat painful joints, tendons, and bones; soreness and numbness of the muscles; motion impairment; and inflammation of the joints. Since the cause of rheumatism is intricate, the method is usually employed in combination with other measures such as warming the channels and dispelling cold from them, eliminating blood stasis or removing intense heat to unblock the channels, and tonifying the liver and kidney to strengthen the tendons and bones.

The rules for using these methods are as follows. In cases with an overabundance of cold and severe pain, drugs for warming and unblocking the channels are added. In those with swelling around the joints, large amounts of drugs for dispelling dampness are given. In those with rigid and persistent joint swelling, drugs for eliminating blood stasis and clearing the channels are added. Drugs for clearing intense heat and unblocking the channels are added if there is heat; drugs for replenishing vital energy and blood are added if there is protracted rheumatism.

Methods of Resuscitation

These methods are used for emergency treatment of unconsciousness due to convulsions, epilepsy, apoplexy, and fever caused by exogenous pathogenic factors. Aromatic stimulants are generally used in this method.

METHODS COMMONLY USED

Removing pathogenic heat to induce resuscitation is applicable chiefly to fever caused by invasion of the nutrient system by exogenous pathogenic factors (marked by high fever, delirium, and convulsions) and to coma resulting from stroke. In the case of high fever that is due to exogenous pathogenic factors, febrifugal and detoxicant drugs and anticonvulsives are added. In stroke, drugs for subduing hyperactivity of the liver and endogenous wind are added.

Clearing phlegm to induce resuscitation is effective in high fever due to exogenous pathogenic factors and marked by coma, wheezing due to excessive phlegm, and thick and slimy tongue coating; in stroke manifested by loss of consciousness, delirium, excessive phlegm, and thick and slimy tongue coating; and in psychosis marked by loss of touch with reality and a thick and slimy tongue coating. Aromatic stimulants, sedatives, and drugs for clearing phlegm are used.

Removing summer heat to induce resuscitation is a method to eliminate summer heat that is marked by sudden distending pain in the chest and abdomen, nausea, loss of consciousness in severe cases, excessive phlegm, and trismus. Aromatic drugs and other medications to stimulate the senses are used.

CAUTIONS

The method is applicable only when pathogenic factors are overabundant and the antipathogenic factor is not impeded. In collapse resulting from loss of vital energy, it is most important to replenish vital energy rather than employ the above resuscitation methods.

This method is only an emergency treatment. The root cause of the disease must be discovered.

Aromatic stimulants are contraindicated in pregnant women to avoid inducing abortion.

Methods of Causing Contraction and Arresting Discharges

These methods check exhaustion and further consumption of vital energy, blood, and body fluid. They are effective against such conditions as spontaneous sweating, night sweats, persistent cough, chronic diarrhea, seminal emission, spermatorrhea, enuresis, uterine bleeding, and morbid leukorrhea. Because the above disorders result from debility, tonics for deficiency are used in addition to astringents and hemostatics.

METHODS COMMONLY USED

Checking profuse sweating is effective in spontaneous sweating and night sweats. The former is due to deficiency of vital energy, and so it is necessary to enhance vital energy and strengthen superficial resistance. The latter is due to deficiency of vital essence, and so it is advisable to replenish vital essence and check profuse sweating. In both conditions, astringents are administered.

Relieving cough with astringent drugs is used to treat persistent unproductive cough. In addition to common antitussives, drugs for consolidating vital energy of the lung to relieve cough should be given. Then cough may be eased and phlegm expectorated. If drugs for consolidating vital energy of the lung are used alone, sometimes cough is relieved but phlegm remains, causing a feeling of oppression in the chest.

The *diarrhea-arresting method* is used to treat fecal incontinence due to chronic diarrhea and to prolapse of the rectum. Styptic or astringent drugs and remedies tonifying the spleen and kidney are employed.

In the *arresting seminal emission method,* seminal emission and spermatorrhea due to hypofunction of the kidney are arrested with styptic or astringent agents.

The *reducing-urination method* is used to treat frequency of urination, enuresis, and urinary incontinence due to deficiency of vital energy of the kidney. Medicines strengthening kidney function and astringent agents to arrest profuse urination are administered.

The *checking-abnormal-menstruation method* temporarily cures severe menstrual bleeding and other uterine bleeding with a few astringent agents in addition to common hemostatics.

The *checking-profuse-leukorrhea method* cures profuse leukorrhea and debility due to deficiency of vital energy. Astringent drugs, as well as remedies replenishing vital energy of the kidney, are used.

Hemostasis is used to cure hemorrhages of various causes. The following measures are often adopted: removing pathogenic heat to stop bleeding, stopping hemorrhage by dispelling pathogenic heat from blood, and replenishing vital energy and invigorating the function of the spleen to stop chronic hemorrhage. The commonly used hemostatics are of cool property and are often carbonized before administration. (Carbonizing introduces a styptic property to the medication.)

CAUTIONS

It is inadvisable to use these methods in the early stage of an illness. In cases with deficiency of the antipathogenic factor and preponderance of the pathogenic factor, these methods should be used with great care. If pathogenic factors and excessive phlegm remain in the lung, the method is unsuitable, for pathogenic factors may be kept inside.

Treating Mental Strain with Tranquilizing Drugs

In these methods, mineral and crustacean drugs are used to cure convulsions, subdue internal wind, and check exuberance of vital function.

METHODS COMMONLY USED

Relieving convulsions and soothing the nerves is applicable to palpitation (including continuous violent palpitation), insomnia, manic-depressive illness, and insanity. Medicines for strengthening vital energy of the heart and for nourishing the heart and blood, sedatives, and drugs for checking hyperactivity are used. If phlegm and heat are present, antipyretics and expectorants are added.

The indications for *checking exuberance of vital function and subduing internal wind* are the following:

- Hyperfunction of the liver leading to stirring of endogenous wind in the liver, with manifestations such as dizziness, headache, irri-

tability, bloodshot eyes, hypertension or convulsions and tremor
in severe cases, facial paralysis, and hemiplegia.
- High fever caused by exogenous pathogenic heat and marked by
delirium, convulsions, and spasms.
- Spasms of the limbs due to injury of vital essence in febrile disease and stirring of endogenous wind.

Strong tranquilizing agents such as anticonvulsants and drugs subduing hyperactivity of the liver and replenishing vital essence of the
liver and kidney are given in these conditions.

Reinforcing the function of the kidney to maintain normal inspiration is
applicable to cases with decreased lung and kidney function leading
to failure of the kidney to maintain normal inspiration. Manifestations of this condition include shortness of breath, asthma upon exertion, uneven breathing (expiration exceeds inspiration), profuse
sweating due to debility, cold limbs, and pale or livid complexion.
Drugs for maintaining normal inspiration, astringent agents for the
lung, and remedies invigorating the function of the kidney are given.

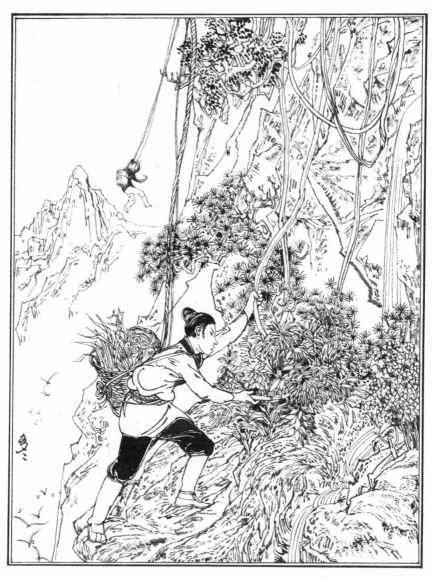

Farmers gathering wild herbs.

Medicinal herbs are prescribed in accordance with several basic concepts. Herbs are categorized as having various properties and flavors; as having ascending, descending, floating, and sinking functions; and as acting on specific organs and channels. These classifications form a basis for deciding which herbs to prescribe. In addition, certain precautions must be taken when prescribing herbs.

CLASSIFICATION OF HERBS

The Properties and Flavors of Medicinal Herbs

All Chinese medicinal herbs have specific properties and flavors that are important signs of their actions. Knowing these properties and flavors helps to guide medical practice.

The properties of herbs—i.e., what sorts of conditions various herbs are useful for treating—have been determined empirically on the basis of clinical effects. Originally the flavors of herbs were discerned by taste, for in ancient times they could not be explained chemically.

In general, each medicinal herb is classified as having one of four properties—cold, hot, cool, or warm—according to its therapeutic effects; warm differs from hot, and cool from cold, only in degree. Within a category such as hot or cold, various degrees also exist. Herbs effective for heat symptom-complexes are said to have cold or cool properties. For example, *Radix Scutellariae* (skullcap root) and *Radix Isatidis* (Dyer's woad root) are effective against fever, thirst, and sore throat and thus are considered cold in property. Conversely, drugs that alleviate or remove cold symptom-complexes are termed warm or hot in property. For instance, *Radix Aconiti Praeparata* (monkshood root) and *Rhizoma Zingiberis* (dried ginger) can warm the stomach, disperse pathogenic cold, and correct a forceless deep pulse. This suggests that they are hot in property.

Traditionally, medicinal herbs are classified as having five basic flavors: pungent, sweet, sour, bitter, and salty. In addition, some herbs are classified as insipid (lacking in flavor) or as producing a puckery feeling. Insipid is generally grouped with sweet and puckery with sour. Pungent, sweet, and insipid are considered to pertain to *yang;* sour, puckery, bitter, and salty pertain to *yin.* As indicated above, practice has proved that the five flavors of herbs are signs of

CHAPTER TWO

———◆·◆———

Chinese Medicinal Herbs:
Basic Concepts
and Common Examples

A S NOTED IN THE PRECEDING CHAPTER, tradit
Chinese medicine contends that disease develops when
ogenic factors disturb the equilibrium of *yin* and *yang* i
human body. Medicinal herbs[1] help to increase body resist
eliminate pathogenic factors, and restore a relative balance bet
yin and *yang*. Thus, harmonious function of the *zang-fu* organs i
restored.

Through centuries of medical practice, knowledge of herbs i
Chinese materia medica has been accrued by repeated observatior
experiment. Each medicinal herb has been shown to have sp
properties and actions. Chinese medicinal herbs have been ana
according to the theories of *yin-yang, zang-fu* organs, channels
collaterals, and principles of treatment.

This chapter begins by discussing basic concepts regarding m
inal herbs. Then information on more than 330 of the most
monly used herbs is presented.

---

1. These include any plant, animal, or mineral products that have therapeutic v
namely, the basic ingredients of medicines. The names of medicinal herbs have beer
cized throughout this book to distinguish them from compound preparations.

the herbs' actions, and different flavors indicate different effects. Also, by virtue of the classification of phenomena in nature according to the theory of the five elements (see volume 1, chapter 2), the five herb flavors correspond to the *zang-fu* organs.

Generally, herbs *pungent* in flavor have a dispersing action, promoting the flow of vital energy and blood. Therefore, these herbs are usually good for exterior symptom-complexes, stagnation of vital energy, and stasis of blood. Some pungent herbs, such as *Semen Cuscutae* (Chinese dodder seed), are tonics. Pungent herbs manifest their therapeutic actions in the lung and large intestine.

Herbs *sweet* in flavor are tonics and manifest their therapeutic action in the spleen and stomach. Thus they regulate the vital function of the stomach and relieve acute symptoms. They are often used to treat debility as well as pain due to spasm of the limbs. Some sweet herbs, such as *Radix Glycyrrhizae* (licorice root), harmonize other herbs' actions.

Herbs *sour* in flavor have astringent actions and arrest discharges. They usually are effective for sweating due to deficiency of vital energy and for diarrhea. Sour herbs manifest their therapeutic action in the liver and gallbladder.

Herbs that are *puckery* have actions similar to those of herbs sour in flavor. They are often used to cure profuse sweating due to deficiency of vital energy, as well as to treat urinary frequency, spermatorrhea, and bleeding.

Herbs *bitter* in flavor eliminate pathogentic damp-heat and manifest their therapeutic action in the heart and small intestine. These herbs are good for constipation and restlessness due to intense heat.

Herbs *salty* in flavor can dispel masses, reduce swellings, and relieve constipation. They are generally used to treat conditions such as tuberculous cervical lymphadenitis, abdominal masses, and constipation due to pathogenic heat. Salty herbs manifest their therapeutic action in the kidney and urinary bladder.

Herbs that are *insipid* dispel pathogenic dampness through diuresis. They are often used to treat edema and difficulty in urination.

The properties and flavors of medicinal herbs must always be considered together. For example, if two herbs are both cold in property but are of different flavors (e.g., one is bitter and the other pungent), they differ in their actions.

The Ascending, Descending, Floating, and Sinking Actions of Medicinal Herbs

Each herb also is classified, according to its direction of action, as one or more of the following: ascending, descending, floating, and sinking. "Ascending" and "descending" pertain explicitly to the direction of action. Herbs that are "floating" are those that can disperse pathogenic factors; those that are "sinking" have, for example, tranquilizing actions.

Generally, herbs with ascending and floating tendencies are used to activate vitality, dispel pathogenic wind and cold, induce vomiting, and cause resuscitation. Herbs with descending and sinking tendencies are used to promote diuresis, clear waste matter from the bowels, dispel intense heat, tranquilize the nerves, check exuberance of vital function, subdue endogenous pathogenic wind, promote digestion, put down the adverse upward flow of vital energy, exert astringent action, and relieve cough and asthma. Depending on which other herbs accompany them in a prescription, some herbs can have either an ascending or a descending action, or either a floating or a sinking action.

The ascending and descending, floating and sinking actions of herbs help the body to restore its normal function and eliminate pathogenic factors. For example, vomiting, asthma, and cough due to the adverse upward flow of vital energy are often treated with antiemetics, antiasthmatics, and antitussives that have descending character. Herbs to strengthen and lift up vital energy are used in treating diarrhea, prolapse of the rectum, and uterine bleeding when these conditions are caused by sinking of vital energy.

The characters of herbs are closely related to the herbs' flavors and properties. Most herbs of ascending and floating character are pungent or sweet in flavor, warm or hot in property. Most herbs descending and sinking in character are sour, bitter, salty, or puckery, as well as cold or cool in property.

Classification of Herbs According to the Organs and Channels on Which They Act

Different herbs act on different organs and channels. For instance, herbs cold or cool in property all clear away intense heat, but some remove the heat from the heart, some from the lung, and some from the liver. Similarly, all tonics are capable of nourishing, but some nourish the lung, some the spleen, and others the kidney.

As discussed in volume 1, any morbid change and its manifestations may be classified as an affliction of a specific channel. For example, cough and asthma suggest a disorder of the Lung Channel; pain in the hypochondria and convulsions are usually seen in disorders of the Liver Channel; insomnia frequently occurs in disorders of the Heart Channel; abdominal distension and loose stools reflect trouble in the Spleen Channel; and soreness in the lumbar region and knees, impotence, seminal emission, and spermatorrhea point to trouble in the Kidney Channel. Thus *Semen Armenicae Amarum* (apricot kernel) is good for cough and asthma, as it acts on the Lung Channel; *Scorpio* (scorpion) is effective for convulsions, as it acts on the Liver Channel; stir-baked jujube is used to treat insomnia, as it acts on the Heart Channel; *Rhizoma Atractylodis Macrocephalae* (large-headed atractylodes rhizome) is used in treating abdominal distension and loose stools, as it acts on the Spleen Channel; and *Fructus Psoraleae* (malaytea scurfpea fruit) is used to treat soreness in the lumbar region and knees, impotence, and seminal emission, as it acts on the Kidney Channel. Knowing on which channels herbs act gives doctors important help in prescribing drugs.

Precautions in Prescribing Medicinal Herbs

Various precautions must be taken when prescribing medicinal herbs. During pregnancy, some herbs should be avoided or only used very carefully. Some foods are prohibited when a patient is taking herbs. Also, as will be discussed in chapter 3, unfavorable interactions of herbs must be considered.

Some drastic or toxic herbs are prohibited during pregnancy, as they have long been known to induce abortion. These herbs include *Fructus Crotonis* (croton fruit), *Semen Pharbitidis* (morning glory seed), *Radix Euphorbiae Pekinensis* (Peking spurge), *Mylabris* (blister beetle), *Radix Phytolaccae* (India pokeberry), *Moschus* (musk), *Rhizoma Sparganii* (burred rhizome), *Rhizoma Zedoariae* (zedoary turmeric rhizome), *Hirudo* (leech), and *Tabanus Bivittatus* (gadfly). In addition, herbs good for stimulating menstrual discharge, removing blood stasis, and promoting the normal flow of vital energy, as well as herbs pungent in flavor, should be used with care during pregnancy because they can also induce abortion. Among these herbs are *Semen Persicae* (peach kernel), *Flos Carthami* (safflower), *Radix et Rhizoma Rhei* (rhubarb root), *Fructus Aurantii Immaturus* (immature bitter orange), *Radix Aconiti Praeparata, Rhizoma Zingiberis,* and *Cortex Cinnamomi* (bark of Chinese cassia tree).

Dietary prohibitions include the following. Foods that counteract the effects of specific herbs must be avoided when taking them. For example, scallion counteracts *Radix Dichroae* (antipyretic dichroa root); scallion, garlic, and radish counteract *Radix Polygoni Multiflori* (multiflower knotweed tuber) and *Radix Rehmannia* (rehmannia root); turtle counteracts *Herba Menthae* (peppermint); vinegar counteracts *Poria* (tuckahoe); amaranth counteracts *Carapax Trionycis* (turtle shell); and honey counteracts scallion. Furthermore, raw, cold, greasy, and irritant foods should be avoided when medication is being administered.

COMMONLY USED MEDICINAL HERBS

Diaphoretics (Herbs Used in Treating Exterior Symptom-complexes)

These herbs dispel pathogenic factors from the exterior of the body by diaphoresis. Some also are effective for cough, asthma, exanthesis in measles, generalized aching, and so on.

DIAPHORETICS PUNGENT IN FLAVOR AND WARM IN PROPERTY

These diaphoretics generally are used in treating exterior symptom-complexes caused by pathogenic wind and cold. They are effective chiefly for conditions marked by aversion to cold, fever, absence of sweat, generalized aching, thin white tongue coating, and floating and tight pulse (e.g., cough and asthma due to superficial affliction, edema, ulcers, rheumatism).

On the basis of experimental results, it is hypothesized that the herbs have two kinds of actions. On the one hand, they may dilate peripheral vessels, improve microcirulation, and induce sweating by stimulating the sweat glands. On the other, they may regulate body temperature and increase the pain threshold so as to alleviate heat and pain.

Medicinal Herb	Property(s)	Flavor(s)	Channel(s) Acted on	Action(s)	Indication(s)	Amount (grams)[2]	Remarks
Herba Ephedrae (Chinese ephedra)	warm	pungent and slightly bitter	Lung and Urinary Bladder	Dispelling pathogenic factors from the exterior of the body; relieving asthma; detumescence through diaphoresis and diuresis	Exterior symptom-complexes caused by pathogenic wind-cold (e.g., cough, asthma)	2–10	Use with care in patients with profuse sweating, insomnia, and hypertension

2. The gram is the unit used throughout this volume. It is now the accepted unit of weight in prescriptions in China. One gram equals ⅓ *qian*.

Medicinal Herb	Property(s)	Flavor(s)	Channel(s) Acted on	Action(s)	Indication(s)	Amount (grams)	Remarks
Ramulus Cinnamomi (cassia twig)	warm	pungent and sweet	Heart, Lung, and Urinary Bladder	Increasing perspiration; dispelling pathogenic factors from the superficial muscles; warming the channels and removing obstruction of the flow of vital energy	Exterior deficiency symptom-complexes caused by pathogenic wind-cold; retention of phlegm and fluid, arthralgia, pectoral pain	3–10	Prohibited in patients with deficiency of vital essence and intense internal heat; use with care in pregnant women and patients with profuse menstrual bleeding
Herba Elsholtziae seu Moslae (Chinese mosla)	moderately warm	pungent	Lung and Stomach	Dispelling pathogenic factors from the exterior of the body through diuresis and diaphoresis	Common cold in summer; diseases caused by dampness	3–10	
Folium Perillae (leaf of purple perilla)	moderately warm	pungent	Lung and Spleen	Dispelling pathogenic cold through diaphoresis	Common cold due to pathogenic wind-cold, vomiting, diarrhea; and food poisoning due to ingestion of spoiled crab and fish	3–10	
Herba Schizonepetae (schizonepeta)	mild	pungent	Lung and liver	Dispelling pathogenic wind and pathogenic factors from the exterior of the body	Common cold caused by pathogenic cold or wind-heat; rubella, fail-	3–10	

Name	Nature	Taste	Channels	Actions	Indications	Dosage	Precautions
				through diaphoresis; arresting bleeding	ure of exanthesis in measles; pharyngitis, tonsillitis, epistaxis, bloody stools, and uterine bleeding		
Radix Ledebouriellae (ledebouriella root)	moderately warm	pungent and sweet	Urinary Bladder, Liver, and Spleen	Dispelling pathogenic wind dampness from the exterior of the body; relieving spasm	Common cold due to pathogenic wind-cold; migraine; arthralgia due to pathogenic wind, cold, and dampness	3–10	Use with care in patients with convulsions due to insufficient blood and vital essence and with intense internal heat
Radix Angelicae Daburicae (dahurian angelica root)	warm	pungent	Lung and Stomach	Dispelling pathogenic wind from the exterior of the body, discharging pus, reducing swelling, and arresting pain	Common cold due to pathogenic wind-cold; frontal headache, toothache, or rhinitis, boils, carbuncles, leukorrhoea	3–10	
Herba Asari (wildginger)	warm	pungent	Lung and Liver	Dispelling pathogenic wind-cold from the exterior of the body; analgesia, reducing copious thin phlegm and arresting pain	Cough and asthma due to pathogenic cold (bronchitis, bronchiectasis); common cold caused by pathogenic wind-cold; headache due to rheumatism or influenza	3–10	

Medicinal Herb	Property(s)	Flavor(s)	Channel(s) Acted on	Action(s)	Indication(s)	Amount (grams)	Remarks
Rhizoma et Radix Ligustici (ligusticum root)	warm	pungent	Urinary bladder	Dispelling pathogenic wind-cold from the exterior of the body; analgesia	Headache due to pathogenic wind-cold or rheumatism	2–10	

DIAPHORETICS PUNGENT IN FLAVOR AND COOL IN PROPERTY

These agents are used to dispel pathogenic wind and cold from the exterior of the body. They are effective chiefly for high fever with mild intolerance of cold, dry throat, thirst, thin yellow tongue coating, floating and rapid pulse; incipient acute febrile disease; and eye troubles due to pathogenic wind and heat.

Medicinal Herb	Property(s)	Flavor(s)	Channel(s) Acted on	Action(s)	Indication(s)	Amount (grams)	Remarks
Herba Menthae (peppermint)	cool	pungent	Lung and Liver	Dispelling pathogenic wind-heat; promoting exanthesis in measles	Incipient acute febrile disease due to pathogenic wind-heat; invasion of the head by pathogenic wind-heat (headache, blood-shot eyes, sore throat); failure of exanthesis in measles	2–10	Added when the decoction is nearly done

Fructus Arctii (great burdock achene)	cold	pungent and bitter	Lung and Stomach	Dispelling pathogenic wind-heat; relieving pyogenic inflammation; promoting exanthesis in measles	Inflammation of the throat (pharyngitis, upper respiratory tract infection); failure of exanthesis in measles; constipation due to pathogenic wind-heat; swelling, unruptured boils	3–10	Use with care in patients having loose stools
Folium Mori (mulberry leaf)	cold	bitter and sweet	Lung and Liver	Dispelling pathogenic wind-heat; quenching fire in the liver; restoring eyesight	Mild cases of exogenous affection by pathogenic wind-heat; impairment of the lung by pathogenic dryness; bloodshot eyes due to invasion of the Liver Channel by pathogenic wind-heat	5–10	
Flos Chrysanthemi (chrysanthemum flower)	moderately cold	pungent, sweet, and bitter	Lung and Liver	Dispelling pathogenic wind-heat; relieving pyogenic inflammation; restoring eyesight	Exogenous affection by pathogenic wind-heat; incipient acute febrile disease; bloodshot painful eyes due to invasion of the Liver Channel by pathogenic wind-heat	10–20	

Medicinal Herb	Property(s)	Flavor(s)	Channel(s) Acted on	Action(s)	Indication(s)	Amount (grams)	Remarks
Radix Puerariae (pueraria root)	cool	sweet and pungent	Spleen and Stomach	Dispelling pathogenic factors from the exterior of the body; invigorating vital function to generate body fluid	Discomfort and pain in the neck and back; incipient measles; diarrhea due to damp-heat (acute enteritis and dysentery); thirst in diabetes	5–20	
Radix Bupleuri (thorowax root)	moderately cold	bitter and pungent	Pericardium, Liver, Triple Burner, and Gallbladder	Expelling pathogenic factors from the exterior of the body; soothing a depressed liver; invigorating vital function	Invasion of the *Shaoyang* Channel by pathogenic factors located between the exterior and interior of the body; remittent fever; prolapse of organs	3–10	

Antipyretics (Herbs for Clearing Away Internal Heat)

These herbs are cool or cold in property and can clear away internal heat. They generally are used in treating febrile or inflammatory conditions, dysentery, and other heat symptom-complexes due to deficiency of vital essence.

HERBS FOR REDUCING INTENSE INTERNAL HEAT

HERBS FOR REMOVING PATHOGENIC HEAT FROM THE VITAL ENERGY SYSTEM

Medicinal Herb	Property(s)	Flavor(s)	Channel(s) Acted on	Action(s)	Indication(s)	Amount (grams)	Remarks
Gypsum Fibrosum (gypsum)	extremely cold	sweet and pungent	Lung and Stomach	Reducing intense internal heat; relieving restlessness and thirst	Acute febrile disease with pathogenic factors in the vital energy system; asthma due to pathogenic heat in the lung; headache caused by pathogenic heat in the stomach; toothache, protracted ulcers, eczema, scalds	15–60	Decocted first
Rhizoma Anemarrhenae (windweed rhizome)	cold	sweet and bitter	Lung, Stomach, and Kidney	Reducing intense internal heat; replenishing vital essence; eliminating pathogenic dryness	Excessive heat in the vital energy system; cough due to pathogenic heat in the lung; dry cough due to want of body fluid; intense heat caused by deficiency of vital essence; hectic fever and night sweats	6–12	Inadvisable in patients having loose stools

Medicinal Herb	Property(s)	Flavor(s)	Channel(s) Acted on	Action(s)	Indication(s)	Amount (grams)	Remarks
Fructus Gardeniae (Cape jasmine fruit)	cold	bitter	Heart, Liver, Lung, Stomach, and Tri-Burner	Reducing intense internal heat through diuresis; relieving restlessness; cooling blood; relieving pyogenic inflammation	Irritability and restlessness due to febrile conditions; epidemic keratoconjunctivitis; jaundice caused by pathogenic damp-heat; hemorrhage, boils and sores	3–10	Appropriate amount for external use

HERBS FOR ELIMINATING PATHOGENIC HEAT AND DAMPNESS

Medicinal Herb	Property(s)	Flavor(s)	Channel(s) Acted on	Action(s)	Indication(s)	Amount (grams)	Remarks
Rhizoma Coptidis (coptis root)	cold	bitter	Heart, Liver, Stomach, and Large Intestine	Clearing away pathogenic damp-heat; removing toxicity	Dysentery due to pathogenic damp-heat (bacillary dysentery); high fever and delirium due to febrile disease; vomiting due to pathogenic heat in the stomach; pyogenic infection of the skin; otitis media	1–5	

Cortex Phelloden-dri (corktree bark)	cold	bitter	Kidney, Urinary Bladder, and Large Intestine	Eliminating damp-heat and toxicity; relieving fever due to deficiency of vital energy or vital essence	Dysentery and urinary disturbance due to pathogenic damp-heat; jaundice; swollen and painful knee joints and feet; intense internal heat caused by deficiency of vital essence; hectic fever and night sweats; leukorrhea; boils or sores	3–10
Radix Scutellariae (baikal skullcap root)	cold	bitter	Lung, Stomach, Gallbladder, and Large Intestine	Clearing away pathogenic dampness; removing toxicity; hemostasis	Diarrhea, dysentery due to pathogenic damp-heat; jaundice; cough caused by pathogenic heat in the lung; bleeding due to intense heat; boils; threatened abortion	3–10
Radix Gentianae (Chinese gentian)	cold	bitter	Stomach, Liver, and Gallbladder	Eliminating intense heat and dampness; reducing pathogenic fire from the liver	Jaundice due to pathogenic damp-heat; convulsions due to flaring up of internal wind in the liver, inflammation of the skin and perineum	3–6

Medicinal Herb	Property(s)	Flavor(s)	Channel(s) Acted on	Action(s)	Indication(s)	Amount (grams)	Remarks
Radix Sophorae Flavescentis (sophora flavescent root)	cold	bitter	Heart, Liver, Stomach, Large Intestine, and Urinary bladder	Eliminating intense heat and dampness; dispelling pathogenic wind; counteracting parasites; causing urination	Dysentery and jaundice due to pathogenic dampheat; dermatitis; boils	3–10	

HERBS FOR ELIMINATING PATHOGENIC HEAT FROM BLOOD

These herbs are used in treating febrile diseases with bleeding symptoms (e.g., hemoptysis, epistaxis, bleeding per rectum, petechial eruptions) due to excessive heat in the blood.

Medicinal Herb	Property(s)	Flavor(s)	Channel(s) Acted on	Action(s)	Indication(s)	Amount (grams)	Remarks
Cornu Rhinoceri (rhinoceros horn)	cold	salty	Heart, Liver, and Stomach	Easing the nerves; relieving convulsions; counteracting toxicity	Loss of consciousness; convulsions; purple rash; erysipelas	1.5–6	Incompatible with *Radix Aconiti* and *Radix Aconiti Kusnezoffii*; use with care in pregnant women
Radix Rehmannia (rehmannia root)	cold	sweet and bitter	Heart, Liver, and Kidney	Eliminating pathogenic heat from the blood; replenishing	Invasion of the *jing* and blood systems by pathogenic heat;	9–30	Amount doubled when used fresh

Herb	Nature	Flavor	Meridians	Actions	Indications	Dosage	Remarks
				vital essence to generate body fluid	persistent mild fever in the advanced stage of febrile disease; internal heat due to deficiency of vital essence; bleeding; nettle rash; injury of body fluid due to excessive heat; constipation		
Radix Scrophulariae (figwort root)	cold	sweet, bitter, and salty	Lung, Stomach, and Kidney	Eliminating pathogenic heat and toxicity; replenishing vital essence; resolving hard lumps in the body	Invasion of the *ying* system by pathogenic heat in acute disease; injury of vital essence; pathogenic dryness in the lung due to deficiency of vital essence; expectoration of sputum; acute swelling and pain in the throat; thromboangiitis obliterans	9–30	Restrains *Radix Veratrum Nigrum*
Cortex Moutan Radicis (tree peony bark)	cold	bitter and slightly pungent	Heart, Liver, and Kidney	Eliminating pathogenic heat; activating blood circulation to remove blood stasis	Invasion of the *ying* system by pathogenic heat due to febrile conditions; hemoptysis; epistaxis; anemia due to pathogenic heat in blood; appendicitis	6–12	Use with care in pregnant women

Medicinal Herb	Property(s)	Flavor(s)	Channel(s) Acted on	Action(s)	Indication(s)	Amount (grams)	Remarks
Radix Arnebiae seu Lithospermi (purple gromwell root)	cold	sweet	Heart and Liver	Eliminating pathogenic heat and toxicity from blood; activating blood circulation; promoting exanthesis in measles	Measles (treatment and prevention) due to febrile conditions; carbuncles, boils, eczema	3–10	Appropriate amount for external use

HERBS FOR CLEARING AWAY FEVER DUE TO DEFICIENCY OF VITAL ENERGY, VITAL ESSENCE, OR BODY FLUID

These herbs relieve fever due to impairment of body fluid in the advanced stage of acute febrile disease. They also relieve hectic fever and night sweats caused by consumptive disease (e.g., tuberculosis).

Medicinal Herb	Property(s)	Flavor(s)	Channel(s) Acted on	Action(s)	Indication(s)	Amount (grams)	Remarks
Cortex Lycii Radicis (wolfberry root-bark)	cold	sweet and insipid	Lung and Kidney	Relieving fever due to deficiency of vital energy; clearing away pathogenic heat from the blood and lung	Mild fever due to deficiency of vital energy, essence, or blood; hectic fever and night sweats; asthmatic cough associated with afternoon fever	6–12	

Radix Stellariae (starwort root)	moderately cold	sweet	Lung and Stomach	Relieving fever due to deficiency of vital energy	Hectic fever and night sweats due to deficiency of vital essence; mild fever due to infantile malnutrition; emaciation	3–10
Rhizoma Picrorrhizae	cold	bitter	Heart, Liver, Stomach, and Large Intestine	Relieving fever due to deficiency of vital energy and expelling damp-heat	Hectic fever and night sweats due to deficiency of vital essence; mild fever due to infantile malnutrition; dysentery caused by pathogenic damp-heat; hemorrhoids	3–10

Herbs for Eliminating Heat-Toxins

These herbs have antipyretic, antibacterial, or antiviral actions. They are effective against carbuncles, erysipelas, rashes, swollen throat, and dysentery due to pathogenic heat-toxins. Some are used in treating pyogenic suppurative infections, as they can relieve pathogenic heat and inflammation.

HERBS FOR TREATING ACUTE FEBRILE CONDITIONS

Medicinal Herb	Property(s)	Flavor(s)	Channel(s) Acted on	Action(s)	Indication(s)	Amount (grams)	Remarks
Flos Lonicerae (honeysuckle flower)	cold	sweet	Lung, Stomach, and Large Intestine	Eliminating heat-toxins	Exogenous affliction by pathogenic wind-heat; incipient acute febrile disease or preponderance of heat-toxins; ulcers and carbuncles; bacterial dysentery and acute enteritis	6–10	
Fructus Forsythiae (forsythia fruit)	moderately cold	bitter	Lung, Heart, and Gallbladder	Eliminating heat-toxins; causing carbuncles to subside	Exogenous affliction by pathogenic heat; incipient acute febrile disease; penetration of pathogenic heat into the pericardium; dark yellow urine and painful urination due to pathogenic fire going downward from the heart into the small intestine; pyogenic infections; tuberculous cervical lymphadenitis; anaphylactoid purpura	6–16	

Folium Isatidis (Dyer's wood leaf)	bitter	extremely cold	Heart, Lung, and Stomach	Removing intense heat from blood and resolving rash	Febrile diseases; viral infections (including mumps, encephalitis B, viral pneumonia, influenza, epidemic meningitis); erysipelas; oral ulcers; swollen and painful throat	10–16	Amount increased to 60, if fresh leaves are used; fresh leaves used for local application
Radix Isatidis (Dyer's wood root)	bitter	cold	Heart and Lung	Eliminating heat-toxins; removing intense heat from blood; easing sore throat pain	Rash in acute febrile diseases; mumps; encephalitis B; erysipelas; acute infectious hepatitis; viral myelitis	15–30	
Rhizoma Paridis (Paris rhizome)	bitter	moderately cold and slightly toxic	Liver	Eliminating heat-toxins; reducing swelling and pain; arresting convulsions	Acute pyogenic inflammations and toxemia; high fever; cancer of uterine cervix; chronic bronchitis; protracted cough in pulmonary tuberculosis; injuries and wounds; snakebite	5–10	

HERBS FOR TREATING SUPPURATIVE INFECTIONS ON THE BODY SURFACE

Medicinal Herb	Property(s)	Flavor(s)	Channel(s) Acted on	Action(s)	Indication(s)	Amount (grams)	Remarks
Herba Violae (Chinese violet)	cold	pungent and bitter	Heart and Liver	Eliminating heat-toxins	Pyogenic infections (especially on the face and back); acute conjunctivitis; sty; snakebite	10–16	
Herba Taraxaci (dandelion herb)	cold	bitter and sweet	Liver and Stomach	Eliminating heat-toxins; removing pathogenic dampness through diuresis	Pyogenic infections; acute mastitis; appendicitis; acute icteric hepatitis; urinary tract infection; acute conjunctivitis; sty	10–30	
Herba Houttuyniae (cordate houttuynia)	moderately cold	pungent	Lung	Eliminating heat-toxins	Pulmonary abscess; pneumonia; acute and chronic bronchitis; enteritis; urinary tract infection; boils and carbuncles	15–30	
Herba Patriniae (patrinia herb)	moderately cold	bitter and pungent	Stomach, Large Intestine, and Liver	Eliminating heat-toxins; reducing inflammation; removing pus and blood stasis; alleviating pain	Appendicitis; lung abscess; boils and carbuncles; painful menstruation due to impeded blood circulation	6–15	

Medicinal Herb	Property(s)	Flavor(s)	Channel(s) Acted on	Action(s)	Indication(s)	Amount (grams)	Remarks
Cortex Dictamni Radicis (ditlany root-bark)	cold	bitter	Spleen and Stomach	Eliminating damp-heat-toxins; dispelling internal pathogenic wind	Pyogenic infections due to pathogenic damp-heat; urticaria; tinea; itching of the skin	4–10	

HERBS FOR TREATING DYSENTERY

Medicinal Herb	Property(s)	Flavor(s)	Channel(s) Acted on	Action(s)	Indication(s)	Amount (grams)	Remarks
Herba Portulacae (purslane)	cold	sour	Large Intestine and Liver	Eliminating heat-toxins to cure dysentery; promoting hemostasis	Dysentery; boils and sores; uterine bleeding, profuse leukorrhea	30–60	
Radix Pulsatillae (pulsatilla root)	cold	bitter	Large Intestine	Eliminating heat-toxins and removing intense heat from blood to cure dysentery	Bacterial and amebic dysentery	6–15	
Cortex Fraxini (ash bark)	cold	bitter	Liver, Gallbladder, and Large Intestine	Eliminating heat-toxins; counteracting dysentery; regulating the liver and improving vision; resolving phlegm	Bloody dysentery; bloodshot eyes due to flaring up of liver fire; chronic bronchitis	1–5	

Herbs for Treating Sore Throat

Medicinal Herb	Property(s)	Flavor(s)	Channel(s) Acted on	Action(s)	Indication(s)	Amount (grams)	Remarks
Radix Sophorae Subprostratae (subprostrate sophora root)	cold	bitter	Lung	Eliminating heat-toxins; easing sore throat pain	Sore throat due to collection of pathogenic heat; hypertension; inhibiting the growth of cancers, e.g., of the lung, throat, and urinary bladder	6–9	
Lasiosphaera seu Calvatia (puffball)	mild	pungent	Lung	Removing pathogenic heat from the lung; easing sore throat; arresting bleeding	Cough due to intense heat in the lung; loss of voice, swollen and painful throat (upper respiratory infection, tonsillitis), bleeding due to injury, frostbite; ulcers of the legs	3–6	

Herbs for Eliminating Intense Heat and Improving Eyesight

These herbs are effective against pathogenic heat from the liver and internal pathogenic wind and heat. They are applicable chiefly to eye troubles due to intense heat in the liver or pathogenic wind-heat. These disorders are characterized by reddened and swollen eyes with excessive tears, crusting, and nebula.

Medicinal Herb	Property(s)	Flavor(s)	Channel(s) Acted on	Action(s)	Indication(s)	Amount (grams)	Remarks
Semen Cassiae (sickle senna seed)	moderately cold	sweet, bitter, and salty	Liver and Large Intestine	Eliminating intense heat; improving eyesight; relaxing the bowels	Pathogenic heat or wind-heat in the liver; reddened eyes with pain and excessive tears; photophobia (epidemic conjunctivitis, keratitis)	9–15	
Spica Prunellae (selfheal spica)	cold	bitter and pungent	Liver and Gallbladder	Quenching liver fire; removing stagnancy; decreasing blood pressure	Reddened and swollen eyes due to flaring up of excessive heat in the liver; tuberculous cervical lymphadenitis; goiter due to phlegm-heat; chronic laryngitis; glossitis	6–10	
Semen Celosiae (feather cockscomb seed)	moderately cold	bitter	Liver	Quenching liver fire; improving eyesight; removing nebula	Reddened eyes due to flaring up of excessive heat in the liver; nebula; dizziness and hypertension	6–10	

Medicinal Herb	Property(s)	Flavor(s)	Channel(s) Acted on	Action(s)	Indication(s)	Amount (grams)	Remarks
Flos Buddleiae (pale butterfly-bush flower)	moderately cold	sweet	Liver	Quenching liver fire; improving eyesight and removing nebula	Reddened and swollen eyes due to excessive heat in the liver; excessive tears, crusting; photophobia; nebula due to chronic conjunctivitis	6–10	

HERBS FOR ELIMINATING PATHOGENIC HEAT AND HEATSTROKE

These herbs promote urination, dispel pathogenic heat, generate body fluid, and relieve thirst. They are effective against acute disease due to summer heat, accompanied by manifestations such as fever, profuse sweating, and thirst.

Medicinal Herb	Property(s)	Flavor(s)	Channel(s) Acted on	Action(s)	Indication(s)	Amount (grams)	Remarks
Folium Nelumbinis (lotus leaf)	mild	bitter	Heart, Liver, and Spleen	Eliminating summer heat; removing blood stasis and stopping bleeding	Illnesses due to summer-heat; diarrhea due to colitis or functional disturbance in the gastrointestinal system; hematuria; bloody stools; postpartum hemorrhaging	15–30	

Medicinal Herb	Property(s)	Flavor(s)	Channel(s) Acted on	Action(s)	Indication(s)	Amount (grams)	Remarks
Semen Phaseoli Radiatus (mung bean)	cold	sweet	Heart and Stomach	Eliminating heat-toxins; relieving summer heat; promoting urination	Prevention of heat-stroke	3–60	Antidote for *Radix* Aconiti Praeparata and *Fructus Cannabis*
Semen Sojae Germinatum (soya bean roll)	mild	sweet	Spleen and Stomach	Removing pathogenic damp-heat through diuresis; expelling pathogenic factors from the exterior of the body	Fever, diminished perspiration, difficulty in urination due to internal accumulation of pathogenic damp-heat; collection of pathogenic damp-heat in the large intestine (e.g., dysentery); common cold in summer	6–18	

Antiperiodics

These herbs prevent malaria, and some can relieve spells of fever and chills. It has been proven that the herbs can counteract malarial parasites.

Medicinal Herb	Property(s)	Flavor(s)	Channel(s) Acted on	Action(s)	Indication(s)	Amount (grams)	Remarks
Herba Artemisiae Chinghao (sweet wormwood)	cold	bitter and pungent	Liver and Gallbladder	Antimalaria; relieving fever due to deficiency of vital energy;	Malaria; acute febrile disease in its later stage; moder-	3–9	20–40 grams used in the treatment of malaria

Medicinal Herb	Property(s)	Flavor(s)	Channel(s) Acted on	Action(s)	Indication(s)	Amount (grams)	Remarks
				eliminating intense heat and summer heat	ate fever of unknown origin; affliction with summer-heat		
Radix Dichroae (antipyretic dichroa)	moderately cold and slightly toxic	bitter and pungent	Lung and Liver	Relieving malaria; inducing expectoration of sputum; producing emesis	Counteracting malaria; promoting expectoration of profuse sputum	4–9	
Fructus Bruceae (brucea fruit)	cold	bitter	Large Intestine and Liver	Eliminating heat-toxins; antimalaria; eroding warts	Tertian or quartan malaria, dysentery, amebic dysentery; corns, common warts; trichomonas vaginitis	10–15 granules[3] per dose; 5% decoction for vaginal douche	Inadvisable to take over a long period as it is harmful to the gastrointestinal tract, liver, and kidney

Expectorants, Antitussives, and Antiasthmatics

PHLEGM-RESOLVING HERBS OF WARM PROPERTY

These herbs dispel pathogenic cold and resolve phlegm. They generally are used to treat diseases caused by cold phlegm or phlegm-dampness.

Medicinal Herb	Property(s)	Flavor(s)	Channel(s) Acted on	Action(s)	Indication(s)	Amount (grams)	Remarks
Rhizoma Arisaematis (jack-in-the-pulpit)	warm and toxic	bitter and pungent	Lung, Liver, and Spleen	Eliminating pathogenic dampness and resolving phlegm; dispelling pathogenic wind from the interior of the body; arresting convulsions	Cough with persistent sputum; apoplexy with excessive sputum; Bell's palsy, epilepsy, tetanus, subcutaneous nodules, carbuncle; cancer of cervix	5–9	Use with care in pregnant women
Rhizoma Pinelliae (pinellia) tuber	warm and toxic	pungent	Spleen, Lung, and Stomach	Eliminating pathogenic dampness and resolving phlegm; stopping vomiting; reducing masses and swellings	Retention of sputum; cough; adverse flow of vital energy; upward disturbance in the functioning of the stomach; nausea, vomiting, and suffocating feeling in the chest; globus hystericus; goiter; nodules, boils, and swellings	5–9	Incompatible with *Radix Aconiti*

3. One granule denotes an individual piece of the fruit (herb).

Medicinal Herb	Property(s)	Flavor(s)	Channel(s) Acted on	Action(s)	Indication(s)	Amount (grams)	Remarks
Semen Sinapis Albae (white mustard seed)	warm	pungent	Lung	Warming the lung to eliminate sputum; reducing masses and swellings	Retention of cold-phlegm; cough, asthma, and stuffy feeling in the chest; pain in the hypochondria; arthralgia due to blockage of the channels by damp-phlegm; deep tuberculous abscess	3–9	Appropriate amount for external use; inadvisable to use in patients susceptible to skin allergy because it induces blisters
Rhizoma Cynanchi Staumtoni (white swallow-wort)	moderately warm	pungent and sweet	Lung	Dispelling phlegm; keeping flow of *qi* going downward; stopping cough	Impairment of lung function; failure to expectorate profuse sputum; asthma due to adverse flow of vital energy; edema	3–9	

PHLEGM-RESOLVING HERBS WITH COLD PROPERTY

These herbs, which are of cold property, dispel pathogenic heat and resolve phlegm. They are usually used to treat manifestations such as asthma resulting from blockage of the lung by phlegm and heat, stuffy feeling in the chest, thick and yellow sputum, and failure of expectoration.

Medicinal Herb	Property(s)	Flavor(s)	Channel(s) Acted on	Action(s)	Indication(s)	Amount (grams)	Remarks
Radix Platycodi (root of balloon-flower)	mild (neutral)	bitter and pungent	Lung	Ventilating and soothing a troubled lung; expelling sputum; draining pus	Cough unproductive of sputum; stuffy feeling in the chest; sore throat; hoarseness; lung abscess; expectoration of pus and blood	3–9	1–1.5 grams in powder form taken with hot water
Bulbus Fritillariae Cirrhosae (tendril-leaved fritillary bulb)	moderately cold	bitter and sweet	Lung and Heart	Resolving phlegm and stopping cough; clearing away pathogenic heat; reducing masses	Cough due to affection by exogenous pathogenic wind-heat; prolonged cough productive of scanty sputum and caused by deficiency of vital energy or vital essence of the lung; dry throat; expectoration of thick yellow sputum due to retention of phlegm-heat; boils; mastitis; lung abscess; thyroma	3–9	Incompatible with *Radix Aconiti*
Bulbus Fritillariae Thunbergii (fritillary bulb)	cold	bitter	Lung and Heart	As above	As above	3–9	Incompatible with *Radix Aconiti*

Medicinal Herb	Property(s)	Flavor(s)	Channel(s) Acted on	Action(s)	Indication(s)	Amount (grams)	Remarks
Radix Peucedani (purple-flowered peucedanum)	moderately cold	bitter and pungent	Lung	Keeping the flow of *qi* going downward; dispelling sputum; expelling pathogenic wind and heat	Cough and asthma due to pathogenic heat in the lung; thick yellow sputum and stuffy feeling in the chest; common cold due to pathogenic wind and heat	3–9	
Fructus Trichosanthis (Mongolian snakegourd fruit)	cold	sweet	Lung, Stomach, and Large Intestine	Resolving phlegm by removing pathogenic heat from the lung; invigorating the smooth flow of vital energy to treat stuffy feeling in the chest; relaxing the bowels	Cough due to pathogenic heat in the lung; angina pectoris; constipation	12–30	Incompatible with *Radix Aconiti*
Folium Eriobotryae (loquat leaf)	mild	bitter	Lung and Stomach	Resolving phlegm; stopping cough; regulating the vital function of the stomach and putting down upward adverse flow of vital energy	Cough due to pathogenic heat in the lung; vomiting due to heat in the stomach	9–15	
Concretio Silicea bambusae (tabasheer)	cold	sweet	Heart, Liver, and Gallbladder	Clearing away pathogenic heat and resolving phlegm; dispelling pathogenic heat	Infantile convulsions produced by phlegm and heat; loss of conscious-	3–9	

Medicinal Herb	Property(s)	Flavor(s)	Channel(s) Acted on	Action(s)	Indication(s)	Amount (grams)	Remarks
				from the heart or pericardium to relieve convulsions	ness in adults due to febrile conditions; stroke		
Sargassum (kelp)	cold	bitter and salty	Liver, Stomach, and Kidney	Clearing phlegm; removing pathogenic dampness through diuresis; reducing hard lumps and enlarged nodes	Goiter and tubercular cervical lymphadenitis; edema and edemic beriberi	9–15	
Thallus Laminariae seu Eckloniae (dried thallus)	cold	salty	Liver, Stomach, and Kidney	As above	As above	9–15	

Antitussives and Antiasthmatics

These are herbs for relieving cough and asthmatic symptoms.

Medicinal Herb	Property(s)	Flavor(s)	Channel(s) Acted on	Action(s)	Indication(s)	Amount (grams)	Remarks
Semen Armeniacae Amarum (bitter apricot kernel)	moderately warm, slightly toxic	bitter	Lung and Large Intestine	Relieving cough and asthma; relaxing the bowels	Any kind of cough or asthma; constipation	3–9	

Medicinal Herb	Property(s)	Flavor(s)	Channel(s) Acted on	Action(s)	Indication(s)	Amount (grams)	Remarks
Radix Asteris (aster root)	mildly warm	bitter, sweet	Lung	Resolving phlegm to relieve cough	Cough and adverse flow of vital energy; expectoration of scanty sputum; chronic cough due to deficiency of vital energy or vital essence of the lung; expectoration of bloody sputum	3–9	
Flos Farfarae; (coltsfoot flower)	warm	pungent	Lung	Moistening the lung and keeping the flow of *qi* going downward; resolving phlegm to relieve cough	Any kind of cough	3–9	
Cortex Mori Radicis (mulberry root-bark)	cold	sweet	Lung	Quenching fire in the lung to relieve asthma; reducing swelling through diuresis	Cough and asthma due to pathogenic heat in the lung; pneumonectasis; acute bronchitis; edema; high blood pressure	9–18	
Semen Lepidii seu Descurainiae (pepperweed or flixweed tansy mustard seed)	extremely cold	bitter and pungent	Lung and Urinary Bladder	As above	Asthmatic cough with excessive phlegm; edema; pleural effusion; ascites; dysuria; cor pulmonale, edema due to heart failure	3–9	

| *Radix Stemonae* (stemona root) | mild (neutral) | bitter and sweet | Lung | Moistening the lung, relieving cough; anthelmintic | Cough (including whooping cough and cough due to tuberculosis); oxyuria; hair and body lice | 3–9 |

Dampness-Resolving Herbs With Fragrant Odor

These herbs reinforce the function of the spleen and dispel pathogenic dampness. They are effective for damp-phlegm symptom-complexes produced by long-standing retention of pathogenic dampness due to deficiency of vital energy of the spleen. They also are useful in treating febrile conditions caused by dampness, as well as in treating infectious febrile disease in summer. The herbs should be used with care in patients deficient in vital energy and vital essence because, being of pungent flavor and warm property, they may injure vital essence.

Most of the herbs reinforce the function of the stomach, and some serve as antibiotics and counteract the influenza virus. Because their active constituents evaporate readily, the herbs should be added when the decoction is nearly done.

Medicinal Herb	Property(s)	Flavor(s)	Channel(s) Acted on	Action(s)	Indication(s)	Amount (grams)	Remarks
Herba Agastachis (wrinkled giant-hyssop)	moderately warm	pungent	Spleen, Stomach, and Lung	Dispelling dampness and pathogenic factors from the exterior of the body; regulating the vital function of the stomach to cure vomiting	Morbid conditions due to summer heat and pathogenic dampness; infectious febrile diseases caused by pathogenic dampness; gathering of pathogenic dampness in the body; stuffy feeling in the chest; poor appetite and nausea; apply locally to treat monilia vaginitis	3–10	Amount doubled when used fresh
Herba Eupatorii (eupatorium)	mild (neutral)	pungent	Spleen and Stomach	Dispelling pathogenic dampness and pathogenic factors from the exterior of the body	Gathering of pathogenic dampness in the body; morbid conditions due to summer-heat and pathogenic dampness	3–10	Amount doubled when used fresh
Rhizoma Acori Graminei (grass-leaved sweetflag rhizome)	warm	pungent	Heart and Stomach	Dispelling pathogenic dampness; causing resuscitation and soothing the nerves	Blockage of the middle burner by pathogenic dampness; impaired consciousness due to infectious febrile conditions; loss of	3–10	

Name				Actions	Indications	Dosage
					consciousness due to penetration of pathogenic heat into the pericardium; manic-depressive insanity; dementia	
Semen Cardamomi Rotundi (round cardamon seed)	warm	pungent	Spleen and Stomach	Removing pathogenic dampness and promoting the normal flow of vital energy, warming the spleen and stomach to stop vomiting	Sensation of gastric fullness; nausea; vomiting; abdominal pain due to obstruction of the middle burner by pathogenic dampness; incipient infectious disease caused by pathogenic dampness	3–10
Rhizoma Atractylodis (atractylodes rhizome)	warm	pungent and bitter	Spleen and Stomach	Eliminating pathogenic dampness to reinforce the function of the spleen; dispelling pathogenic wind to remove dampness	Dyspepsia due to collection of pathogenic dampness in the middle burner; diarrhea in summer; pain due to rheumatism; night blindness; and softening of the cornea	3–10

Stomachics and Evacuants

These herbs whet the appetite and promote digestion. They generally are used in treating dyspepsia or indigestion. Most of these herbs stimulate secretion of gastric juice and peristalsis of the stomach and intestines.

Medicinal Herb	Property(s)	Flavor(s)	Channel(s) Acted on	Action(s)	Indication(s)	Amount (grams)	Remarks
Fructus Crataegi (hawthorn fruit)	moderately warm	sour and sweet	Spleen, Stomach, and Liver	Improving digestion; reinforcing the function of the stomach; activating the blood circulation to eliminate blood stasis	Dyspepsia or retension of fatty food; postpartum blood stasis; abdominal pain; hepatosplenomegaly; distending pain of hernia	10–15 (30–120 if necessary)	
Fructus Hordei Germinatus (malt)	mild (neutral)	sweet and sour	Spleen and Stomach	Improving digestion, reinforcing the function of the stomach; arresting the secretion of milk	Dyspepsia induced by cereal food or excessive consumption of fruit; early stage of mastitis and stopping breast feeding	10–15	(30–120 fresh for stopping breast feeding)
Massa Fermentata Medicinalis (medicated leaven)	warm	sweet and pungent	Spleen and Stomach	Improving digestion and reinforcing the function of the stomach	Food retention; abdominal distension; poor appetite and diarrhea	3–9	
Endothelium Corneum Gigeriae Galli (membrane	mild (neutral)	sweet	Spleen, Stomach, Small Intes-	Improving digestion, stopping enuresis, resolving stone	Retention of food due to weakened functioning of the	3–9	3 grams taken in powder form

			tine, and Urinary Bladder		spleen; enuresis in children; nocturnal emission; tuberculosis; urinary stone	
Semen Raphani (radish seed)	mild (neutral)	pungent and sweet	Lung, Spleen, and Stomach	Improving digestion and removing abdominal distension, expelling phlegm and keeping the flow of *qi* going downward	Dyspepsia; stagnation of vital energy; stuffy feeling in the chest and abdominal distension; belching and acid regurgitation; diarrhea; profuse phlegm, cough, asthma	6–12

Carminatives (Herbs for Regulating the Flow of Vital Energy)

Most of these herbs are aromatic in odor, pungent in flavor, and warm in property. They promote the normal flow of vital energy, and they remove obstruction or stagnation of vital energy in the spleen, stomach, liver, and lung. Some can reinforce the function of the stomach, dispel phlegm, and dispel masses. Modern research has shown that these herbs help to regulate the functioning of the digestive tract and stimulate contraction of the smooth muscle of the stomach and intestines, so as to evacuate accumulated gas. It has been shown that they also promote secretion of gastric juice to improve digestion; strengthen the functioning of the spleen; whet the appetite; or inhibit peristalsis of the intestines to alleviate spasm and pain. They also promote the secreting function of the bronchi to loosen phlegm. These herbs must be used with care in patients deficient in vital energy and vital essence, since they are of pungent and dry property and easily injure vital essence.

Medicinal Herb	Property(s)	Flavor(s)	Channel(s) Acted on	Action(s)	Indication(s)	Amount (grams)	Remarks
Pericarpium Citri Reticulatae (dried orange peel)	warm	pungent and bitter	Spleen and Lung	Promoting the normal flow of vital energy and reinforcing the function of the spleen; eliminating phlegm; putting down the adverse flow of vital energy to stop vomiting	Abdominal distension and pain due to stagnation of vital energy of the spleen and stomach; asthmatic cough and oppressed feeling in the chest caused by accumulation of phlegm and pathogenic dampness; hiccups and vomiting due to dysfunction of the stomach in sending down food	3–9	
Fructus Aurantii Immaturus (immature citron)	moderately warm	bitter, pungent, and slightly sour	Spleen and Stomach	Promoting the normal flow of vital energy to remove sputum; dispelling lumps	Stagnation of vital energy of the spleen and stomach; retention of phlegm and fluid; pectoral pain (coronary heart disease—e.g., angina pectoris); constipation due to collection of pathogenic heat; abdominal distension with pain; prolapse of uterus or rectum; gastroptosis; shock	see Remarks column	3–9 grams used in treating prolapse of uterus or rectum; 12–30 grams used in treating shock (intravenous drip or injection)

Cortex Magnoliae Officinalis (magnolia bark)	warm	bitter and pungent	Spleen, Stomach, Lung, and Large Intestine	Promoting the normal flow of vital energy; eliminating pathogenic dampness; alleviating asthma by putting down adverse flow of vital energy	Obstruction of the middle burner by pathogenic dampness; stagnation of vital energy; abdominal distension with pain; asthmatic cough due to retention of phlegm and pathogenic dampness	3–9
Radix Aucklandiae (costus root)	warm	pungent and bitter	Spleen, Stomach, Large Intestine, and Gallbladder	Promoting the normal flow of vital energy to kill pain	Stagnation of vital energy of the spleen and stomach; abdominal distension with pain; dyspepsia and stuffiness and fullness sensation in the chest and abdomen due to hypofunction of the spleen and stomach; dysentery or stagnation of vital energy of the liver and gallbladder due to pathogenic dampness and heat; dysentery; biliary colic	3–9; 9–15 grams used in treating gallbladder pain

Medicinal Herb	Property(s)	Flavor(s)	Channel(s) Acted on	Action(s)	Indication(s)	Amount (grams)	Remarks
Rhizoma Cyperi (nutgrass flatsedge)	mild (neutral)	pungent and slightly bitter	Liver and Stomach	Restoring the normal function of a depressed liver; regulating menstruation to relieve mentrual pain	Pain caused by melancholy and stagnation of vital energy; stagnation of vital energy of the liver; menstrual irregularities; painful menstruation	6–12	
Radix Linderae (spicebush root)	warm	pungent	Stomach, Kidney, and Urinary Bladder	Promoting the normal flow of vital energy to disperse pathogenic cold and alleviate pain	Stagnation of vital energy associated with pain caused by accumulation of pathogenic cold; frequent urination, or urinary incontinence due to deficiency of vital energy and to pathogenic cold	3–12	
Pericarpium Arecae (areca peel)	moderately warm	pungent	Spleen, Stomach, Large and Small Intestines	Promoting the normal flow of vital energy to relieve dyspepsia; removing pathogenic dampness and edema through diuresis	Abdominal distension due to retention of undigested food and obstruction of vital energy; retention of fluid and pathogenic dampness; edema; tinea of the foot	3–9	

Purgatives

These herbs promote defecation to remove undigested food from the stomach and intestines. They also remove excessive pathogenic heat and expel retained water through purgation. They are used in treating dyspepsia, constipation due to collection of excessive pathogenic heat or cold, and retention of water.

Modern study of these herbs has revealed that they act as follows. First, they stimulate the digestive tract locally and promote intestinal movement. Second, some purgatives stimulate the secretion of bile, which gives rise to contraction of the gallbladder and diastole of the sphincter of Oddi, so as to treat gallbladder disorders. Third, some of the herbs counteract inflammation. Fourth, some may promote the absorptive function of the peritoneum, help the tissue water enter the intestines, and thus aid in removal of ascites.

DRASTIC PURGATIVES

Most of these herbs are bitter in flavor and cold in property. They are very effective for dyspepsia and constipation because they can reduce intense internal heat. Drastic purgatives are often given together with carminatives to enhance the action and remove abdominal distension. To treat constipation due to collection of pathogenic cold, some of the herbs are used with other herbs warm in property.

Medicinal Herb	Property(s)	Flavor(s)	Channel(s) Acted on	Action(s)	Indication(s)	Amount (grams)	Remarks
Radix et Rhizoma Rhei (rhubarb)	cold	bitter	Spleen, Stomach, Large Intestine, Liver, and Pericardium	Clearing away stagnant food; reducing intense heat and cooling blood; activating blood circulation to eliminate blood stasis; arresting gallbladder pain and clearing away jaundice	Constipation due to excessive pathogenic heat in the stomach and intestines or due to pathogenic cold; dysentery caused by pathogenic dampness and heat; jaundice due to dampheat; bleeding; boils and scalds	3–12	Use with care in pregnant or menstruating women
Natrii Sulfas (sodium sulfate)	cold	bitter and salty	Stomach and Large Intestine	Eliminating constipation; reducing intense internal heat	Constipation due to excessive pathogenic heat; acute intestinal obstruction; acute pharyngitis	10–15	Taken mixed with herb decoction or hot water; prohibited in pregnant women; use with care in the aged
Folium Sennae (senna leaf)	cold	sweet and bitter	Large Intestine	Clearing away excessive pathogenic heat and undigested food	Constipation due to intense internal heat; abdominal distension; ascites	3–6	Prohibited in pregnant women; overdose induces nausea, vomiting, and abdominal pain

MILD LAXATIVES

These purgatives contain oil components that aid defecation. They are especially effective for constipation in the aged and debilitated, as well as in postpartum women afflicted with deficiency of blood or in patients suffering from injury of essence or from hemorrhage.

Medicinal Herb	Property(s)	Flavor(s)	Channel(s) Acted on	Action(s)	Indication(s)	Amount (grams)	Remarks
Fructus Cannabis (hemp seed)	mild (neutral)	sweet	Spleen, Stomach, and Large Intestine	Moistening the intestine to relieve constipation; replenishing vital energy and vital essence	Chronic constipation caused by deficiency of vital energy; constipation due to febrile conditions that injure vital essence; senile constipation; constipation in postpartum women	9–30	
Semen Pruni (bushcherry seed)	mild (neutral)	sweet and bitter	Large and Small Intestines	Moistening the intestines to relieve constipation; reducing edema through diuresis	Stagnation of vital energy in the large intestine; constipation due to pathogenic dryness of the large intestine; edema due to beriberi; difficulty in urination	3–12	Intoxication occurs when 60–120 grams are given

Medicinal Herb	Property(s)	Flavor(s)	Channel(s) Acted on	Action(s)	Indication(s)	Amount (grams)	Remarks
Mel (honey)	mild (neutral)	sweet	Lung, Spleen, and Large Intestine	Moistening the intestines to relieve constipation; arresting cough; nourishing the stomach and spleen	Constipation in the aged and debilitated; injury of essence after febrile disease; cough; application locally for scalds and boils	15–30	

HYDROGOGUES

These drastic purgatives, which cause diarrhea and urination, are used to remove excess water from the body. They are used in treating edema, accumulation of pathogenic water in the chest and abdomen, asthma due to retention of phlegm and fluid, and ascites occurring in late-stage schistosomiasis. The herbs are often toxic, and it is inadvisable to take them for a long period.

Medicinal Herb	Property(s)	Flavor(s)	Channel(s) Acted on	Action(s)	Indication(s)	Amount (grams)	Remarks
Radix Euphorbiae Kansui (kansui root)	cold and toxic	bitter	Lung, Kidney, and Large Intestine	Expelling retained water; relieving edema and constipation	Ascites due to schistosomiasis or cirrhosis; exudative pleurisy; constipation due to accumulation of heat; swelling due to damp-heat	0.5–1.0	Used in bolus or powder form; incompatible with *Radix Glycyrrhizae*; prohibited in pregnancy; raw herb for external use only

Name	Nature	Taste	Meridian	Function	Indications	Dosage	Notes
Radix Euphorbiae Pekinensis (Peking spurge root)	cold and toxic	bitter	Lung, Kidney, and Large Intestine	Removing pathogenic dampness through diuresis; relieving edema; dispelling lumps	Hydrothorax and ascites; apply locally to treat boils, swelling and lumps due to accumulation of phlegm	1.5–3	1 gram used in powder mixtures; incompatible with Radix Glycyrrhizae: prohibited in pregnancy
Flos Genkwa (lilac daphne flower)	warm and toxic	pungent	Lung, Kidney, and Large Intestine	Eliminating retained water; clearing away phlegm to stop coughing; killing tinea and worms	Hydrothorax (in exudative pleurisy); ascites (in cirrhosis); coughing and asthma; intractable tinea; frostbite	1.5–3	0.6 gram used in powder mixtures; incompatible with Radix Glycyrrhizae: prohibited in pregnancy
Semen Pharbitidis (pharbitis seed)	cold and toxic	bitter	Lung, Kidney, and Large Intestine	Inducing diarrhea and urination in order to expel undigested food and retained water; anthelmintic	Constipation due to intense heat in the stomach and intestines; edema; ascites (in cirrhosis)	3–9	1.5–3 grams used in powder mixtures; prohibited during pregnancy

Anthelmintics

These herbs are used to combat intestinal parasites such as roundworms and tapeworms. It is advisable to take them with purgatives before meals. Because the herbs are somewhat toxic, excessive amounts should not be given. In pregnant women, the aged, and the debilitated, the herbs must be administered with care.

Medicinal Herb	Property(s)	Flavor(s)	Channel(s) Acted on	Action(s)	Indication(s)	Amount (grams)	Remarks
Fructus Quisqualia Indica (guisqualis fruit)	warm	sweet	Spleen and Stomach	Eliminating intestinal parasites and treating the resulting malnutrition	Roundworm; pinworm; oxyuriasis	6–12 (roasted)	For children, 1.5 granules per day for 3–4 successive days (total amount not over 20 granules); overdose causes dizziness, hiccups, and vomiting
Omphalia Lapidescens (omphalia)	cold and slightly toxic	bitter	Stomach and Large Intestine	Eliminating intestinal parasites	Tapeworm; hookworm; roundworms	3–6	Taken in powder form
Semen Cucurbita Moschata (pumpkin seed)	warm	sweet	Stomach and Large Intestine	As above	Tapeworm; late-stage schistosomiasis	60–120	Taken in powder form followed after two hours by 180–360 grams. Decoction of *Semen Arecae*; half an hour later 15 grams *Nutrii Sulfas* is given to expel the parasites from the body
Semen Arecae (betel nut)	warm	pungent and bitter	Stomach and Large Intestine	Eliminating intestinal parasites and relieving dyspepsia	Tapeworm; liver fluke; dyspepsia; abdominal distension; constipation, tenesmus dysentery	6–15	60–120 grams used in treating parasitoses

Aromatic Stimulants

Most herbs causing resuscitation are pungent in flavor and warm in property. They are used in treating sudden loss of consciousness due to such conditions as epilepsy and apoplexy.

Medicinal Herb	Property(s)	Flavor(s)	Channel(s) Acted on	Action(s)	Indication(s)	Amount (grams)	Remarks
Moschus (musk)	warm	pungent	Heart and Spleen	Causing resuscitation; invigorating blood circulation and removing stagnation; inducing abortion	Loss of consciousness due to high fever; stroke; convulsions; epilepsy; boils; amenorrhea; abdominal masses; trauma; arthralgia, angina pectoris; death of fetus or retention of placenta	0.10–0.15	Used in powder mixtures; prohibited in pregnancy
Borneolum (borneol)	moderately cold	pungent and bitter	Heart, Spleen, and Lung	Causing resuscitation; clearing away pathogenic heat and alleviating pain	Loss of consciousness and convulsions; sudden onset of coma due to excessive pathogenic cold in the interior of the body; boils and canker sores or sore throat; eye diseases	0.03–0.10	Used in powder mixtures

Herbs for Dispelling Internal Cold

These herbs are warm or hot in property. They warm the stomach and spleen and dispel pathogenic cold from them, or they reinforce vital function. They are used in treating symptom-complexes of internal cold due to direct attack of the interior of the body by exogenous pathogenic cold or due to hypofunction of the spleen and stomach or the heart and kidney. Use of these herbs is inadvisable in patients deficient in vital essence.

Medicinal Herb	Property(s)	Flavor(s)	Channel(s) Acted on	Action(s)	Indication(s)	Amount (grams)	Remarks
Radix Aconitii Praeparata (monkshood root)	extremely hot, toxic	pungent and sweet	Heart, Kidney, Spleen	Restoring vital function from collapse, warming the kidney and invigorating the vital function of the kidney, dispelling pathogenic cold to kill pain	Deficiency of vital function of the spleen and kidney; shock and prostration; edema due to deficiency of spleen and kidney *yang*; arthralgia due to cold-damp	3–15	Prohibited in pregnancy; avoid overdose and poisoning
Rhizoma Zingiberis (dried ginger)	hot	pungent	Heart, Lung, Spleen, and Stomach	Restoring vital function and warming the spleen and stomach; warming the lung to resolve phlegm	Hypofunction of the spleen and stomach with cold manifestations (e.g., chronic gastritis, chronic colitis, dyspepsia); cough and expectoration of profuse sputum due to pathogenic cold in the lung; collapse	3–9	

Herb	Nature	Taste	Channels	Function	Indications	Dosage	Cautions
Cortex Cinnamomi (cinnamon bark)	extremely hot	pungent and sweet	Kidney, Spleen, Heart, and Liver	Warming the spleen and stomach to reinforce their vital function; dispelling pathogenic cold to kill pain	Hypofunction of the spleen and kidney; gastro-abdominal pain due to pathogenic cold; lumbago and dysmenorrhea due to obstruction of the flow of vital energy and to pathogenic cold; abscess due to pathogenic cold	2–5	Inadvisable in pregnancy
Fructus Evodiae (evodia fruit)	hot, slightly toxic	pungent and bitter	Liver, Spleen, Stomach, and Kidney	Warming the spleen and stomach to kill pain; putting down upward adverse flow of vital energy to stop vomiting	Stomachache due to deficiency of vital energy and to pathogenic cold; pain in the hypochondria; vomiting; acid regurgitation caused by disharmony of the liver and stomach; chronic diarrhea and diarrhea occurring before dawn daily	2–5	Inadvisable in pregnancy; overdose causes visual trouble
Flos Caryophylii (cloves)	warm	pungent	Spleen, Stomach, and Kidney	Warming the spleen and stomach to put down upward adverse flow of vital energy; warming the kidney to reinforce its vital function	Hiccups, vomiting, or diarrhea due to pathogenic cold in the stomach; impotence due to hypofunction of the kidney	2–5	Restrains *Radix Curcumae*

Herbs for Subduing Hyperactivity of the Liver

HERBS FOR SUBDUING HYPERACTIVITY OF THE LIVER AND ENDOGENOUS PATHOGENIC WIND

These herbs are also known as anticonvulsives. Some control hyperactivity of the liver and dispel pathogenic heat from the liver.

Medicinal Herb	Property(s)	Flavor(s)	Channel(s) Acted on	Action(s)	Indication(s)	Amount (grams)	Remarks
Cornu Antelopis (antelope horn)	cold	salty	Liver and Heart	Subduing hyperactivity of the liver and endogenous pathogenic wind; quenching fire; improving eyesight	Convulsions due to stirring up of internal pathogenic heat in febrile conditions; infantile convulsions; epilepsy; dizziness resulting from hyperactivity of the liver; headache and bloodshot eyes due to flaring up of excessive heat in the liver	1–3	0.3–0.5 gram used in powder form; decocted separately and then mixed with the rest of the decoction
Calculus Bovis (ox gallstone)	cold	bitter and sweet	Liver and Heart	Subduing intense endogenous pathogenic wind to relieve convulsions; clearing away phlegm to cause resuscitation	Convulsions due to high fever in febrile disease; penetration of pathogenic heat into the pericardium; apoplexy; infantile convulsions;	0.15–0.3	Used in powder mixtures or boluses; prohibited in pregnancy

					epilepsy; obstruction of the Heart Channel by phlegm due to intense heat; severe sore throat or boils		
Lumbricus (earthworm)	cold	salty	Liver, Spleen, and Urinary Bladder	Clearing away intense internal heat to subdue endogenous pathogenic wind; inducing diuresis	Irritability, restlessness, and convulsions due to high fever; urinary disturbance due to pathogenic heat in the urinary bladder; asthma; arthritis; hypertension	5–15	
Ramulus Uncariae cum Uncis (uncaria stem with hooks)	moderately cold	sweet	Liver and Pericardium	Subduing endogenous pathogenic wind to relieve convulsions; clearing away intense heat to relieve hyperactivity of the liver	Convulsions due to high fever in febrile disease; hypertensive vertigo; infantile convulsions, epilepsy	10–15	Decocted for a short time
Rhizoma Gastrodiae (gastrodia tuber)	mild (neutral)	sweet	Liver	Subduing endogenous pathogenic wind to relieve hyperactivity of the liver	Convulsions, epilepsy due to stirring up of endogenous pathogenic wind; vertigo and headache caused by hyperactivity of the liver; arthritis and numbness of limbs	3–9	1–1.5 grams taken in powder form

Medicinal Herb	Property(s)	Flavor(s)	Channel(s) Acted on	Action(s)	Indication(s)	Amount (grams)	Remarks
Scorpio (scorpion)	mild (neutral) and toxic	pungent	Liver	Subduing endogenous pathogenic wind to stop convulsions; relieving pyogenic inflammation; dispelling masses; removing obstruction in the channels to kill pain	Convulsions due to high fever; acute or chronic infantile convulsions; stroke, Bell's palsy; tetanus; suppurative infection of the body surface; migraine, arthralgia	2–5	
Scolopendra (centipede)	warm	salty	Liver	Subduing endogenous pathogenic wind to stop convulsions; relieving pyogenic inflammation; removing obstruction in the channels to kill pain	Acute or chronic infantile convulsions; spasm due to tetanus; infection on the body surface; protracted headache; rheumatic arthritis	1–3	

HERBS FOR SEDATING EXUBERANCE OF VITAL FUNCTION OF THE LIVER

Some of these herbs quench pathogenic fire in the liver and soothe the nerves. They are used in treating exuberance of vital function due to deficiency of vital essence.

Medicinal Herb	Property(s)	Flavor(s)	Channel(s) Acted on	Action(s)	Indication(s)	Amount (grams)	Remarks
Concha Haliotidis (sea-ear shell)	cold	salty	Liver	Checking exuberance of vital function of the liver; quenching fire in the liver to improve eyesight	Dizziness or hypertension caused by exuberance of vital function of the liver due to deficiency of vital essence of the liver and kidney; acute conjunctivitis due to flaring up of excessive heat of the liver; nebula due to intense pathogenic heat and wind; blurred vision due to deficiency of liver blood	15–20	
Ochra (red ochre)	cold	bitter	Heart and Liver	Checking exuberance of vital function of the liver; putting down upward adverse flow of vital energy to arrest bleeding	Exuberance of vital function of the liver; marked by dizziness and headache; vomiting and hiccups due to upward flow of stomach *qi*; asthma due to adverse flow of lung *qi* or deficiency of the kidney; hemoptysis, epistaxis, uterine bleeding due to pathogenic heat in the blood	10–30	

Medicinal Herb	Property(s)	Flavor(s)	Channel(s) Acted on	Action(s)	Indication(s)	Amount (grams)	Remarks
Concha Margaritifera Usta (pearl shell)	cold	salty	Liver and Heart	Checking exuberance of vital function of the liver; quenching fire in the liver to improve eyesight	Dizziness, tinnitus caused by exuberance of vital function of the liver due to deficiency of vital essence of the liver and kidney; blurred vision, night blindness due to deficiency of vital essence of the liver; bloodshot eyes and photophobia caused by intense heat in the liver	15–60	
Radix Paeoniae Alba (white peony root)	moderately cold	bitter and sour	Liver	Checking exuberance of vital function of the liver; nourishing blood and consolidating vital essence and body fluid; killing pain by soothing the liver	Dizziness, tinnitus caused by deficiency of vital essence and exuberance of vital function of the liver; spontaneous perspiration caused by derangement of constructive energy and defensive energy; night sweats due to deficiency of vital essence; pain	9–18	

					in the hypochondria resulting from stagnation of vital energy of the liver; disharmony of the liver and stomach or of the liver and spleen; dysmenorrhea, irregular menstruation due to deficiency of the blood	
Os Draconis (dragon's bone)	moderately cold	sweet and puckery	Heart and Liver	Checking exuberance of vital function of the liver; easing the nerves; causing contraction and arresting discharges	Dizziness, irritability, and restlessness caused by deficiency of vital essence of the liver and exuberance of vital function of the liver; disturbed mind, palpitation, and insomnia due to deficiency of vital energy and blood of the heart; epilepsy; mania; spermatorrhea; leukorrhea; rashes; protracted ulcers	15–30

Medicinal Herb	Property(s)	Flavor(s)	Channel(s) Acted on	Action(s)	Indication(s)	Amount (grams)	Remarks
Concha Ostreae (oyster shell)	moderately cold	salty	Liver and Kidney	Checking exuberance of vital function; softening and dispelling hard lumps; causing contraction and arresting discharges	Dizziness, irritability, and restlessness due to hyperactivity of vital function and deficiency of vital essence; injury of vital essence; stirring up of endogenous pathogenic wind and convulsions; enlargement of the liver and spleen; spontaneous perspiration; spermatorrhea; leukorrhea, uterine bleeding	15–30	

Sedatives and Tranquilizers

These herbs are used in treating such conditions as nervousness and excitement, palpitation, insomnia, excessive dreaming during sleep, infantile convulsions, epilepsy, and psychosis. Pharmacologic experiments have shown that they have sedative and hypnotic effects on the central nervous system.

Medicinal Herb	Property(s)	Flavor(s)	Channel(s) Acted on	Action(s)	Indication(s)	Amount (grams)	Remarks
Cinnabaris (cinnabar)	cold and toxic	sweet	Heart	Dispelling pathogenic heat from the heart or pericardium; relieving convulsions and pyogenic inflammation; soothing the nerves	Convulsions, insomnia due to flaring up of pathogenic fire of the heart; palpitation; epilepsy; suppurative infection on the body surface	0.3–1	Taken in powder form; excessive use causes mercury poisoning
Succinum (amber)	mild (neutral)	sweet	Heart, Liver, and Urinary Bladder	Relieving convulsions and soothing the nerves; promoting blood circulation to correct stasis; promoting urination	Convulsions and epilepsy; insomnia and excessive dreaming during sleep; absence of menstruation due to blood stasis; abdominal masses; dysuria, hematuria, scanty urination due to urinary tract infection	1.5–3	

Medicinal Herb	Property(s)	Flavor(s)	Channel(s) Acted on	Action(s)	Indication(s)	Amount (grams)	Remarks
Semen Ziziphi Spinosae (wild jujube seed)	mild (neutral)	sweet and sour	Heart and Liver	Nourishing the heart and liver; soothing the nerves and arresting perspiration	Insomnia, palpitation due to deficiency of heart blood; restlessness, insomnia, palpitation, and amnesia caused by breakdown of the normal coordination between the heart and kidney; spontaneous perspiration or night sweats due to debility	9–18	1.5 grams taken in powder form at bedtime
Cortex albiziae (albizia bark)	mild (neutral)	sweet	Heart and Liver	Soothing the nerves; promoting blood circulation to remove swellings	Insomnia and amnesia due to neurasthenia; injuries and wounds; hematomas; painful swellings	9–15	
Ganoderma Lucidum (lucid ganoderma)	moderately warm	sweet and slightly bitter	Heart, Spleen, Lung, Liver, and Kidney	Replenishing the heart and soothing the nerves; reinforcing vital energy and enriching blood; stopping cough and asthma	Deficiency of both blood and vital energy of the heart; asthmatic cough due to lowered functioning of the liver and kidney; debility due to protracted illness	9–15	

Diuretics and Hydrogogues

These herbs are used in treating edema and difficulty in urination.

HERBS TO PROMOTE DIURESIS AND TREAT EDEMA

Medicinal Herb	Property(s)	Flavor(s)	Channel(s) Acted on	Action(s)	Indication(s)	Amount (grams)	Remarks
Poria (poria)	mild (neutral)	insipid and slightly sweet	Heart, Lung, Spleen, and Urinary Bladder	Reinforcing the function of the spleen and removing pathogenic dampness through diuresis; easing the nerves	Edema or abundant dampness due to deficiency of vital energy of the spleen; abdominal distension and loose stools; palpitation and insomnia	6–18	
Polyporus Umbellatus (umbellate porefungus)	mild (neutral)	insipid and sweet	Kidney and Urinary Bladder	Removing pathogenic dampness through diuresis	Edema; difficulty in urination; pain during urination; hematuria; distension of the lower abdomen due to retention of pathogenic dampness	6–18	

Medicinal Herb	Property(s)	Flavor(s)	Channel(s) Acted on	Action(s)	Indication(s)	Amount (grams)	Remarks
Rhizoma Alismatis (water plantain tuber)	cold	insipid and sweet	Kidney and Urinary Bladder	Removing pathogenic dampness and heat through diuresis	Edema, difficulty in urination due to retention of pathogenic dampness; morbid leukorrhea caused by pathogenic dampness and heat; oliguria	3–9	
Semen Phaseoli (phaseolus seed)	mild (neutral)	sour and sweet	Spleen, Heart, and Small Intestine	Eliminating edema and promoting detoxication through diuresis	Edema due to nephritis or malnutrition; edema in the legs due to beriberi; apply locally to treat boils and sores	9–30	Appropriate amount for local application
Stigma Maydis (corn stigma)	(neutral)	sweet	Urinary Bladder, Liver, and Gallbladder	Relieving edema through diuresis; subduing jaundice by removing pathogenic dampness from the gallbladder; stopping hemorrhage; reducing blood pressure	Nephritic edema; ascites due to cirrhosis; painful urination due to accumulation of pathogenic heat in the urinary bladder; jaundice due to hepatitis; diabetes; cholecystitis; hypertension; epistaxis; bleeding of the gums	15–60	

Herbs to Increase Urinary Flow and Eliminate Urinary Disturbances

This category consists of herbs cold in property that increase excretion of urine and correct urinary disturbances.

They are used in treating continuous dripping of urine, frequent urination, concentrated urine, pain during urination, hematuria, cloudy urine, and retention of urine.

Medicinal Herb	Property(s)	Flavor(s)	Channel(s) Acted on	Action(s)	Indication(s)	Amount (grams)	Remarks
Semen Plantaginis (plantain seed)	moderately cold	sweet	Lung, Urinary Bladder, Small Intestine, Kidney, and Liver	Increasing excretion of urine to eliminate urinary disturbances; clearing away intense heat to improve eyesight	Urinary disturbances due to pathogenic dampness and heat (acute urethritis, cystitis); nephritic edema; reddened and painful eyes due to collection of pathogenic wind-heat in the channels; cough due to pathogenic heat of the lung	3–12	

Medicinal Herb	Property(s)	Flavor(s)	Channel(s) Acted on	Action(s)	Indication(s)	Amount (grams)	Remarks
Caulis Clematidis Armandii (Si-chuan clematis stem)	cold	bitter	Heart, Small Intestine, and Urinary Bladder	Increasing excretion of urine to clear away pathogenic heat; promoting the secretion of milk; stimulating menstrual discharge	Flaring up of pathogenic fire of the heart; urinary disturbance due to pathogenic dampness and heat (e.g., acute urethritis); nephritic edema; edema of the legs; absence of lactation; amenorrhea due to blood stasis	3–9	
Talcum (talc)	cold	sweet and insipid	Stomach and Urinary Bladder	Increasing urinary excretion to eliminate urinary disturbances; clearing away summer heat	Urinary disturbances due to pathogenic dampness and heat (acute urethritis, cystitis); heatstroke; apply externally to treat eczema and impetigo	6–18	
Herba Polygoni Avicularis (common knot-grass)	moderately cold	bitter	Urinary Bladder	Increasing excretion of urine to eliminate urinary disturbances; killing worms; relieving itching	Urinary disturbances due to pathogenic dampness and heat; calculi in the urinary tract and hematuria (e.g., urethritis,	9–15	Appropriate amount for external use

Herba Dianthi (pink)	cold	bitter	Heart, Small Intestine, and Urinary Bladder	Increasing urinary excretion to clear away pathogenic heat; eliminating urinary disturbances	Urinary disturbances due to pathogenic dampness and heat; hematuria (found in acute urethritis, cystitis) stone in the bladder); chyluria; apply externally to treat eczema and trichomonas vaginitis	6–12
Folium Perillae (purple perilla leaf)	moderately cold	bitter	Lung and Urinary Bladder	Increasing urinary excretion to eliminate urinary disturbances; removing intense heat from blood and stopping hemorrhage	Painful urination due to pathogenic dampness and heat; hematuria; stone in the bladder; nephritis	9–15

HERBS TO SUBDUE JAUNDICE THROUGH DIURESIS

These herbs act on the gallbladder to subdue jaundice.

Medicinal Herb	Property(s)	Flavor(s)	Channel(s) Acted on	Action(s)	Indication(s)	Amount (grams)	Remarks
Herba Artemisiae Scopariae (oriental wormwood)	moderately cold	bitter	Spleen, Stomach, Liver, and Gallbladder	Removing pathogenic dampness and heat through diuresis; subduing jaundice	Jaundice due to pathogenic dampness and heat (icteric hepatitis)	9–15	
Herba Lysimachiae (loosestrife)	mild	slightly salty	Liver, Gallbladder, Kidney, and Urinary Bladder	Removing pathogenic dampness and jaundice; increasing urinary excretion; clearing away pathogenic heat to relieve edema	Jaundice and urinary disturbances due to pathogenic dampness and heat; calculi of the urinary tract, including bladder and kidney stones; gallstones	30–60	

Antirheumatics

These herbs dispel pathogenic wind and dampness from the channels, joints, and muscles to relieve arthritis, activate blood circulation, and cause the muscles and joints to relax. Some of the herbs reinforce the functioning of the liver and kidney to some extent and strengthen muscles and bones. They are used mainly in treating such conditions as rheumatic and rheumatoid arthritis, pain and numbness in the limbs, motion impairment of the joints, contracture of the muscles, and pain in the back and knees.

HERBS FOR RELIEVING RHEUMATISM AND PAIN

Medicinal Herb	Property(s)	Flavor(s)	Channel(s) Acted on	Action(s)	Indication(s)	Amount (grams)	Remarks
Radix Angelicae Pubescentis (pubescent angelica root)	moderately warm	pungent and bitter	Kidney and Urinary Bladder	Expelling pathogenic wind and dampness; alleviating pain	Arthralgia due to pathogenic wind, cold, and dampness; affliction by pathogenic wind, cold, and dampness; toothache due to pathogenic wind and heat	3–9	
Radix Gentianae Macrophyllae (large-leaf gentian root)	moderately cold	bitter and pungent	Stomach, Liver, and Gallbladder	Relieving rheumatism and fever due to deficiency of vital energy or vital essence	Arthralgia due to pathogenic wind, cold, and dampness; rheumatic or rheumatoid arthritis; hemiplegia; hectic fever due to deficiency of vital essence	6–12	
Radix Clematidis (clematis root)	warm	pungent	the twelve channels	Relieving rheumatism; removing obstruction of the channels to alleviate pain	Arthralgia due to pathogenic cold; chronic rheumatic arthritis; numbness of the limbs; contracture of the muscles; obstruction of the throat or the upper esophagus by fishbone	3–12	Soak in vinegar to soften fish bone

Medicinal Herb	Property(s)	Flavor(s)	Channel(s) Acted on	Action(s)	Indication(s)	Amount (grams)	Remarks
Radix Stephaniae Tetrandrae (tetrandra root)	cold	bitter and pungent	Lung, Spleen, and Urinary Bladder	Relieving rheumatism; killing pain; increasing urinary excretion	Generalized aches due to rheumatism; rheumatic or rheumatoid arthritis; edema and difficulty in urination	6–12	

HERBS FOR ACTIVATING *Qi* AND BLOOD CIRCULATION AND CAUSING THE MUSCLES AND JOINTS TO RELAX

Medicinal Herb	Property(s)	Flavor(s)	Channel(s) Acted on	Action(s)	Indication(s)	Amount (grams)	Remarks
Fructus Chaenomelis (Chinese flowering quince)	warm	sour	Liver and Spleen	Activating blood circulation and causing the muscles and joints to relax; regulating the function of the stomach and expelling dampness	Rheumatic pains; edema and pain in the legs; muscle spasms; abdominal pain and diarrhea due to summer heat affecting the spleen	6–12	
Caulis Trachelospermi (Chinese starjasmine stem)	moderately cold	bitter	Heart, Liver, and Kidney	Expelling pathogenic wind from the channels; removing pathogenic heat from the blood	Rheumatic pain; globus hystericus	6–15	

Medicinal Herb	Property(s)	Flavor(s)	Channel(s) Acted on	Action(s)	Indication(s)	Amount (grams)	Remarks
Retinervus Luffae Fructus (vegetable sponge)	mild	sweet	Lung, Stomach, and Liver	Expelling pathogenic wind from the channels; promoting blood circulation	Rheumatic pain; pain in the thorax and hypochondria; muscle spasms	3–12	
Herba Siegesbeckieae (common St. Paulswort)	moderately warm	pungent and bitter	Liver and Heart	Relieving rheumatism; unblocking the channels; promoting detoxication	Limb numbness due to rheumatism; painful muscles and joints; hemiplegia; boils	10–15	
Ancistrodon Acutus (long-noded pit viper)	warm and toxic	sweet and salty	Liver	Expelling pathogenic wind from the channels; relieving convulsions	Intractible arthralgia due to pathogenic wind and dampness; hemiplegia; spasms or convulsions; protracted ulcers or abscesses	3–10	

HERBS FOR STRENGTHENING MUSCLES AND BONES

Medicinal Herb	Property(s)	Flavor(s)	Channel(s) Acted on	Action(s)	Indication(s)	Amount (grams)	Remarks
Cortex Acanthopanacis Radicis (acanthopanax bark)	warm	pungent	Liver and Kidney	Relieving rheumatism; strengthening the muscles and bones	Arthralgia due to pathogenic dampcold; difficulty in urination	9–15	

Medicinal Herb	Property(s)	Flavor(s)	Channel(s) Acted on	Action(s)	Indication(s)	Amount (grams)	Remarks
Rhizoma Drynariae (drynaria rhizome)	warm	bitter	Liver and Kidney	Strengthening the function of the kidney; curing bone fractures; promoting blood circulation	Lumbago and pain in the knees due to deficiency of vital energy of the kidney and liver; weakness of the lower limbs; toothache; tinnitus; bone fracture with pain and swelling	9–15	
Radix Dipsaci (dipsacus root)	warm	bitter	Liver and Kidney	Strengthening the function of the kidney, muscles, and bones; stopping hemorrhage and preventing miscarriage; promoting blood circulation	Lumbago and pain in the knees due to deficiency of vital energy of the liver and kidney; arthralgia; uterine bleeding; vaginal bleeding in pregnancy; threatened abortion; injuries and wounds; fractures	9–15	
Ramulus Loranthi (parasitic loranthus)	mild (neutral)	bitter	Liver and Kidney	Strenthening the function of the kidney and liver; relieving rheumatism; nourishing blood and preventing miscarriage	Arthralgia associated with impairment of the liver and kidney; uterine bleeding; vaginal bleeding in pregnancy; threatened abortion; hypertension; coronary heart disease	9–18	

Hemostatics

These herbs promote coagulation and keep blood flowing within the vessels in order to arrest all kinds of bleeding. They include astringents, cooling agents, hemostatics eliminating blood stasis, and agents invigorating blood circulation to eliminate blood stasis.

ASTRINGENT HEMOSTATICS

Medicinal Herb	Property(s)	Flavor(s)	Channel(s) Acted on	Action(s)	Indication(s)	Amount (grams)	Remarks
Herba Agrimoniae (hairyvein agrimony)	mild (neutral)	puckery and bitter	Lung, Liver, and Spleen	Arresting bleeding through astringency; detoxication; killing worms; treating boils	All kinds of bleeding; dysentery; malaria; trichomonas vaginitis; abscesses or boils; hemorrhoids	10–15 to 30–60	
Rhizoma Bletillae (bletilla tuber)	moderately cold	bitter, sweet, and puckery	Lung, Liver, and Stomach	Arresting bleeding; reducing swelling and healing wounds	Bleeding of the lung and stomach; traumatic bleeding; ulcers and inflammation; anal fistula; scalds	5–15	2–5 grams taken in powder form
Crinis Carbonisatus (carbonized hair)	mild (neutral)	bitter	Liver and Stomach	Arresting bleeding and removing stasis; promoting urination and replenishing vital essence	All kinds of bleeding; dysuria	6–10	1.5–3 grams taken in powder form

Medicinal Herb	Property(s)	Flavor(s)	Channel(s) Acted on	Action(s)	Indication(s)	Amount (grams)	Remarks
Petiolus Trachy-carpi Carbonisatus (carbonized petiole of windmill-palm)	mild (neutral)	bitter and puckery	Lung, Liver, and Large Intestine	Arresting bleeding through astringency	Epistaxis; hemoptysis; passage of bloody stools; uterine bleeding	5–15	1–2 grams taken in powder form

Herbs for Removing Pathogenic Heat from the Blood to Stop Bleeding

Medicinal Herb	Property(s)	Flavor(s)	Channel(s) Acted on	Action(s)	Indication(s)	Amount (grams)	Remarks
Herba seu Radix Cirsii Japonici (Japanese thistle)	cool	sweet	Heart and Liver	Expelling intense heat from blood to stop bleeding; reducing swelling through urination	Bleeding due to febrile conditions; hematemesis; hematuria; inflammations; jaundice due to pathogenic damp-heat; nephritis; hypertension	10–15	Up to 60 grams of fresh herb may be taken
Herba Cephalano-ploris (field thistle)	cool	sweet	Heart and Liver	As above	As above	10–15	As above

Name	Property	Taste	Channels	Functions	Indications	Dosage	External use
Radix Sanguisorbae (burnet garden root)	moderately cold	bitter and sour	Liver, Stomach, and Large Intestine	Expelling intense heat from blood to stop bleeding; detoxication and arresting discharge	Bloody stools due to hemorrhoids; uterine bleeding due to excessive heat in the blood; dysentery with frequent bloody stools; hematuria; scalds	10–15	Appropriate amount for external use
Cacumen Biotae (biota tops)	moderately cold	bitter and puckery	Lung, Liver, and Large Intestine	Expelling intense heat from blood to stop bleeding; arresting cough; promoting hair regeneration	All kinds of bleeding due to febrile conditions; scalds; cough due to pathogenic heat of the lung	10–15	Appropriate amount for external use
Rhizoma Imperatae (imperata rhizome)	cold	sweet	Stomach, Lung, and Urinary Bladder	Expelling intense heat from blood to stop bleeding; promoting urination by dispelling pathogenic heat	Hematemesis; epistaxis; hematuria due to febrile conditions; acute urinary tract infection; edema; jaundice, dysuria due to pathogenic heat	15–30	
Flos Sophorae (sophora flower)	moderately cold	bitter	Large Intestine and Liver	Expelling intense heat from blood to stop bleeding; reducing high blood pressure	Passage of bloody stools; hemorrhoid bleeding due to febrile conditions; hypertension	8–16	

Medicinal Herb	Property(s)	Flavor(s)	Channel(s) Acted on	Action(s)	Indication(s)	Amount (grams)	Remarks
Radix Boehmeriae (ramie root)	cold	sweet	Heart, Liver, Kidney, and Urinary Bladder	Stopping bleeding and miscarriage, promoting urination by dispelling pathogenic heat	Hemoptysis, hematemesis, hematuria, excessive menstrual bleeding, other uterine bleeding, purpura due to febrile conditions; traumatic bleeding; miscarriage; hematuria; skin inflammation; acute urinary-tract infection; edema due to nephritis or during pregnancy	10–30	

HERBS FOR ELIMINATING BLOOD STASIS

Medicinal Herb	Property(s)	Flavor(s)	Channel(s) Acted on	Action(s)	Indication(s)	Amount (grams)	Remarks
Radix Notoginseng (pseudoginseng)	warm	slightly bitter, and sweet	Liver and Stomach	Removing blood stasis to arrest bleeding; reducing swelling and alleviating pain	All kinds of bleeding associated with stasis and painful swellings; contused wounds; trauma; angina pectoris	2–5	Taken in powder form

Pollen Typhae (cattail pollen)	mild (neutral)	sweet	Liver and Heart	Stopping bleeding and activating blood circulation; promoting urination	All kinds of bleeding, including traumatic bleeding, hematuria, and postpartum hemorrhage; postpartum abdominal pain due to stasis; dysmenorrhea	5–10	Decocted wrapped in gauze; appropriate amount for external use
Radix Rubiae (rubia root)	cold	bitter	Liver	Expelling intense heat from the blood to stop bleeding; activating blood circulation; dispersing blood stasis	All kinds of bleeding due to excessive pathogenic heat in the blood; traumatic bleeding; contused wounds; amenorrhea due to blood stasis; trauma; arthralgia	10–15	As above
Folium Artemisiae Argyi (Chinese mugwort leaf)	warm	pungent and bitter	Liver, Spleen, and Kidney	Warming the channels to arrest bleeding and expelling cold to arrest pain	Excessive menstrual bleeding; vaginal bleeding in pregnancy due to deficiency of vital energy and to pathogenic cold; dysmenorrhea or abdominal pain	3–8	

Medicinal Herb	Property(s)	Flavor(s)	Channel(s) Acted on	Action(s)	Indication(s)	Amount (grams)	Remarks
Rhizoma Zingiberis praeparata (stir-baked ginger)	warm	bitter and puckery	Spleen and Liver	Warming the channels to arrest bleeding and warming the middle-burner to arrest pain	Hematemesis; passage of bloody stools and uterine bleeding due to deficiency of vital energy and to pathogenic cold; postpartum abdominal pain due to deficiency of blood and cold in the interior	3–6	

Herbs for Invigorating Blood Circulation to Eliminate Blood Stasis

These herbs generally are used in treating diseases caused by impeded blood circulation or by blood stasis. Pharmacologic experiments have shown that the herbs can dilate the vessels, improve microcirculation, counteract inflammation, and reverse the development of hyperplasia.

Medicinal Herb	Property(s)	Flavor(s)	Channel(s) Acted on	Action(s)	Indication(s)	Amount (grams)	Remarks
Rhizoma Ligustici Chuanxiong; (chuanxiong rhizome)	warm	pungent	Liver, Gallbladder, and Pericardium	Invigorating blood circulation and promoting the flow of vital energy; expel-	Irregular menstruation, amenorrhea, dysmenorrhea due to stagnation of vi-	3–9	

				...ling pathogenic wind to arrest pain	tal energy and blood; postpartum abdominal pain due to blood stasis; contused wounds, skin inflammation		
Radix Salviae Miltiorrhizae (red sage root)	moderately cold	bitter	Invigorating blood circulation to eliminate blood stasis; expelling intense heat from the body and subduing swelling; calming the mind	Heart, Pericardium, and Liver	Many kinds of blood stasis and pain; hepatosplenomegaly; boils and carbuncles; severest stages of febrile disease	3–15	Incompatible with *Radix Veratrum Nigrium*
Herba Leonuri (mother-wort)	moderately cold	pungent and bitter	Invigorating blood circulation and eliminating blood stasis; promoting urination and detoxication	Liver, Heart, and Urinary Bladder	Amenorrhea due to impeded blood circulation; dysmenorrhea; postpartum abdominal pain due to blood stasis; abdominal masses; nephritic edema; boils and itching	10–30	Use with care in pregnancy

Medicinal Herb	Property(s)	Flavor(s)	Channel(s) Acted on	Action(s)	Indication(s)	Amount (grams)	Remarks
Radix Cyathulae (cyathula root)	mild	bitter and sour	Liver and Kidney	Invigorating blood circulation and eliminating blood stasis; causing the blood to flow downward; promoting urination by reinforcing the kidney and liver	Amenorrhea due to blood stasis; dysmenorrhea; postpartum abdominal pain due to blood stasis; hematemesis; epistaxis; hematuria; arthralgia and immobility of the waist and knees; aphtha due to flaring up of pathogenic fire; hypertension; urinary tract infection	6–15	
Flos Carthami (safflower)	moderately warm	pungent	Liver and Heart	Invigorating blood circulation and eliminating blood stasis; regulating menstruation	Dysmenorrhea due to blood stasis; amenorrhea; postpartum abdominal pain due to blood stasis; abdominal masses; contused wounds; hematoma; arthralgia	3–9	Contraindicated in pregnant women and in women with excessive menstrual bleeding
Semen Persicae (peach kernel)	mild (neutral)	bitter and pungent	Liver, Lung, and Large Intestine	Invigorating blood circulation and eliminating blood stasis; relaxing the bowels	Dysmenorrhea due to blood stasis; amenorrhea; abdominal masses; constipation	6–9	Contraindicated in pregnancy and hemoptysis

Name	Nature	Taste	Channels	Actions	Indications	Dosage	Remarks
Radix Curcumae (curcuma root)	cold	pungent and bitter	Heart, Liver, and Gallbladder	Promoting the flow of vital energy; eliminating blood stasis and relieving pain; dispelling pathogenic heat from the heart; eliminating jaundice	Pain in the chest or costal region due to stagnation of vital energy and blood stasis; dysmenorrhea; amenorrhea; jaundice; inducing resuscitation by dispelling pathogenic heat from the heart	3–9	
Rhizoma Sparganii (burreed tuber)	mild (neutral)	pungent and bitter	Liver and Spleen	Eradicating blood stasis; promoting the flow of vital energy to relieve pain	Amenorrhea, postpartum abdominal pain due to blood stasis; abdominal masses; abdominal pain due to retention of food	3–9	Contraindicated in pregnant women and in women with excessive menstrual bleeding
Squama Manitis (pangolin scales)	moderately cold	salty	Liver and Stomach	Promoting menstruation; eliminating blood stasis; promoting lactation; dispersing lumps; reducing swelling by draining pus	Amenorrhea, abdominal masses; inadequacy of lactation; tuberculosis of the cervical lymph nodes; boils and ulcers	3–9	1–1.5 grams taken in powder form

Antineoplastics

These herbs are used in treating tumors (especially malignant ones). Pharmacologic experiments have shown that some of them contain components active against cancer and a few impede the metabolism of malignant cells and inhibit their growth. Thus they may lessen symptoms, reduce tumor size, and prolong the patient's life.

Medicinal Herb	Property(s)	Flavor(s)	Channel(s) Acted on	Action(s)	Indication(s)	Amount (grams)	Remarks
Flos Vinca (vinca rosea)	cool and toxic	bitter	—	Treating tumors by preventing their growth and spread; reducing hypertension	Acute lymphocytic leukemia; choriocarcinoma; breast cancer; Hodgkin's disease	9–15	Appropriate amount for external use
Fructus et Radix Camptotbeca Acuminate	cold and toxic	bitter	—	Treating tumors by preventing their growth and spread	Stomach cancer; cancer of the esophagus or colon; choriocarcinoma; chronic granulocytic leukemia; lung cancer; cancer of the urinary bladder; cancer of the head and neck; psoriasis	3–9	Ointment containing 20% *Fructus Camptotheca Acuminata* used externally
Rhizoma Zedoariae (zodoary)	warm	pungent and bitter	Liver and Spleen	Eradicating blood stasis; promoting the normal flow of vital energy and alleviating pain	Cancer of the uterine cervix, skin cancer; abdominal masses; abdominal distension due to retention of food or gas	3–9	Contraindicated in pregnancy; appropriate amount for external use to treat skin cancer

Herba Crotalariae (crotalaria)	mild and toxic	bitter	—	Treating tumors by preventing their growth and spread; removing pathogenic heat; detoxication	Skin cancer; cancer of the uterine cervix, esophagus, or rectum; dysentery; boils and skin inflammation	9–15	Appropriate amount for external use; injections now available
Bulbus Cremastrae (edible tulip bulb)	warm and toxic	bitter	—	Treating tumors by preventing their growth and spread	Breast cancer; nasopharyngeal carcinoma; cancer of the esophagus or uterine cervix; skin cancer	0.6–0.9	Appropriate amount for external use
Nidus Vespae (cells in a honeycomb)	mild and toxic	pungent	Liver and Stomach	Dispelling wind to arrest pain	Breast cancer; cancer of the esophagus; stomach cancer; nasopharyngeal carcinoma; mastitis; tuberculosis of the cervical lymph nodes; boils; rashes; toothache	3–12	As above
Mylabris (blister beetle)	warm and toxic	pungent	Liver and Stomach	Treating tumors; dispersing masses; cauterizing abscesses	Cancer of the liver, esophagus, or lung; stomach cancer; breast cancer; abdominal masses; necrosing abscesses; protracted itching disorders	0.03–0.06	In powder mixture; appropriate amount for external use

Medicinal Herb	Property(s)	Flavor(s)	Channel(s) Acted on	Action(s)	Indication(s)	Amount (grams)	Remarks
Semen Strychni (vomiting nut)	cold and toxic	bitter	Liver and Stomach	Treating tumors; dispersing masses; activating the circulation of *qi* through the channels and arresting rheumatic pain	Stomach cancer; cancer of the esophagus, liver, or lung; breast cancer; skin cancer, tuberculosis of the lymph nodes; abscesses; trauma; rheumatic arthralgia; numbness and paralysis of limbs	0.3–0.9	Overdose causes intoxication; prohibited in pregnancy
Herba Oldenlandiae (olden landia)	cold	sweet and bitter	Stomach, Large and Small Intestine	Treating tumors; expelling pathogenic heat and toxin; removing dampness through diuresis	Stomach cancer; cancer of the esophagus or rectum; appendicitis; boils; sore throat; snakebite; acute urinary tract infection	15–60	Appropriate amount for external use
Radix Actinidiae (actinida)	cold	sweet and sour	Liver, Stomach, and Urinary Bladder	Treating tumors; expelling pathogenic heat and toxin; removing damp-wind; promoting urination	Stomach cancer; cancer of the esophagus; arthralgia; dysuria due to damp-heat; jaundice	15–30	
Herba Scutellariae Barbatae (sunplant)	cold	pungent and slightly bitter	Liver, Lung, and Stomach	Activating the flow of blood	Cancer of the lung or liver; stomach cancer; boils; snakebite; lung abscess; sore throat; chronic hepatitis; ascites due to cirrhosis	15–60	

Anesthetics and Analgesics

These herbs are used to relieve all kinds of pain. Herbs for promoting the flow of vital energy and blood circulation are also prescribed to help pain.

Medicinal Herb	Property(s)	Flavor(s)	Channel(s) Acted on	Action(s)	Indication(s)	Amount (grams)	Remarks
Radix Aconiti (monkshood root)	hot and extremely toxic	pungent and bitter	Heart, Liver, and Spleen	Warming the channels to kill pain; expelling pathogenic wind	Pain in the chest and abdomen due to abundant endogenous pathogenic cold; arthralgia and numbness due to pathogenic wind and cold; pain caused by injuries or wounds; headache, including migraine	3–9	Prohibited in pregnancy; incompatible with *Rhizoma Pinelliae, Fructus Trichosanthis,* and *Rhizoma Bletillae*; inadvisable to take over a long period; apply only externally in fresh condition; inadvisable to use on broken skin
Rhizoma Corydalis (corydalis tuber)	warm	pungent and bitter	Liver and Spleen	Invigorating blood circulation and promoting the flow of vital energy	Pain caused by stagnation of blood and vital energy; bruises and pain due to injury	3–9	

Medicinal Herb	Property(s)	Flavor(s)	Channel(s) Acted on	Action(s)	Indication(s)	Amount (grams)	Remarks
Flos Daturae Stramonii (jamestownweed flower)	warm and toxic	pungent	Heart, Liver, and Spleen	Alleviating pain; arresting cough and asthma; stopping convulsions	Pain in the chest and abdomen due to pathogenic cold; arthralgia; injuries and wounds; epilepsy; recurrent convulsions and spasms; cough and asthma with scanty sputum	0.3–0.9 (*Florus,* Folium) 0.3–0.5 (Fructus)	Appropriate amount for external use; overdose causes intoxication

Tonics

These herbs, which have tonifying actions, are used in treating debility.

VITAL ENERGY TONICS

These are herbs that reinforce the vital functions of the spleen, lung, and heart in order to treat deficiency symptom-complexes.

Medicinal Herb	Property(s)	Flavor(s)	Channel(s) Acted on	Action(s)	Indication(s)	Amount (grams)	Remarks
Radix Ginseng (ginseng root)	mild (neutral)	sweet and slightly bitter	Spleen, Lung, and Heart	Reinforcing vital energy; strengthening the function of the lung and spleen; promoting the secretion of body fluid and relaxing the nerves	Collapse due to deficiency of vital energy; prostration of vital energy after great loss of blood; hypofunction of the cardiovascular system, lung, or stomach; peripheral circulatory failure; diabetes mellitus; impairment of body fluid due to febrile conditions; decreased sexual function due to neurological disorders	3–9	30 grams for emergency treatment; incompatible with *Veratrum Nigrum* (drought onion)
Radix Codonopsis Pilosulae (pilose asiabell root)	mild (neutral)	sweet	Lung and Spleen	Invigorating the function of the stomach and spleen and replenishing vital energy	Deficiency of vital energy of the spleen and lung; deficiency of both vital energy and blood	9–15	Incompatible with *Veratrum Nigrum*

Medicinal Herb	Property(s)	Flavor(s)	Channel(s) Acted on	Action(s)	Indication(s)	Amount (grams)	Remarks
Fructus Schisandrae (magnolia-vine fruit)	warm	sour and sweet	Lung, Heart, and Kidney	Reinforcing vital energy and promoting the secretion of body fluid; strengthening the function of the kidney and heart; arresting perspiration and spermatorrhea	Impairment of body fluid due to deficiency of vital energy; asthma due to weakness of the lung and kidney; palpitation; amnesia; neurasthenia; spontaneous perspiration; night sweats due to debility; spermatorrhea; chronic diarrhea	3–9	
Radix Astragali (astraglus root)	moderately warm	sweet	Spleen and Lung	Reinforcing vital energy to invigorate vital function and check perspiration; discharging pus and promoting the growth of new tissue; reducing swelling through diuresis	Deficiency of vital energy; debility due to chronic disease; prolapse of the rectum or uterus due to sinking of vital energy of the spleen; profuse perspiration due to debility; edema and albuminuria due to chronic nephritis; hemiplegia; protracted ulcer	9–15, or up to 30	
Rhizoma Atractylodis Macrocephalis	warm	bitter and sweet	Spleen and Stomach	Invigorating the function of the spleen	Poor appetite, abdominal distension,	3–12	

alae (white atractylodes rhizome)				and reinforcing vital energy; removing pathogenic dampness through diuresis; arresting profuse perspiration	loose stools due to deficiency of vital energy of the spleen and stomach; retention of phlegm and fluid; spontaneous sweating; miscarriage		
Fructus Ziziphi Jujubae (red date)	mild (neutral)	sweet	Spleen and Stomach	Invigorating the function of the spleen and reinforcing vital energy; enriching the blood and relaxing the nerves	Hypofunction of the spleen and stomach; menopause syndromes	3–10 dates	
Radix Glycyrrhizae (licorice root)	mild (neutral)	sweet	Heart, Lung, Spleen, and Stomach	Invigorating the function of the spleen and stomach; reinforcing vital energy; arresting cough by expelling sputum; spasmolytic to alleviate pain; detoxicant for drug poisoning	All kinds of deficiency of vital energy, e.g., ulcers, boils, sore throat; food or drug poisoning; cough and asthma; peptic ulcer; Addison's disease; viral hepatitis	3–9	Incompatible with *Radix Euphorbiae Pekinensis, Flos Genkwa, Radix Euphorbiae Kan Sui*

Yang TONICS

These herbs reinforce vital function, especially kidney function, which is the foundation of the native constitution. (The vital function of the kidney is believed to be the source of heat energy of the body.) The herbs are used chiefly in treating conditions marked by fatigue, cold limbs, weakness in the back and knees, frequency of urination, enuresis, impotence, spermatorrhea, deep pulse, dizziness, and tinnitus, as well as in treating maldevelopment of infants and treating infertility. It has now been shown experimentally that these herbs regulate adrenocortical function, adjust energy metabolism, increase or restore physical and mental tone, improve sexual ability, promote development and growth, and enhance body resistance.

Medicinal Herb	Property(s)	Flavor(s)	Channel(s) Acted on	Action(s)	Indication(s)	Amount (grams)	Remarks
Cornu Pantotrichum (pilose deer horn)	warm	salty and sweet	Kidney and Liver	Reinforcing the vital function of the kidney; enriching vital essence and blood; strengthening muscles and bones	Lowered vital function of the kidney and insufficient vital essence and blood; maldevelopment of infants; uterine bleeding; penetrating ulcers causing insufficiency of blood and vital energy	0.5–1	Taken in powder form or mixed in a bolus
Fructus Psoraleae (psoralea fruit)	extremely warm	pungent and bitter	Kidney and Spleen	Reinforcing the vital function of the kidney; warming the spleen to stop diarrhea	Impotence, spermatorrhea due to insufficient vital function of the kidney; chronic diarrhea occurring daily just before dawn and due to hypofunction of the spleen and kidney	3–9	

							Appropriate amount for external use
Fructus Cnidii (cnidium fruit)	warm	pungent and bitter	Kidney	Warming the kidney to reinforce its vital function; used externally for drying oozing and killing worms	Impotence; weakness in the back and knees; infertility due to lowered vital function of the kidney; leukorrhea; pruritus of pudendum; eczema of the scrotum; rashes	6–15	Appropriate amount for external use
Radix Morindae (morinda root)	moderately warm	pungent and sweet	Kidney and Liver	Reinforcing vital function of the kidney; strengthening the muscles and bones; expelling pathogenic wind-dampness	Impotence, spermatorrhea; premature ejaculation, and weakness in the back and knees, all due to lowered vital function of the kidney; flaccidity of extremities due to hypofunction of the liver and kidney; arthralgia due to wind-dampness; edema due to beriberi	6–15	
Herba Epimedii (epimedium)	warm	pungent	Kidney and Liver	Arresting cough and asthma	Impotence due to lowered vital function of the kidney; infertility in women; arthralgia; infantile paralysis; cough and asthma due to deficiency of vital essence; hypertension during menopause	9–15	

Medicinal Herb	Property(s)	Flavor(s)	Channel(s) Acted on	Action(s)	Indication(s)	Amount (grams)	Remarks
Rhizoma Curculiginis (curculigo rhizome)	warm and slightly poisonous	pungent	Kidney, Spleen, and Liver	Reinforcing the vital function of the kidney and spleen; strengthening the muscles and bones; expelling pathogenic cold and dampness	Impotence, enuresis due to lowered vital function of the kidney; abdominal pain and diarrhea due to hypofunction of the spleen and kidney; cold sensation of the waist and knees; arthralgia due to cold-damp	3–9	
Hippocampus (sea horse)	warm	sweet and salty	Kidney and Liver	Reinforcing the vital function of the kidney	Weakness in the back and knees, impotence, frequency of urination due to lowered vital function of the kidney; abdominal masses; trauma; goiter; deep abscess	1–1.5	Taken in powder form
Cortex Eucommiae (eucommia bark)	warm	sweet	Kidney and Liver	Strengthening the function of the kidney, liver, muscles, and bones; preventing miscarriage; reducing blood pressure	Aching back and weakness of the lower limbs; hypertension due to deficiency of vital energy or vital essence of the kidney or liver; threatened abortion	9–15	

Fructus Corni; (dogwood fruit)	warm	sweet and sour	Kidney and Liver	Strengthening the function of the liver and kidney; arresting profuse perspiration and spermatorrhea	Weakness of the back and knees, impotence, frequency of urination due to deficiency of vital energy or vital essence of the kidney and liver; hypertension resulting from hypofunction of the liver and kidney; spermatorrhea; spontaneous perspiration; night sweats; profuse menstrual and other uterine bleeding	6–12, or up to 30
Herba Cistanchis (cistanche)	warm	sweet and salty	Kidney and Large Intestine	Reinforcing the vital function of the kidney; relieving constipation	Impotence; premature ejaculation; infertility in women; constipation due to deficiency of blood or body fluid after childbirth; senile constipation	9–18

Medicinal Herb	Property(s)	Flavor(s)	Channel(s) Acted on	Action(s)	Indication(s)	Amount (grams)	Remarks
Herba Cynomorii (cynomorium)	warm	sweet	Liver, Kidney, and Large Intestine	Strengthening the function of the liver and kidney, relieving constipation	Impotence, spermatorrhea due to hypofunction of the kidney; weakness of the muscles and bones due to deficiency of vital essence of the liver and kidney; constipation due to deficiency of body fluid and blood	9–15	
Semen Astragali Complanati (flattened milkvetch seed)	warm	sweet	Liver and Kidney	Strengthening the function of the liver and kidney; arresting spermatorrhea and improving eyesight	Backache, spermatorrhea, premature ejaculation due to hypofunction of the kidney; neurasthenia; blurred vision due to weakened liver and kidney	9–15	
Semen Cuscutae (dodder seed)	mild (neutral)	pungent and sweet	Liver and Kidney	Strengthening the function of the kidney and enriching vital essence; invigorating the function of the liver to improve eyesight; promoting sleep	Deficiency of vital function and vital essence of the kidney; blurred vision, loose stools, or diarrhea due to weakened kidney and liver; threat-	9–15	

Herb	Nature	Taste	Meridian	Actions	Indications	Dosage	Administration
					ened abortion due to deficiency of vital function of the kidney		
Cordyceps (Chinese caterpillar fungus)	warm	sweet	Lung and Kidney	Strengthening the function of the lung and kidney; relieving asthma	Impotence, spermatorrhea due to deficiency of vital essence of the kidney; cough and asthma due to deficiency of vital function of the lung and kidney	6–15	1.5–3 grams taken in powder form
Gecko (gecko)	mild (neutral)	salty	Lung and Kidney	Strengthening the function of the lung and kidney; maintaining normal inspiration of the lung and kidney to relieve asthma	Asthma, cough, shortness of breath due to deficiency of vital function of the kidney and lung; expectoration of bloody sputum; impotence and frequent urination due to deficiency of vital function of the kidney	1–1.5	Taken in powder form
Placenta Hominis (dried human placenta)	warm	sweet and salty	Heart, Lung, and Kidney	Strengthening the function of the kidney and enriching vital essence and vital energy to nourish blood	Generalized weakness; fatigue; pulmonary tuberculosis; neurasthenia; anemia; albuminuria due to chronic nephritis	1.5–3	In bolus or powder mixture

BLOOD TONICS

These herbs are used to treat deficiency of blood. They are effective for pale complexion and lips, dizziness, tinnitus, blurred vision, palpitation, insomnia, amnesia, and delayed or absent menstruation. Most of them improve the function of the hematopoietic system and nourish the body to promote health. The herbs also protect the liver (which stores blood) and have a sedative action.

Medicinal Herb	Property(s)	Flavor(s)	Channel(s) Acted on	Action(s)	Indication(s)	Amount (grams)	Remarks
Radix Angelicae Sinensis (Chinese angelica)	warm	sweet and pungent	Liver, Heart, and Spleen	Nourishing the blood and regulating menstruation; activating blood circulation to alleviate pain; relieving constipation	Deficiency of blood; abdominal pain due to insufficient blood; irregular or painful menstruation, absence of menstruation; trauma, arthralgia; boils; angina pectoris; constipation due to deficiency of blood	3–12	
Caulis Spatholobi (spatholobus stem)	warm	sweet and pungent	Liver	Invigorating blood circulation and nourishing the blood; activating channels and tendons	Deficiency of blood manifested by absence of menstruation, delayed menstruation, painful menstruation; dizziness; numbness of the body and limbs; arthralgia	9–30	

Name	Property	Taste	Channels	Functions	Indications	Dosage	Remarks
Radix Rehmanniae Praeparata (prepared rehmannia root)	moderately warm	sweet	Heart, Liver, and Kidney	Nourishing the blood and replenishing vital essence	All kinds of deficiency of blood; deficiency of vital essence of the liver and kidney	9–30	
Colla Corii Asini (donkey-hide gelatin)	mild (neutral)	sweet	Lung, Liver, and Kidney	Nourishing the blood and stopping bleeding; replenishing vital essence and moistening the lung	Deficiency of blood; hemorrhage such as hemoptysis; bleeding due to miscarriage, other uterine bleeding; insomnia and irritability due to deficiency of essence; cough without sputum due to deficiency of essence of the lung	6–15	Taken dissolved in hot water
Radix Polygoni Multiflori (multiflower knotweed tuber)	moderately warm	sweet, bitter, and puckery	Liver, Heart, and Lung	Replenishing vital essence of the liver and kidney; nourishing the blood and essence; relieving constipation and promoting detoxication	Deficiency of vital essence of the liver and kidney; reduced blood volume; hypertension; coronary heart disease; neurasthenia; urticaria; senile constipation	9–25	

Yin Tonics

These herbs replenish vital essence and fluids. They are used in treating deficiency of vital essence, especially that of the lung, stomach, or liver.

Medicinal Herb	Property(s)	Flavor(s)	Channel(s) Acted on	Action(s)	Indication(s)	Amount (grams)	Remarks
Radix Glehniae (glehnia root)	moderately cold	sweet	Lung and Stomach	Replenishing vital essence of the lung and stomach; promoting the secretion of body fluid	Dryness of the lung due to deficiency of vital essence; impairment of vital essence of the lung and stomach due to excessive pathogenic heat	9–10	Incompatible with *Veratrum Nigrum*
Fructus Lycii (wolfberry fruit)	mild (neutral)	sweet	Liver and Kidney	Replenishing vital essence to improve eyesight; nourishing blood	Deficiency of vital essence of the liver and kidney; lack of blood; blurred vision; diabetes	6–15	
Radix Ophiopogonis (lily-turf root)	moderately cold	sweet and slightly bitter	Heart, Lung, and Stomach	Replenishing vital essence of the stomach and lung; clearing pathogenic fire of the heart	Impairment of body fluid due to excessive pathogenic heat; dryness of the lung resulting from deficiency of vital essence; restlessness, insomnia caused by deficiency of vital essence of the heart	3–9	

Radix Asparagi (asparagus root)	cold	sweet and bitter	Lung and Stomach	Replenishing vital essence to clear pathogenic heat; moistening the lung and nourishing the kidney	Dryness of the lung due to deficiency of vital essence; hectic fever; night sweats; spermatorrhea and weakness of the legs; dryness of the intestines and constipation in late-stage febrile disease	6–18
Rhizoma Polygonati Odorati (fragrant solomonseal rhizome)	moderately cold	sweet	Lung and Stomach	Replenishing vital essence of the lung and stomach; invigorating the secretion of body fluid	Impairment of vital essence and body fluid due to pathogenic dry-heat in the lung and stomach; angina pectoris	9–30
Rhizoma Polygonati (siberian solomonseal rhizome)	mild (neutral)	sweet	Lung, Kidney, and Spleen	Replenishing vital essence of the lung; nourishing the spleen; reinforcing the spleen	Dry cough due to deficiency of vital essence of the lung; debility after an illness; reduced blood volume; loss of appetite and lassitude due to deficiency of spleen and stomach	9–30

Medicinal Herb	Property(s)	Flavor(s)	Channel(s) Acted on	Action(s)	Indication(s)	Amount (grams)	Remarks
Herba Dendrobii (dendrobium)	moderately cold	sweet and insipid	Lung, Stomach, and Kidney	Invigorating secretion of body fluid and nourishing the stomach; replenishing vital essence to clear away pathogenic heat	Deficiency of vital essence of the stomach and flaring up of pathogenic fire due to deficiency of vital essence of the kidney; thirst and spontaneous perspiration in late-stage febrile disease	9–20	
Fructus Ligustri Lucidi (glossy privet fruit)	cool	bitter and sweet	Liver and Kidney	Nourishing the liver and kidney to improve eyesight	Dizziness, blurred vision, weakness of the back and knees due to deficiency of vital essence of the liver and kidney; early cataract; premature greying; central angiospastic retinitis	9–15	
Plastrum Testudinis (tortoise plastron)	mild	salty and sweet	Liver and Kidney	Replenishing vital essence to check hyperactivity of the liver; nourishing the kidney and strengthening the bones	Hectic fever and night sweats; seminal emission due to deficiency of vital essence of the kidney; dizziness, tinnitus caused by deficiency of vital essence; impairment	9–30	

of vital essence due to febrile conditions; stirring up of endogenous pathogenic wind due to deficiency of vital essence; weakness of the back and legs due to deficiency of vital essence of the liver and kidney; profuse menstrual and other uterine bleeding caused by deficiency of vital essence and excessive pathogenic heat in the blood

Carapax Trionycis (turtle shell)	cold	salty	Liver and Kidney	Replenishing vital energy to check hyperactivity of the liver; softening hard lumps and dispelling masses	Hectic fever, night sweats due to deficiency of vital essence; consumption of vital essence in late-stage febrile disease; convulsions due to stirring up of endogenous pathogenic wind; abdominal masses; hepatosplenomegaly	9–30

Astringents

These are herbs sour and puckery in flavor that arrest or reduce perspiration, diarrhea, spermatorrhea, frequent urination, and leukorrhea.

ANHIDROTICS

These herbs strengthen superficial resistance and check perspiration. They are used in treating spontaneous sweating and night sweats.

Medicinal Herb	Propery(s)	Flavor(s)	Channel(s) Acted on	Action(s)	Indication(s)	Amount (grams)	Remarks
Radix Ephedrae (ephedra root)	mild (neutral)	sweet	Heart and Lung	Checking the secretion of sweat	Spontaneous perspiration due to deficiency of vital energy; night sweats due to deficiency of vital essence	3–9	
Fructus Tritici Levis (blighted wheat)	cool	sweet	Heart	As above	Spontaneous perspiration and night sweats	9–30	

ANTIDIARRHEALS

These herbs are used mainly in treating chronic diarrhea and dysentery.

Medicinal Herb	Property(s)	Flavor(s)	Channel(s) Acted on	Action(s)	Indication(s)	Amount (grams)	Remarks
Halloysitum Rubrum (red kaolin)	warm	sweet and puckery	Stomach and Large Intestine	Counteracting diarrhea; arresting bleeding and healing wounds	Chronic diarrhea associated with hemorrhage, bloody stools, profuse menstrual bleeding due to deficiency of vital energy and to pathogenic cold; protracted ulcers or unhealed wounds	6–24	Appropriate amount for external use; inadvisable in dysentery caused by pathogenic dampness
Semen Myristicae (nutmeg)	warm	pungent	Spleen, Stomach, and Large Intestine	Arresting diarrhea; warming the stomach and spleen, and promoting the normal flow of vital energy	Chronic diarrhea and diarrhea occurring before dawn daily, both conditions caused by deficiency of vital essence and excessive pathogenic cold of the spleen and kidney; abdominal pain, loss of appetite, or vomiting because of hypofunction of the spleen and stomach due to cold	3–9	

Medicinal Herb	Property(s)	Flavor(s)	Channel(s) Acted on	Action(s)	Indication(s)	Amount (grams)	Remarks
Fructus Chebulae (chebula fruit)	mild (neutral)	bitter, sour, and puckery	Lung and Large Intestine	Counteracting diarrhea; easing the pain of sore throat	Chronic dysentery, diarrhea; asthma due to deficiency of vital essence of the lung; persistent cough and hoarseness	3–9	
Pericarpium Granati (pomegranate bark)	warm	sour and puckery	Large Intestine	Counteracting diarrhea; killing parasites	Chronic diarrhea and dysentery; bloody stools or prolapse of the rectum; roundworms; tapeworms; pinworms	4–10	
Galla Chinensis (Chinese gall)	cold	sour and puckery	Lung, Large Intestine, and Stomach	Bringing excessive fire of the lung downward; counteracting diarrhea and checking the abnormal secretion of sweat; arresting bleeding	Persistent cough; cough with expectoration of sputum due to pathogenic heat in the lung; chronic diarrhea; spontaneous perspiration and night sweats; spermatorrhea; prolapse of the rectum or uterus; apply externally for boils and ulcers with profuse pus	0.5–1.5	Taken in powder form; for external use, apply appropriate amount

HERBS FOR CHECKING SPERMATORRHEA, FREQUENT URINATION, AND EXCESSIVE LEUKORRHEA

Medicinal Herb	Property(s)	Flavor(s)	Channel(s) Acted on	Action(s)	Indication(s)	Amount (grams)	Remarks
Fructus Rosae Laevigatae (cherokee rose fruit)	mild (neutral)	sweet and puckery	Kidney and Urinary Bladder	Arresting spermatorrhea and reducing urination; antidiarrheal	Spermatorrhea due to lowered functional activity of the kidney; frequent urination; whitish and turbid urine; excessive discharge of leukorrhea due to deficiency of vital energy of the spleen and kidney; protracted diarrhea	6–18	
Oötheca Mantidis (mantis egg-case)	mild (neutral)	sweet, salty, and puckery	Liver and Kidney	Nourishing the kidney to reinforce its vital function; arresting spermatorrhea and reducing urination	Frequent urination; fecal incontinence; spermatorrhea; premature ejaculation due to lowered functional activity of the kidney; infantile enuresis; impotence caused by deficiency of vital energy of the kidney	3–9	

Medicinal Herb	Property(s)	Flavor(s)	Channel(s) Acted on	Action(s)	Indication(s)	Amount (grams)	Remarks
Fructus Alpiniae Oxyphyllae (galangal fruit)	warm	pungent	Spleen and Kidney	Nourishing the kidney to arrest spermatorrhea; reducing urination; arresting diarrhea by warming the spleen	Spermatorrhea; premature ejaculation; frequent urination;; whitish and turbid urine; diarrhea and abdominal cold and pain due to deficiency of vital energy with symptoms of cold	3–9	
Os Sepiae (cuttlefish bone)	moderately warm	salty and puckery	Liver and Stomach	Arresting spermatorrhea and excessive leukorrhea; stopping bleeding; used as an antacid	All kinds of hemorrhage (e.g., pulmonary, gastric, and intestinal bleeding, hematuria, and uterine bleeding); excessive leukorrhea; spermatorrhea; peptic ulcer	6–12	Smaller amount in powder form
Semen Euryales (euryale seed)	mild (neutral)	sweet and puckery	Spleen and Kidney	Reinforcing vital function of the spleen and kidney to stop diarrhea and arrest spermatorrhea and excessive leukorrhea	Chronic diarrhea due to deficiency of vital energy of the spleen; spermatorrhea or premature ejaculation due to weakened functional activity of the kidney; frequent urination or	9–15	

Semen Nelumbinis (lotus seed)	mild (neutral)	sweet and puckery	Spleen, Kidney, and Heart	Nourishing the spleen to stop diarrhea; reinforcing the function of the kidney to arrest spermatorrhea	Diarrhea due to deficiency of vital energy of the spleen; breakdown of the normal physiologic coordination between the heart and kidney; spermatorrhea, frequent urination or leukorrhea due to deficiency of vital energy of the kidney; insomnia, irritability, and palpitation due to deficiency of the heart	9–18
					discharge of turbid urine; leukorrhea due to pathogenic damp-heat or deficiency of vital energy of the spleen and kidney	
Fructus Rubi (raspberry fruit)	moderately warm	sweet and sour	Liver and Kidney	Nourishing the liver and kidney; arresting seminal emission; improving eyesight; reducing urination	Frequent urination; spermatorrhea; enuresis; blurred vision due to deficiency of the liver and kidney	9–15

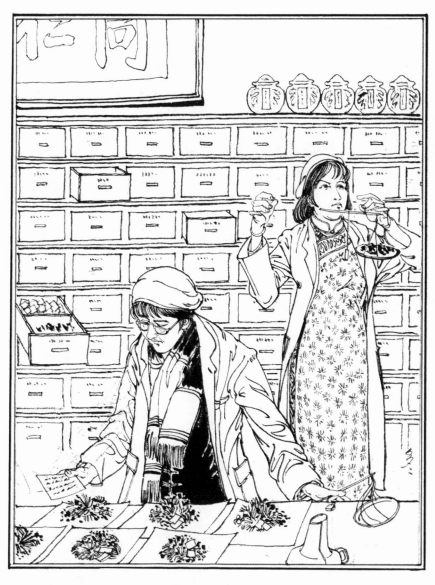

Herbal pharmacists reading a prescription and dispensing herbs.

CHAPTER THREE

An Introduction to
Traditional Chinese Prescriptions

I N TRADITIONAL CHINESE MEDICINE, prescriptions, which
are composed of various herbs according to the principles discussed below, are often considered the major means of treating
disease. Since ancient times, physicians have summarized the experience in this field. Many effective prescriptions have thus been ver-
ified and handed down. For instance, 10,000 prescriptions are listed
in *Peaceful Holy Benevolent Prescriptions,* which was compiled in A.D.
992. About 20,000 prescriptions are contained in the *General Collection of Wise Healing,* which was also written during the Song Dynasty
(in 1111–1117). Many of these prescriptions are still being used.

The use of various herbs together has several benefits. Primarily,
it improves the curative effect by allowing the ingredients' actions
full play. Also, the use of several ingredients together permits effective treatment of relatively complicated diseases. Finally, it allows
the toxic actions of some herbs to be reduced or neutralized.

INTERACTION OF INGREDIENTS IN A PRESCRIPTION

Before exploring how a prescription is composed and modified, it
is necessary to know how the ingredients interact. Thus, the following concepts should be considered.

A single ingredient is administered if it is good for a specific mild disease. However, two herbs with similar properties are sometimes used together to reinforce each other's actions; this is called *mutual reinforcement.* An example is *Radix et Rhizoma Rhei* and *Natrii Sulfas,* which administered together effectively expel intense heat through strong purgation.

Sometimes when two or more ingredients are combined in a prescription, one is the principal substance and the others play a subsidiary role, reinforcing its action; this is termed *assistance.* For example, when *Radix Scutellariae* and *Radix et Rhizoma Rhei* are administered together, the latter enhances the former's action of reducing intense heat.

Various herbs can weaken or neutralize each other's toxicity. This is known as *restraint* or *neutralization.* For instance, *Rhizoma Zingiberis recens* can relieve or neutralize the toxicity of *Rhizoma Pinelliae* and *Rhizoma Arisaematis.* Thus it is said that the latter two ingredients are restrained by the former. "The nineteen medicaments of restraint" (table 3.1) are well known in traditional Chinese medicine.

One ingredient can weaken the action of another ingredient or even render it ineffective. This is called *counteraction.* For example, the action of *Rhizoma Zingiberis recens* is counteracted by *Radix Scutellariae,* and that of *Radix Ginseng* is counteracted by *Semen Raphani.* Some of the nineteen medicaments of mutual restraint also counteract each other.

TABLE 3.1.   Nineteen Medicaments of Restraint

Restraining Compound	*Restrained Compound*
Sulfur	Crude mirabilite
Mercury	Arsenic
Radix Euphorbiae Ebracteolatae (ebracteolate euphorbia root)	*Lithargyrum litharge*
Fructus Crotonis	*Semen Pharbitides*
Flos Caryophylli (clove flower)	*Radix Curcumae*
Natrii Sulfas (sodium sulfate)	*Rhizoma Sparganii*
Radix Aconiti and *Radix Aconiti Kusnezaffii*	*Cornu Rhinoceri*
Radix Ginseng	*Faeces Trogopterorum* (flying squirrel feces)
Cortex Cinnamomi	*Halloystitum Rubrum*

TABLE 3.2.   Eighteen Incompatible Medicaments

Radix Glycyrrhizae	incompatible with	*Radix Euphorbiae Kansui*
		Radix Euphoribiae Pekinensis
		Flos Genkwa
		Sargassum
Radix Aconiti	incompatible with	*Bulbus Fritillariae*
		Fructus Trichosanthis
		Rhizoma Pinelliae
		Radix Ampelopsis (Japanese ampelopsis)
		Rhizoma Bletillae
Radix Veratri nigri	incompatible with	*Radix Ginseng*
		Radix Codopsis Pilosulae
		Radix Scrophulariae
		Radix Salviae Miltiorrhizae
		Herba Asari
		Radix Paeoniae Alba

In addition, some combinations of two ingredients can give rise to serious side effects or even toxicity. This is termed *incompatibility*. Among these combinations are the "eighteen incompatible medicaments" (table 3.2). The herbs of each combination should not be given together.

In summary, the following principles should be adhered to: herbs that are mutually reinforcing or that assist other herbs should be used to full advantage; those that in certain combinations restrain or counteract may be used effectively as antidotes under potentially toxic circumstances; and herbs that are incompatible should not be used together at all.

PRINCIPLES OF COMPOSING AND MODIFYING A PRESCRIPTION

A prescription is not a simple arbitrary mixture of medicinal substances. Nor is it even a carefully composed mixture of ingredients with merely additive actions. Rather, it is a combination of ingredients in proper amounts in accordance with specific principles for combining herbs as appropriate to the stage of disease and the differentiation of symptom-complexes.

Composition of Prescriptions

A prescription normally contains four categories of ingredients: principal, adjuvant, auxiliary and/or correctant, and conductant. The *principal* ingredient plays the leading role in counteracting the disease. An *adjuvant* ingredient strengthens the principal ingredient's action. An *auxiliary* ingredient relieves secondary symptoms, and a *correctant* ingredient either tempers the action of the principal ingredient if the latter is too potent or checks any potential toxic side effects. A *conductant* ingredient directs the action to the affected channel or site.

The relative amounts of ingredients in a prescription are related to the ingredients' roles. Li Dongyuan (1180–1252), a notable physician of the Jin Dynasty, stated in the *Treatise on Spleen and Stomach:* "In amount, the order is as follows: the principal, adjuvant, auxiliary, and conductant ingredients." The amount of the principal ingredient can never be exceeded by that of the adjuvant ingredient. Only when the principal ingredient plays the leading role and its action is modulated by the other ingredients can the patient's disorder be cured.

It is clear, then, that the ingredients in a prescription are in close cooperation with one another to exert their due effect. All prescriptions that have proved effective are, without exception, characterized by their clear aim and precise formulation. Consider, for example, Decoction of Ephedra (described later in this chapter), the ingredients of which are:

Herba Ephedrae	9 grams	
Ramulus Cinnamomi	6	"
Semen Armeniacae Amarum	9	"
Radix Glycyrrhizae	3	"

The indication for this prescription is exterior affection by pathogenic wind and cold. In this condition, the lung is invaded by cold; hence it is necessary to use herbs pungent in flavor and warm in property to expel pathogenic factors from the lung through perspiration. Therefore, *Herba Ephedrae* serves as the principal ingredient to dispel pathogenic wind and cold from the body and to relieve asthmatic cough by ventilating the lung and smoothing the flow of vital energy; *Ramulus Cinnamomi* is the adjuvant ingredient that aids *Herba Ephedrae* in diaphoresis and warms and clears the channels to relieve pains over the limbs and the body; *Semen Armeniacae Amarum* serves as the auxiliary ingredient to relieve asthma by ventilating the lung; and *Radix Glycyrrhizae* serves as the conductant ingredient to harmonize the action of all the other ingredients and direct them to their proper channels.

All prescriptions contain a principal ingredient. However, some prescriptions may lack one or more of the other categories. For example, Decoction of Ginseng, which is used to treat collapse, has only one ingredient—*ginseng.* In some prescriptions, the principal or adjuvant ingredient may also serve as the auxiliary or conductant ingredient: Pills of Coptis and Evodia for exuberant fire in the Liver Channel are composed only of *Rhizoma Coptidis,* which is the principal ingredient, and *Fructus Evodiae,* the auxiliary; and Jade Screen Powder (described later in this chapter) consists of three ingredients: *Radix Astragali,* the principal, *Rhizoma Atractylodis Macrocephalae,* the adjuvant, and *Radix Ledebouriellae,* the auxiliary.

Modification of Prescriptions

In composing a prescription, the following factors should be considered: the disease condition, the constitution and age of the patient, the season, and the geographical environment. Xu Lintai (1693–1771), a physician of the Qing Dynasty, states in *On the Origin and Source of Medicine* that "When trying to use an old handed-down prescription, you must first determine whether all the symptoms and signs of the patient you are treating are consistent with those described in that prescription and whether every ingredient is good for the case. If not, you must make the proper modifications or, if it is impossible to do so, choose another recipe."

As indicated by the above quotation, the composition of a prescription is sometimes modified. *Modification* means that the principal ingredient remains the same but that other ingredients are added or

deleted according to the signs and symptoms present and the stage
of the disease. In Chinese medicine, this is known as "modification
based on the disease condition." For example, Powder of *Lonicera* and
Forsythia (described later in this chapter) is good for exterior heat
symptom-complexes due to pathogens. But if the condition is associated with severe thirst due to impairment of fluid, *Radix Trichosanthis* (snakegourd root) is added to generate fluid and relieve thirst.
If it is associated with a swollen sore throat due to accumulation of
pathogenic heat, *Herba Schizonepetae* and *Semen Sojae Praeparatum* should
be replaced by *Lasiosphaera seu Calvatia, Radix Scrophulariae,* and *Radix Isatidis* to clear away the heat and ease the throat. And if it is
associated with epistaxis due to a circulatory disorder caused by pathogenic heat, *Rhizoma Imperatae* and *Cacumen Biotae* (arbovitae twig)
should be used instead of *Herba Schizonepetae,* in order to cool the
blood and stop bleeding. These examples show that it is not always
necessary to follow the set formula. On the contrary, variations should
be made according to the patient's condition.

Relative amounts of ingredients can also be varied. Prescriptions
consisting of the same substances in different proportions have different effects. For example, Decoction of Artemisiae is especially effective for jaundice due to pathogenic damp-heat. In severe jaundice,
a large amount of *Herba Artemisiae Scopariae* is used. If there is no
marked dyspepsia, the amount of *Radix et Rhizoma Rhei* in this prescription may be reduced. Such variation sometimes changes the relationship between the principal and subordinate ingredients. As a
result, the effect of and indications for the prescription change. For
example, Minor Purgative Decoction and Decoction of Magnoliae
with Two Other Herbs both consist of *Radix et Rhizoma Rhei, Fructus
Aurantii Immaturus,* and *Cortex Magnoliae Officinalis.* But whereas the
former prescription contains 12 g, 12 g, and 6 g of the three ingredients, respectively, the latter contains 12 g, 12 g, and 24 g. Thus,
in the former prescription, *Radix et Rhizoma Rhei* is the principal
ingredient, *Fructus Aurantii Immaturus* is the adjuvant ingredient, and
Cortex Magnoliae Officinalis serves as the auxiliary and conductant ingredient. Therefore, this prescription is used to relieve constipation
due to pathogenic heat through purgation. In the latter prescription,
however, the principal ingredient is *Cortex Magnoliae Officinalis;* the
adjuvant is *Fructus Aurantii Immaturus,* and *Radix et Rhizoma Rhei*
becomes the auxiliary and conductant. This prescription, then, is

used to promote the flow of vital energy and relieve abdominal distension due to stagnancy of vital energy.

Drug Forms: Their Administration and Actions

The major forms of drugs include decoctions, powders, pills, capsules, and honey boluses. Powders, pills, and capsules are similar to their equivalents in western medicine. Decoctions and honey boluses are prepared as described below.

DECOCTIONS

"The curative effects of a prescription depend on the appropriate method of making a decoction." *(On the Origin and Source of Medicine).*

The decoction is the main form of administering a prescription. Throughout history, Chinese practitioners have attached great importance to the decoction process.

The decoction is a form of medicinal preparation in which herbs are boiled in order to extract their chemically effective contents. An earthen pot with a cover should be used during the decoction process because metal may induce undesirable chemical reactions. The pot should be clean and oil-free. The herbs are placed in the pot and first steeped in tap water that just covers the herbs (about 200–300 ml water per 30 g herbs), so that the active constituents may be dissolved into the liquid.

Duration and degree of heating: "Make a decoction over a strong fire first and a slow fire later, and no one will fail to respond to the prescription," wrote Li Shizhen (1518–1593) in *Compendium of Materia Medica.*

The pot is first put over high heat, and when the contents boil, the heat is turned down to prevent boiling over or burning of the herbs. Diaphoretic or antipyretic preparations should be decocted over high heat for a short period (10–15 minutes) to prevent evaporation of the effective constituents of the herbs. Conversely, tonics should be simmered for at least half an hour so that all the effective constituents are fully dissolved. The toxicity of herbs such as aconites is decreased through prolonged simmering (45–60 minutes). Strongly volatile (e.g., mint) or heat-sensitive substances are added just before the end of the process in order to preserve their integrity. Herbs with cilia (fine hair-like structures) should be wrapped in tight-woven gauze because the cilia may float to the surface of the decoction and upon swallowing induce coughing. Powdered herbs that settle rapidly and may burn, as well as seeds (e.g., Asiatic plantain seed), should also be wrapped in gauze. Costly ingredients (e.g., musk, bear's gallbladder, pearl) of which small amounts are required are first powdered and then mixed into the finished decoction. Highly volatile or soluble ingredients (e.g., honey) are also added to the finished decoction. Fresh ingredients (e.g., watermelon, pear) are first dejuiced, and the juice is then added at the end of the decoction process.

DOSAGE AND ADMINISTRATION. A single prescription package is usually decocted twice, and the fluid from both decoctions (~200ml)

TABLE 3.3. Commonly Used Herbs Prepared by Special Techniques

Decocted first	*Concha Haliotidis, Concha Ostreae, Os Draconis, Dens Draconis* (dragon's teeth), *Plastrum Testudinis, Carapax Trionycis, Ochra, Gypsum Fibrosum* (gypsum), *Calcitum* (calcite), *Magnetitum* (magnetite), *Cornu Antelopis, Os Tigris* (tiger bone), *Concha Meretricis seu Cyclinae* (clam shell), *Cornu Bubali* (buffalo horn), *Cornu Rhinoceri*
Decocted later	*Herba Menthae, Radix Aucklandiae, Fructus Amomi* (amomum fruit), *Semen Cardamomo Rotundi, Lignum Aquilariae Resinatum* (eagle wood), *Herba Artemisiae Chinghao, Herba Elsholtzia seu Moslae*
Decocted wrapped in a gauze packet	*Halloysitum, Flos Inulae* (inula flower), *Semen Plantaginis*
Simmered separately	*Ginseng, Radix Ginseng Americana* (American ginseng), *Cornu Cervi Pantotrichum*
Melted in Decoction	*Colla Corii Asini, Colla Plastri Testudinis* (glue of tortoise plastron), *Colla Cornus Cervi, Maltose, Colla Os Tigris*
Dissolved in boiling water before taking	*Powder of Calculus Bovis, Powder of Cinnabaris, Powder of Succinum, Natrii Sulfas, Powder of Radix Notoginseng, Succus Rhizoma Zingiberis, Succus Nelumbinis Rhizomatis, Succus Bambusae* (bamboo juice), honey

is mixed together before administration. The dregs are discarded. The decoction is divided into two equal doses, one taken in the morning and one in the evening. In children or the severely ill, the decoction may be divided into smaller doses and given at shorter intervals throughout the day. For chronic conditions or for some tonic prescriptions, a single package may be decocted three times and taken in large doses.

Special techniques for preparing herbs for use in decoctions are listed in table 3.3.

BOLUSES

When the term "bolus" is mentioned, it refers to the honey bolus, a kind of traditional Chinese medicinal pill consisting of powdered herbs bound together with honey. Honey contains a large amount of sugar as well as proteins and vitamins. Not only does honey improve the flavor of the bolus; it also arrests cough, relieves constipation, and has detoxifying and tonifying actions. Therefore, the honey bolus is widely used in traditional Chinese medicine, primarily to treat chronic diseases and disorders of deficiency.

The three basic ingredients of the bolus are: processed honey, medicinal herbs, and a lubricant. The honey is prepared by heating it to a temperature that preserves both its sticky consistency and an 11–15 percent water content. The herbs are weighed according to the given prescription and then dried, pulverized, sifted together and then mixed with the honey. The lubricant, which is formed from a 3:7 mixture of beeswax and sesame oil, is added to the honey mixture to prevent it from sticking to the utensils during processing. After the ingredients are thoroughly mixed together by kneading, individual boluses (large spherical pills) are formed and immediately wrapped in wax paper or encased in plastic containers to preserve their moisture content. In order to be taken, each bolus is made into several smaller boluses, which are then swallowed with tepid water.

Different drug forms have different actions. For example, Bolus to Regulate the Functioning of the Spleen and Stomach is used to dispel cold from the spleen and stomach and restore their normal functioning. In bolus form, the action is slow. When a decoction of the same ingredients is used instead, a quicker response is obtained. Therefore the decoction form is more appropriate than the bolus in serious or critical conditions. Another example is Decoction of Aurantii and Atractylodis, which is used to remove retained fluid and dispel abdominal masses. The bolus made of the same ingredients has a milder action and is used for dyspepsia due to a weakened spleen and stomach.

THE CLASSIFICATION OF PRESCRIPTIONS

The earliest recorded classification of prescriptions is in the *Classic of Internal Medicine*. In this work, prescriptions are divided along four lines: as major or heavy prescriptions (consisting of numerous or strong ingredients or large amounts of ingredients) versus minor prescriptions (consisting of a few or mild ingredients or small amounts of ingredients), slow-acting versus quick-acting prescriptions, prescriptions with ingredients odd in number versus those with ingredients even in number, and compound prescriptions (those composed of more than one prescription) versus simple prescriptions.

In his work *Annotated Collection of Prescriptions,* Wang Ang (1682– ?), a physician of the Qing Dynasty, assigned prescriptions to twenty-two classes (tonics, emetics, purgatives, etc.) on the basis of their actions. This classification is convenient in clinical work and is easy to remember. Classifications based on actions are useful in practice because treatment is decided by differentiation of symptom-complexes.

COMMONLY USED PRESCRIPTIONS

The rest of this chapter presents the prescriptions that are most in use in traditional Chinese medicine. Sixteen categories, based on the prescriptions' actions, are included; for each, the most common prescriptions are provided. In general, the first ingredient listed for each prescription is the principal, and the auxiliary follows.

Diaphoretic Prescriptions

PRESCRIPTIONS FOR DISPELLING PATHOGENIC FACTORS FROM THE EXTERIOR OF THE BODY

These prescriptions contain ingredients that are warm in nature and are used to induce perspiration and dispel pathogenic wind and cold.

Prescription	Composition	Amount (grams)	Action(s)	Indication(s)	Remarks
Decoction of Ephedra	Herba Ephedrae Ramulus Cinnamomi Semen Armeniacae Amarum Radix Glycyrrhizae Praeparata	9 6 9 3	Expelling pathogenic cold through sweating; relieving asthma by ventilating a disturbed lung	Symptom-complexes showing attack of the external part of the body by pathogenic wind and cold (common cold, influenza, bronchitis, asthmatic bronchitis)	After taking the decoction, keep warm to induce sweating
Decoction of Ramulus Cinnamomi	Ramulus Cinnamomi Radis Paeoniae Radix Glycyrrhizae Praeparata Rhizoma Zingiberis recens (ginger rhizoma) Fructus Ziziphi Jujubae (Chinese date)	9 9 6 9 4 dates	Dispelling pathogenic factors from the superficial part of the body; harmonizing the nutrient (*ying*) and defensive (*wei*) systems	Exterior symptom-complexes with lowered superficial resistance due to exogenous wind and cold (marked by fever, headache, aversion to wind, profuse perspiration); disharmony of the nutrient and defensive systems	After taking the decoction, consume a little hot rice porridge or hot water and keep warm to induce a little sweating

Prescription	Composition	Amount (grams)	Action(s)	Indication(s)	Remarks
Antiphlogistic Powder of Schizonepeta and Ledebouriella	Herba Schizonepetae	9	Promoting diaphoresis to expel pathogenic factors from the superficial part of the body, dispelling pathogenic wind and dampness	Exterior symptom-complexes in which the external part of the body is attacked by pathogenic wind, cold, and dampness (upper respiratory tract infection, acute tonsillitis, dysentery, incipient boils or ulcers, eczema with cold symptom-complex on the exterior of the body	Administered as a decoction
	Radix Ledebouriellae (ledebouriella root)	6			
	Rhizoma seu Radix Notopterygii (notopterygium root or rhizome)	9			
	Radix Angelicae Pubescentis (angelica root)	6			
	Radix Bupleuri	6			
	Radix Peucedani (root of purple-flowered peucedanum)	6			
	Fructus Aurantii (fruit of citron)	6			
	Poria (tuckahoe)	9			
	Rhizoma Ligustici Chuanxiong (chuanxiong rhizome)	6			
	Radix Glycyrrhizae Praeparate	6			
Decoction of Nine Herbs Including Notopterygium	Rhizoma seu Radix Notopterygii	6	Expelling pathogenic dampness through perspiration; clearing away pathogenic heat	Exterior symptom-complexes in which the external part of the body is attacked by pathogenic dampness; influenza;	
	Radix Ledebourielae	6			
	Rhizoma Atracty-	6			

Prescription	Ingredients	Amount	Actions	Indications	Remarks
	Iodis (Chinese atractylodes rhizome)		from the interior of the body	rheumatic arthritis due to pathogenic wind, cold, and dampness, with accumulation of pathogenic heat in the interior of the body	
	Herba Asari (wildginger)	2			
	Rhizoma Ligustici Chuanxiong	3			
	Radix Angelicae Dahuricae (dahurian angelica root)	3			
	Radix Rehmanniae	3			
	Radix Scutellariae	3			
	Radix Glycyrrhizae	1			
Pulvis Elsholtzia	*Herba Elsholtziae seu Orthodon*	480	Dispelling pathogenic cold from the superficial part of the body; removing pathogenic dampness and regulating the function of the stomach and spleen	Affection by pathogenic cold in the exterior of the body and invasion of the interior by pathogenic dampness in summer; common cold; gastroenteritis; dysentery in summer or autumn	3 grams of powder per dose
	Semen Dolichoris Album (bean of white hyacinth dolichos)	240			
	Cortex Magnoliae Officinalis	240			
Minor Blue Dragon Decoction	*Herba Ephedrae*	9	Dispelling pathogenic cold from the superficial part of the body; removing retained fluid by warming the lung	Affection by pathogenic wind-cold on the exterior of the body and retention of water; chronic tracheitis or bronchitis; bronchial asthma; senile emphysema	Prescription may be modified to treat acute bronchitis
	Radix Paeoniae	9			
	Herba Asari	9			
	Rhizoma Zingiberis	9			
	Radix Glycyrrhizae	9			
	Ramulus Cinnamomi	9			
	Fructus Schisandrae (fruit of Chinese magnolia vine)	9			
	Rhizoma Pinelliae (pinella tuber)	9			

DIAPHORETIC PRESCRIPTIONS COMPOSED OF MEDICINAL INGREDIENTS PUNGENT IN FLAVOR AND WARM IN NATURE

These prescriptions are effective for symptom-complexes in which the external part of the body is attacked by pathogenic wind and heat.

Prescription	Composition	Amount (grams)	Action(s)	Indication(s)	Remarks
Decoction of Mori and Chrysanthemi	*Folium Mori* (white mulberry leaf)	8	Dispelling pathogenic wind and heat; ventilating a disturbed lung to stop coughing	Exterior symptom-complexes in which the external part of body is attacked by pathogenic wind, marked by coughing, feverishness, and slight thirst (influenza, acute bronchitis, acute tonsillitis, epidemic conjunctivitis caused by pathogenic wind and heat)	Taken cold
	Flos Chrysanthmii (chrysanthemum)	6			
	Semen Armeniacae Amarum	6			
	Fructus Forsythiae	6			
	Herba Menthae (peppermint herb)	3			
	Radix Platycodi (root of balloon flower)	6			
	Radix Glycyrrhizae	3			
	Rhizoma Phragmitis (common reed rhizome)	6			
Powder of Lonicera and Forsythia	*Fructus Forsythiae*	30	Dispelling pathogenic wind and heat; eliminating toxic heat	Incipient acute febrile disease (measles, influenza, acute tonsillitis, encephalitis B,	
	Flos Lonicerae	30			
	Radix Platycodi	18			

Prescription	Components		Action	Indication
	Herba Menthae	18		mumps; incipient suppurative infection on the body surface with heat symptom-complex on the exterior of the body
	Herba Lophatheri (henon bamboo leaf)	12		
	Radix Glycyrrhizae	15		
	Spica Schizonepetae (spike of schizonepeta)	12		
	Semen Sojae Praeparatum	15		
	Fructus Arctii	18		
Decoction of Ephedra, Armeniacae, Gypsum, and Glycyrrhizae	*Herba Ephedra*	6	Clearing away pathogenic heat from the lung to relieve asthma	Exogenous affection by pathogenic wind, with accumulation of pathogenic heat in the lung (marked by fever, thirst; sweat may be present or absent; asthmatic cough); acute bronchitis; pneumonia
	Semen Armeniacae Amarum	9		
	Gypsum Fibrosum (plaster)	24		
	Radix Glycyrrhizae	6		
Decoction of Cimicifuga and Puerariae	*Radix Puerariae* (root of kudzu-vine)	9	Dispelling pathogenic factors from the muscles; promoting exanthesis in measles	Failure of exanthesis in measles; acute febrile disease
	Rhizoma Cimicifugae (skunk bugbane rhizome)	3		
	Radix Paeoniae	4		
	Radix Glycyrrhizae Praeparata	3		
Renewed Decoction of Elsholtzia	*Herba Elsholtziae seu Orthodon*	9	Dispelling summer heat from the superficial part of the body; clearing away pathogenic heat	Affection by summer-heat associated with pathogenic dampness
	Flos Lonicerae	9		
	Fructus Forsythiae	9		
	Flos Dolichoris (flower of hyacinth dolichos)	6		

PRESCRIPTIONS FOR STRENGTHENING BODY RESISTANCE AND DISPELLING PATHOGENIC FACTORS FROM THE EXTERIOR OF THE BODY

These prescriptions, which contain ingredients pungent in flavor and warm in property, are used for exogenous affection by pathogenic cold and wind in cases with debility.

Prescription	Composition	Amount (grams)	Action(s)	Indication(s)	Remarks
Pulvis Ginseng for Relieving Inflammation	Radix Bupleuri	30	Reinforcing vital energy while expelling pathogenic factors from the body surface; dispelling pathogenic wind and dampness	Exogenous affection by pathogenic wind and cold, with lowered body resistance; incipient suppurative infection on the body surface; dysentery with exogenous affection	Amounts of ingredients decreased while fresh ginger and peppermint are added
	Radix Peucedani	30			
	Rhizoma Ligustici Chuanxiong	30			
	Fructus Aurantii	30			
	Rhizoma sue Radix Notopterygii	30			
	Radix Angelicae Pubescentis	30			
	Poria	30			
	Radix Platycodi	30			
	Radix Ginseng	30			
	Radix Glycyrrhizae	15			
Decoction of Ginseng and Perillae	Radix Ginseng	30	Invigorating vital energy while expelling pathogenic factors from the body surface; regulating the flow of vital energy and resolving phlegm	Exogenous affection by pathogenic wind and cold, with retention of phlegm and dampness, in weak patients	Amounts of ingredients adjusted according to patient's condition
	Folium Perrilae (leaf of purple perilla)	30			
	Radix Puerariae	30			
	Radix Peucedani	30			
	Fructus Aurantii	30			
	Radix Platycodi	30			

	Pericarpium Citri Reticulatae	30	
	Rhizoma Pinelliae Praeparata	30	
	Poria	30	
	Radix Glycyrrhizae	15	
	Radix Aucklandiae (costus root)	30	
	Rhizoma Zingiberis Recens	30	
	Fructus Ziziphi Jujubae	30	
Decoction of Polygonatum Odoratum with Modifications	Rhizoma Polygonali Odorati Recens	9	Replenishing vital essence and expelling pathogenic factors from the body surface	Affection by exogenous pathogenic wind and heat in patients with deficiency of vital essence
	Caulis Allii Fistulosi (green onion stalk)	3 inches	
	Radix Platycodi	5	
	Radix Cynanchi Atrati (swallow wort root)	3	
	Semen Sojae Praeparatum	12	
	Herba Menthae	5	
	Radix Glycyrrhizae	2	
	Fructus Ziziphi Jujubae	2 dates	

Purgative Prescriptions

COLD PURGATIVE PRESCRIPTIONS

These prescriptions contain cool-natured purgatives and medicinal ingredients that promote the normal flow of vital energy. They usually are used in treating accumulations of endogenous pathogenic heat.

Prescription	Composition	Amount (grams)	Action(s)	Indication(s)	Remarks
Drastic Purgative Decoction	*Radix et Rhizoma Rhei*	12	Purging accumulated pathogenic heat from the exterior of the body	Excessive internal pathogenic heat in the intestines, marked by constipation or loose stools; coma, convulsions, or mania due to excessive internal heat; acute intestinal obstruction without complications; adhesive intestinal obstruction or intestinal obstruction due to ascariasis; acute cholecystitis; acute appendicitis	The *Natrii Sulfas* is added after the decoction is nearly done and the dregs are removed
	Cortex Magnoliae Officinalis	15			
	Fructus Aurantii Immaturus	15			
	Natrii Sulfas (mirabilite)	9			
Decoction of Rhei and Cortex Moutan	*Radix et Rhizoma Rhei*	18	Purging internal pathogenic heat and removing blood stasis, lumps, or swellings	Incipient intestinal abscess, pain and tenderness in the right lower abdomen; acute appendicitis; inflammation of the uterine appendages; pelvic inflammation due to internal excess heat; cholelithiasis	
	Cortex Montan Radicis (root-bark of peony)	9			
	Semen Persicae (peach kernel)	12			

Prescription	Composition	Amount (grams)	Action(s)	Indication(s)	Remarks
	Semen Benincasae (Chinese waxgourd seed)	30			
	Natrii Sulfas	9			
Biliary Lithagogue	*Herba Lysimachiae* (loosestrife whole plant)	30	Expelling calculi from the bile duct; clearing away internal pathogenic heat and dampness	Cholelithiasis	
	Herba Artemisiae Scopariae	12			
	Radix Curcumae	9			
	Fructus Aurantii	9			
	Radix Aucklandiae	9			
	Radix et Rhizoma Rhei	9			

WARM PURGATIVE PRESCRIPTIONS

These prescriptions contain purgatives together with herbs warm in nature. They are used to remove accumulated pathogenic cold in the internal organs.

Prescription	Composition	Amount (grams)	Action(s)	Indication(s)	Remarks
Decoction of Rhei and Aconiti	*Radix et Rhizoma Rhei*	9	Warming the interior of the body and dispelling cold; promoting defecation and alleviating pain	Accumulated pathogenic cold	
	Radix Aconiti Praeparata (monkshood root)	12			
	Herba Asari	6			

Prescription	Composition	Amount (grams)	Action(s)	Indication(s)	Remarks
Pills of Tree Herbs for Emergency	Radix et Rhizoma Rhei Rhizoma Zingiberis Semen Crotonis (croton fruit)	30 30 30	Purging accumulated pathogenic cold	Accumulation of cold, marked by abrupt pain and distension in the stomach and abdomen, trismus, and syncope; food poisoning; acute uncomplicated intestinal obstruction due to accumulation of cold	The pills are ground into fine powder and taken (0.3–1.5 grams per dose) with rice soup or warm boiled water

MILD PURGATIVE PRESCRIPTIONS

These prescriptions contain moistening medicinal ingredients and purgatives. They are used to relieve constipation due to debility and due to insufficiency of body fluid.

Prescription	Composition	Amount (grams)	Action(s)	Indication(s)	Remarks
Semen Cannabis Bolus	Semen Cannabis (cannabis seed) Radix Paeoniae Fructus Aurantii Immaturus Radix et Rhizoma Rhei	50 200 250 500	Moistening the intestines and promoting defecation	Constipation and frequent urination due to pathogenic dry-heat in the intestines and stomach; senile constipation due to intestinal dryness; chronic constipation	Boluses, prepared by grinding the ingredients into a powder and mixing with honey, given

	Ingredient	Amount	Action	Indication	Notes
	Cortex Magnoliae Officinalis	250			once or twice daily; 9 grams per dose; for decoction, amounts of ingredients are reduced, but the proportions are kept the same
	Semen Armeniacae Amarum	250			
Decoction for Constipation Due to Hypofunction of the kidney	Radix Angelicae Sinensis	9–5	Serving as mild laxative	Constipation due to hypofunction of the kidney	
	Radix Achyranthis Bidentalae (ackyranthes root)	6			
	Herba Cistanchis (cistanche)	6–9			
	Rhizoma Alsmatis (oriental water plantain tuber)	4			
	Rhizoma Cimicijugae	15–3			
	Fructus Aurantii	3			

WATER-ELIMINATING PRESCRIPTIONS

These prescriptions are used to remove water or fluid retained in the chest or abdomen; they are also effective for edema. They are used with care because they are toxic.

Prescription	Composition	Amount (grams)	Action(s)	Indication(s)	Remarks
Decoction of Ten Jujubes	*Flos Genkwa* (flower of lilac daphne) *Radix Euphorbiae Kansi* (euphorbia gansui root) *Radix Euphorbiae Pekinensis*	In equal proportions	Eliminating retained water and fluid	Exudative pleurisy; edema; hydrothorax; ascites or generalized edema due to cirrhosis or chronic nephritis	1.5–3 grams mixed in with ten jujube decoction and taken before breakfast
Ship and Cart Pills	*Semen Pharbitidis* (morning glory seed)	120	Promoting the normal flow of vital energy to eliminate retained water	Edema and abdominal distension; ascites due to cirrhosis	Prepared with rice paste; 3–6 grams taken before breakfast
	Radix Euphorbiae Kansui (coated with wheat paste and baked before use)	30			
	Flos Genkwa	30			
	Radix Euphorbiae Pekinensis	30			
	Radix et Rhizoma Rhei	60			
	Pericarpium Citri Reticulatae Viride (dried green orange peel)	15			
	Pericarpium Citri Reticulatae (dried old orange peel)	15			
	Radix Auklandiae	15			
	Semen Arecae (betel nut)	15			
	Calomelas (calomel)	3			

PURGATIVE AND TONIC PRESCRIPTIONS

Prescription	Composition	Amount (grams)	Action(s)	Indication(s)	Remarks
Yellow Dragon Decoction	Radix et Rhizoma Rhei	9	Reinforcing the body resistance and purging	Deficiency of vital energy and blood; constipation or loose stools due to excessive pathogenic heat in the interior of the body	Decocted together with the following herbs: *Radix Platycodi* 3 g, *Rhizoma Zingiberis Recens* 9 g, *Fructus Ziziphi Jujubae* 2 pcs
	Natrii Sulfas	12			
	Fructus Aurantii Immaturus	6			
	Cortex Magnoliae Officinalis	3			
	Radix Glycyrrhizae	3			
	Radix Angelicae Sinensis (Chinese angelica root)	9			
	Radix Ginseng	6			
Purgative Decoction for Enriching the Body Fluid	Radix Scrophulariae	30	Replenishing vital essence to promote secretion of fluid; eliminating internal heat to relieve constipation	Impairment of vital essence due to accumulated heat in the stomach and intestines, marked by lowered body resistance, constipation, dry stools, persistent hemorrhoids	The decoction is divided into three portions and taken three times per day
	Radix Ophiopogonis (tuber of dwarf lilyturf)	24			
	Radix Rehmannia	24			
	Radix et Rhizoma Rhei	9			
	Natrii Sulfas	4.5			
Spleen Warming Decoction	Radix et Rhizoma Rhei	9	Warming the spleen and invigorating its function; eliminating accumulated pathogenic cold through purgation	Constipation due to excessive internal cold; dysentery with abdominal pain and cold extremities	
	Radix Ginseng	6			
	Radix Glycyrrhizae	3			
	Rhizoma Zingiberis	6			
	Radix Aconiti Praeparata	9			

Regulating (Mediation) Prescriptions

PRESCRIPTIONS FOR REGULATING THE SHAOYANG CHANNEL

These prescriptions combat pathogenic factors lingering in the Shaoyang Channel or the Gallbladder Channel, common manifestations of which include bitter taste in the mouth, dizziness, alternate spells of chills and fever, fullness in the chest and costal region, restlessness, nausea, anorexia, and taut pulse.

Prescription	Composition	Amount (grams)	Action(s)	Indication(s)	Remarks
Minor Decoction of Bupleurum	Radix Bupleuri	12	Regulating the function of the Gallbladder Channel	Disease located in the Gallbladder Channel; in women febrile disease manifested by invasion of the uterus by pathogenic heat; malaria; jaundice associated with disorders in the Gallbladder Channel	
	Radix Scutellaria	9			
	Radix Ginseng	9			
	Radix Glycyrrhizae	6			
	Rhizoma Zingeberis Recens	9			
	Rhizoma Pinelliae Praeparata	9			
	Fructus Ziziphi Jujubae	4 pcs			
Major Decoction of Bupleurum	Radix Bupleuri	9	Regulating the function of the Gallbladder Channel; eliminating accumulated pathogenic heat by purgation	Diseases located in the Gallbladder and Stomach Channels (uncomplicated acute pancreatitis; acute cholecystitis or cholelithiasis)	
	Radix Scutellariae	9			
	Radix Paeoniae	9			
	Rhizoma Pinelliae Praeparath	9			
	Fructus Aurantic Immaturus	9			
	Rhizoma Zingiberis Recens	12			

	Radix et Rhizoma Rhei	6
	Fructus Ziziphi Jujubae	4 pcs
Decoction of Chinghao and Scutellariae for Gallbladder Clearing	*Herba Artemisiae Chinghao* (sweet wormwood)	4.5–6
	Caulis Bambusae in Taenis (bamboo shavings)	9
	Rhizoma Pinelliae Praeparata	4.5
	Poria Rubra	9
	Radix Scutellariae	4.5–9
	Fructus Aurantii	4.5
	Paracarpium-Citri Reticulatae	4.5
	Jade Powder (Talcum, *Radix Glycyrrhizae*, and *Indigo Naturalis* in 6:1:0.5 portions, wrapped in gauze packet)	9

Actions: Clearing away pathogenic damp-heat from the gallbladder; regulating the function of the stomach and resolving phlegm

Indications: Pathogenic damp-heat in the Gallbladder Channel (acute cholecystitis, acute gastritis, chronic pancreatitis)

LIVER-SPLEEN REGULATING PRESCRIPTIONS

These prescriptions regulate the function of the spleen and stomach. They are used to restore the function of the spleen and stomach when these organs are troubled by stagnancy of vital energy of the liver.

Prescription	Composition	Amount (grams)	Action(s)	Indication(s)	Remarks
Powder for Cold Limbs	*Radix Bupleuri* *Radix Paeoniae* *Fructus Aurantii Immutrus* *Radix Glycyrrhizae Praeparata*	in equal portions	Dispersing accumulated pathogenic heat to regulate the flow of vital energy of the liver and the spleen	Collapse due to pathogenic heat, marked by cold limbs, pain in the stomach and abdomen, diarrhea, or tenesmus	Amount of ingredients decided by doctor
Ease Powder	*Radix Angelicae sinensis* *Poria* *Rhizoma Atractylodis Macrocephalae* *Radix Bupleuri* *Radix Glycyrrhizae Praeparata*	30 30 30 30 15	Resolving stagnancy of liver *qi*; invigorating spleen function and nourishing the blood	Functional disorders of the spleen and stomach caused by stagnancy of vital energy of the liver and deficiency of blood; chronic hepatitis	6–9 g of powder administered per dose with decoction of a small amount of *Rhizoma Zingeberis Recens* and *Herba Menthae*; for decoction form, amounts of ingredients reduced but proportions kept the same
Pulvis Atractylodes and Paeoniae	*Rhizoma Atractylodis Macrocephalae Praeparata* *Rhizoma Paeoniae Alba Praeparata* *Pericarpium Citri Reticulatae* *Radix Ledebouriellae*	90 60 45 60	Promoting the normal flow of vital energy of the liver and restoring the function of the spleen	Stagnancy of vital energy of the liver and hypofunction of the spleen (marked by abdominal pain accompanied by borborygmus or by diarrhea)	6–9 g of powder per dose; for decoction form, amounts of ingredient reduced but proportions kept the same

GASTROINTESTINAL REGULATION PRESCRIPTIONS

These prescriptions contain ingredients cold or hot in nature and pungent or bitter in flavor.

Prescription	Composition	Amount (grams)	Action(s)	Indication(s)	Remarks
Decoction of Pinelliae for Dispelling Pathogenic Heat from the Heart	*Rhizoma Pinelliae Praeparata*	12	Regulating the vital function of the stomach and relieving nausea and vomiting	Functional disorders of the stomach, marked by fullness in the stomach, nausea, vomiting, borborygmus, and diarrhea; acute gastritis	
	Radix Scutellariae	9			
	Radix Zingiberis	9			
	Radix Ginseng	9			
	Radix Glycyrrhizae	6			
	Rhizoma Coptidis	3			
	Fructus Ziziphi Jujubae	3 dates			

Febrifugal Prescriptions

PRESCRIPTIONS FOR ELIMINATING INTERNAL HEAT FROM THE VITAL ENERGY SYSTEM

Prescription	Composition	Amount (grams)	Action(s)	Indication(s)	Remarks
White Tiger Decoction	Gypsum Fibrosum	30	Clearing internal pathogenic heat and promoting fluid generation	Intense heat in the Stomach Channel; heatstroke; encephalitis B or epidemic meningitis due to intense heat in the vital energy system	
	Rhizoma Anemarrhenae	9			
	Radix Glycyrrhizae	3			
	Semen Oryzae Nonglutinosae (nonglutinous rice)	9			
Decoction of Lophatheri and Gypsum	Herba Lophatheri	9	Clearing internal pathogenic heat and promoting fluid generation; reinforcing vital energy and regulating the function of the stomach	Impairment of vital energy and vital essence as a result of pathogenic heat remaining in the body after recovery from a febrile disease; illness caused by summer heat resulting in impairment of vital energy and fluid	
	Gypsum Fibrosum	30			
	Rhizoma Pinelliae praeparata	9			
	Radix Ophiopogonis	18			
	Radix Ginseng	5			
	Radix Glycyrrhizae praeparata	3			
	Semen Oryzae Nonglutinosae	8			

PRESCRIPTIONS FOR ELIMINATING PATHOLOGICAL HEAT FROM THE NUTRIENT AND BLOOD SYSTEMS

Prescription	Composition	Amount (grams)	Action(s)	Indication(s)	Remarks
Nutrient System Clearing Decoction	Cornu Rhinoceri Radix Rehmannia Radix Scrophulariae Herba Lophatheri Budded Radix Ophiopogonis Radix Salvia Miltiorrhizae Rhizoma Coptidis Flos Lonicerae Fructus Forsythiae	2 15 9 3 9 6 5 9 6	Eliminating toxic heat from the nutrient system and replenishing vital essence	Invasion of the nutrient system by pathogenic heat (marked by feverishness that is worse at night, occasional delirium, insomnia with restlessness, indistinct maculopapular rash); encephalitis B, epidemic meningitis, or septicemia due to intense heat in the nutrient system	
Decoction of Rhinoceros Cornu and Rehmannia	Pulvis Cornu Rhinoceri Radix Rehmannia Cortex Moutan Radicis	1.5–3 12 9	Eliminating toxic heat from the blood system	Epistaxis, hematemesis, hematuria, and hematochezia due to intense heat in the blood system; acute leukocythemia; acute hepatodystrophy; hepatic coma; uremia; septicemia; boils or carbuncles	Administered with Pulvis Cornu Rhinoceri

TOXIC HEAT ELIMINATION PRESCRIPTIONS

These prescriptions are used in treating epidemic infectious diseases, toxic heat, pyogenic infections, and ulcers due to intense heat.

Prescription	Composition	Amount (grams)	Action(s)	Indication(s)	Remarks
Detoxicant Decoction of Coptidis	Rhizoma Coptidis Radix Scutellariae Cortex Phellodendri Fructus Gardeniae	9 6 6 9	Eliminating toxins by purgation of pathogenic heat	Exuberant heat in the triple-burner; carbuncles or boils	
Detoxicant Decoction for Universal Relief	Radix Scutellariae Rhizoma Coptidis Perecarpium Criti Reticulatae Radix Clycyrrhizae Radix Bupleuri Radix Scrophulariae Radix Platycodi Fructus Forsythiae Radix Isatidis Lasiosphaera seu Calvatia Fructus Arctii Herba Menthae Bombyx Batryticatus (batryticated silkworm) Rhizoma Cimicifugae	15 15 6 6 6 6 6 3 3 3 3 3 2 2	Clearing heat toxins and eliminating pathogenic wind	Erysipelas on the face; carbuncles and boils on the head; mumps; acute tonsillitis; lymphadenitis accompanied by disturbance in the circulation of lymph	
Magic Decoction for Rescuing Life	Radix Angelicae dahuricae Bulbus Fritillariae Thunbergii Radix Ledebouriellae Radix Paeonia Rubra (red peony)	3 3 3 3	Clearing heat toxins, dispelling pus of ulcers, and reducing swellings; activating blood circulation to eliminate pain	Incipient suppurative infection on the body surface, marked by red swelling, throbbing pain, mild fever, and aversion to cold; pustules; furuncles; cellulitis; mastitis; suppurative tonsillitis	Decocted with water, or with a mixture of half water and half wine

Prescription	Ingredients		Action	Indications	Administration
	End of Radix Angelicae Sinensis	3			Decoction mixed with 1–2 spoonfuls of wine; taken with herb dregs
	Radix Glycyrrhizae	3			
	Spine Gleditsiae (honeylocust thorn)	3			
	Squama Manitis (pangolin scale)	3			
	Radix Trichosanthis	3			
	Resina Olibani (olibanum)	3			
	Resina Myrrhae (myrrh)	3			
	Flos Lonicerae	9			
	Perecarpium Criti Reticulatae	9			
Decoction of Five Detoxicants	Flos Lonicerae	15	Clearing heat toxins	Acute surgical (noninternal) infections, such as acute mastitis, cellulitis, and suppurative inflammation of the fingers	
	Flos Chrysanthemi Indici (mother chrysanthemus)	15			
	Herba Taraxaci	15			
	Herba Violae	15			
	Radix Semiaquilegiae (semiaquilegia root)	6			
Decoction of Four Miraculous Herbs for Relief of Disorders	Flos Lonicerae	30	Clearing heat toxins, invigorating blood circulation, and alleviating pain	Gangrene due to heat toxins (e.g., thromboangiitis obliterans)	
	Radix Scrophulariae	30			
	Radix Angelicae Sinensis	15			
	Radix Glycyrrhizae	10			

Prescription	Composition	Amount (grams)	Action(s)	Indication(s)	Remarks
Pills of Rhinoceros Gallstone	Calculus Bovis (Rhinoceri) Morschus (musk) Resina Olibani Resina Myrrhae Glutinous Millei (cooked miller)	1 5 15 15 15	Clearing heat toxins; dispelling masses; invigorating blood circulation to eliminate blood stasis	Breast cancer; tubercular cervical lymphadenitis; wandering abscesses (e.g., in lymphadenitis, cystic mastoplasia, multiple abscesses, medullitis)	3 g three times per day

INTERNAL HEAT ELIMINATION PRESCRIPTIONS

These prescriptions are used to remove exuberant pathogenic heat from specific internal organs.

Prescription	Composition	Amount (grams)	Action(s)	Indication(s)	Remarks
Powder for Dispelling Heat from the Heart Channel	Radix Rehmannia End of Radix Glycyrrhizae Caulis Akebiae (fiveleaf akebia) Herba Lophatheri	9 9 9 6	Clearing pathogenic heat from the heart and increasing urine flow	Exuberant pathogenic heat in the Heart Channel, marked by a hot sensation in the chest, ulcers in the mouth and/or on the tongue, and burning pain on urination (e.g., acute urinary tract infection)	
Decoction of Gentianae to Purge the Liver	Radix Gentianae Radix Bupleuri Rhizoma Alismatis Semen Plantaginis	6 6 12 9	Removing excessive pathogenic heat and damp-heat from the liver and gallbladder	Flaring up of liver fire; damp-heat of the Liver Channel (e.g., acute conjunctivitis or otitis media, furuncular swell-	

Prescription	Ingredients	Dose	Action	Indications
	Caulis Akebiae	9		ing of the vestibule of the nose or furuncular otitis, hypertension, acute icteric hepatitis, acute cholecystitis, herpes zoster, acute pyelonephritis, cystitis, acute pelvic inflammation, prostatitis)
	Radix Rehmannia	9		
	End of Radix-Angelicae Sinensis	3		
	Fructus Gardeniae	9		
	Radix Scutellariae	9		
	Radix Glycyrrhizae	6		
Powder for Clearing Away Stomach Heat	Radix Angelicae Sinensis	6	Clearing pathogenic heat from the stomach and blood	Accumulation of pathogenic heat in the stomach and flaring up of collected fire, marked by swelling, pain, and bleeding of the gingiva or by swelling and pain of the lips, tongue, and cheeks
	Rhizoma Coptidis	5		
	Radix Rehmannia	12		
	Cortex Moutan Radicis	6		
	Rhizoma Cimicifugae (skunk bugbane)	6		
Jade Goddess Decoction	Gypsum Fibrosum	15–30	Clearing pathogenic heat from the stomach and replenishing vital essence	Impairment of fluids and deficiency of vital essence that are caused by pathogenic heat in the stomach (e.g., stomatitis or glossitis marked by ulcers in the mouth or on the tongue)
	Radix Rehmannia Praeparata	9–30		
	Radix Ophiopogonis	6		
	Rhizoma Anemarrhenae (rhizome of wind-weed)	4.5		
	Radix Achyranthis Bidentatae (achyranthes root)	4.5		

Prescription	Composition	Amount (grams)	Action(s)	Indication(s)	Remarks
Decoction of Caulis Phragmitis	*Caulis Phragmitis* (reed rhizome) *Semen Coicis* (Job's tears seed) *Semen Benincasea* (Chinese wax gourd seed) *Semen Persicae*	30 30 24 9	Eliminating heat and resolving phlegm; removing stasis and draining pus	Lung abscess marked by expectoration of foul-smelling purulent yellow and bloody sputum and by chest pain; bronchitis; lobar pneumonia; pertussis; cough due to pathogenic heat in the lung	
Decoction of Pulsatilla	*Radix Pulsatillae* *Cortex Phellodendri* *Rhizoma Coptidis* *Cortex Fraxini*	15 12 6 12	Eliminating pathogenic heat toxins from the intestines and cooling the blood to relieve dysentery	Dysentery (either acute bacterial or amebic)	

SUMMER-HEAT ELIMINATION PRESCRIPTIONS

These prescriptions are used in treating excessive thirst, sweating, fatigue, and weak pulse due to summer heat. Because summer-heat with dampness often injures vital energy, they also eliminate dampness and invigorate vital energy.

Prescription	Composition	Amount (grams)	Action(s)	Indication(s)	Remarks
Six to One Powder	*Talcum* *Radix Glycyrrhizae*	180 30	Clearing summer heat and eliminating pathogenic dampness	Exogenous affection by summer heat and pathogenic dampness (marked by fever,	9 g powder per dose; for decoction form,

			amounts of ingredients reduced but proportions kept the same
		thirst, difficulty in urination, vomiting, diarrhea, brown urine discharged with difficulty and pain, urinary system stones)	
Decoction for Eliminating Summer Heat and Invigorating Vital Energy	*Radix Ginseng Americana* (root of American ginseng) — 5 *Herba Dendrobii* — 15 *Radix Ophiopogonis* — 9 *Rhizoma Coptidis* — 3 *Herba Lophatheri* — 6 *Petiolus Nelumbinis* (lotus petiole) — 15 *Rhizoma Anemarrhenae* — 6 *Radix Glycyrrhizae* — 3 *Nonglutinous rice* — 15 *Exocarpium Citrulli* (water melon peel) — 30	Clearing summer heat and invigorating vital energy; replenishing vital essence to generate fluids	Exogenous affection by summer heat, resulting in impairment of both vital energy and vital essence

PRESCRIPTIONS FOR CLEARING AWAY FEVER DUE TO DEFICIENCY OF VITAL ENERGY

These prescriptions contain febrifuges and herbs replenishing vital essence. They are used in treating growth of internal heat caused by deficiency of vital energy due to consumption of fluid.

Prescription	Composition	Amount (grams)	Action(s)	Indication(s)	Remarks
Decoction of Chinghao et Carapax Trionycis	Herba Artemisiae Qinghao	6	Replenishing vital essence and clearing pathogenic heat	Advanced infectious febrile diseases in which vital essence has been impaired (manifested by undulating low fever or by fever at night and subsidence of fever in the morning); pyelonephritis; tuberculosis of the kidney with persistent low fever and heat sensation in the palms and soles	
	Carapax Trionycis (turtle shell)	15			
	Fine Radix Rehmannia	12			
	Rhizoma Anemarrhenae	6			
	Cortex Moutan Radicis	9			
Powder for Removing Heat from the Bones	Herba Artemisiae Qinghao	3	Clearing pathogenic heat due to deficiency of vital energy to relieve hectic fever and night sweats	Consumptive disease marked by hectic fever and night sweats or by persistent low fever	
	Radix Stellariae (starwort root)	5			
	Rhizoma Picrorrhizae	3			
	Radix Gentianae Macrophyllae (root of largeleaf gentian)	3			
	Carapax Trionycis	3			
	Radix Glycyrrhizae	2			
	Cortex Lycii Radicis (root-bark of Chinese wolfberry)	3			

Warming Prescriptions

These prescriptions consist chiefly of ingredients warm or hot in nature and pungent in flavor. They are used to warm the interior and expel cold or to restore vital function from collapse. In using these prescriptions, it is important to differentiate true cold from pseudo-cold. In collapse that is due to excessive pathogenic heat but in which pseudo-cold symptoms are present, these prescriptions are strictly prohibited.

STOMACH-WARMING PRESCRIPTIONS

Prescription	Composition	Amount (grams)	Action(s)	Indication(s)	Remarks
Bolus to Regulate the Functioning of the Spleen and Stomach	*Radix Ginseng* *Rhizoma Zingiberis* *Rhizoma Atractylodis Macrocephalae*	90 90 90	Warming the spleen and stomach and dispelling cold from them; invigorating the vital function of the spleen and stomach	Retention of cold due to hypofunction of the spleen and stomach; hemorrhage due to lowered vital function; chronic infantile convulsions; acute or chronic gastroenteritis; gastroduodenal ulcer; gastrectasis; gastroptosis	9–12 g of pills per dose; for decoction form, amounts of ingredients reduced but proportions kept the same
Decoction of Evodiae	*Fructus Evodiae* (evodia fruit) *Radix Ginseng* *Rhizoma Zingiberis Recens* *Fructus Ziziphi Jujubae*	9 9 18 4 dates	Warming the liver and stomach; bringing down the upward adverse flow of vital energy to stop vomiting	Vomiting due to pathogenic cold in the stomach; vomiting due to stomach dysfunction caused by cold in the liver; vomiting and diarrhea due to affection of the spleen by pathogenic cold in the kidney	

Prescription	Composition	Amount (grams)	Action(s)	Indication(s)	Remarks
Minor Decoction for Functional Restoration of the Spleen and Stomach	Ramulus Cinnamomi Radix Glycyrrhizae Praeparata Fructus Ziziphi Jujubae Radix Paeoniae Rhizoma Zingiberis Recens malt extract	6 3 4 pcs 12 9 18	Warming and reinforcing the stomach and spleen, relieving abdominal pain	Abdominal pain due to deficiency of vital energy and accumulation of cold; palpitation and restlessness due to general debility; fever due to deficiency of vital function caused by consumption	
Magnolia Decoction to Warm the Spleen and Stomach	Cortex Magnoliae Officinalis Praeparata Pericarpium Citri Reticulatae Radix Glycyrrhizae Semen Alpiniae Katsumadai (katsumadai seed) Poria Radix Aucklandiae Rhizoma Zingiberis	30 30 15 15 15 15 2	Warming the stomach and spleen to regulate their function; eliminating dampness and relieving fullness sensation	Pathogenic cold and dampness in the stomach and spleen; abdominal and gastric distension; gastric and abdominal pain caused by exogenous pathogenic cold; chronic enteritis; morbid leukorrhea	

PRESCRIPTIONS FOR WARMING THE CHANNELS AND DISPELLING COLD

Prescription	Composition	Amount (grams)	Action(s)	Indication(s)	Remarks
Angelica Decoction for Treating Cold Limbs	*Radix Angelicae sinensis*	9	Warming the channels and dispelling pathogenic cold from them; nourishing blood and promoting blood circulation	Cold limbs with severe pain due to blood deficiency and affection by cold; thromboangiitis obliterans	
	Ramulus Cinnamomi	9			
	Radix Paeoniae	9			
	Herba Asari	6			
	Radix Glycyrrhizae Praeparata	6			
	Caulis Akebiae	6			
	Fructus Ziziphi Jujubae	5 pcs			
Vital Function Regulation Decoction	*Radix Rehmanniae Praeparata*	30	Activating vital function and tonifying the blood; dispelling pathogenic cold and removing stagnancy	Suppurative infection due to cold accumulation and blood deficiency (e.g., bone tuberculosis, peritoneal tuberculosis, chronic osteomyelitis, osteoperiostitis, chronic lymphadenitis, rheumatoid arthritis, suppurative infection deep in the muscles); chronic bronchitis; chronic bronchial asthma; menorrhagia; chronic rheumatic arthritis	
	Cortex Cinnamomi	3			
	Herba Ephedrae	2			
	Colla Cornus Cervi (deer horn glue)	9			
	Semen Sinapis Albae (white mustard seed)	6			
	Carbonized Rhizoma Zingiberis	2			
	Radix Glycyrrhizae	3			

RESUSCITATION PRESCRIPTIONS

Prescription	Composition	Amount (grams)	Action(s)	Indication(s)	Remarks
Decoction for Prostration with Cold Limbs	Radix Aconiti Praeparata Rhizoma Zingiberis Radix Glycyrrhizae	9 9 12	Restoring vital function from collapse	Excessive endogenous cold damaging vital function (marked by cold limbs, and by lying with the body curled up, aversion to cold, vomiting with abdominal pain, diarrhea with fluid stools containing undigested food)	
Decoction of Ginseng and Aconiti	Radix Ginseng Radix Aconiti Praeparata	12 9	Restoring vital function from collapse and reinforcing vital energy	Sudden failure of vital function due to severe consumption of vital energy (marked by cold limbs, sweating, and respiratory failure); shock or heart failure	
Decoction for Controlling Water	Radix Aconiti Praeparata Poria Radix Paeoniae Rhizoma Atractylodis Macrocephalae Rhizoma Zingiberis Recens	9 9 9 6 9	Invigorating vital function and relieving water retention	Internal retention of water due to functional decline of the kidney (e.g., edema due to chronic nephritis or heart failure); hyperaldosteronism; hypothyroidism; chronic enteritis; intestinal tuberculosis caused by deficiency of vital energy of the spleen and kidney	

Tonifying Prescriptions

These prescriptions are used to correct deficiencies of energy, blood, and essence or to reinforce vital function.

VITAL-ENERGY REINFORCING PRESCRIPTIONS

Prescription	Composition	Amount (grams)	Action(s)	Indication(s)	Remarks
Decoction of Four Noble Ingredients	Radix Ginseng	12	Reinforcing vital energy and invigorating vital function of the middle burner; tonifying the spleen and stomach	Deficiency of vital energy of the spleen and stomach; chronic gastroenteritis; anemia; pulmonary tuberculosis; chronic nephritis and other chronic consumptive diseases marked by anorexia, emaciation, and lassitude	
	Rhizoma Atractylodis Macrocephalae	9			
	Poria	9			
	Radix Glycyrrhizae Praeparata	4.5			
Decoction for Reinforcing Vital Energy and Strengthening the Spleen and Stomach	Radix Astragali Praeparata	15	Reinforcing vital energy to generate fluids; exerting an astringent action on vital essence to arrest sweating	Prolapse of the uterus or anus; gastroptosis; protracted diarrhea or dysentery due to sinking or deficiency of vital energy of the stomach and spleen	
	Radix Ginseng	10			
	Radix Angelicae Sinensis	10			
	Pericarpium Citri Reticulatae	6			
	Rhizoma Cimicifugae	3			
	Radix Bupleuri	3			
	Rhizoma Atractylodis Macrocephalae	10			
	Radix Glycyrrhizae Praeparata	5			

Prescription	Composition	Amount (grams)	Action(s)	Indication(s)	Remarks
Decoction for Invigorating the Pulse Beat	Radix Ginseng Radix Ophiopogonis Fructus Schisandrae	10 15 6	As above	Deficiencies of both vital energy and vital essence in the later stages of febrile disease; pulmonary tuberculosis; chronic bronchitis; neurasthenia; heart failure; arrhythmia	

BLOOD-TONIFYING PRESCRIPTIONS

Prescription	Composition	Amount (grams)	Action(s)	Indication(s)	Remarks
Decoction of Four Herbs	Radix Angelicae Sinensis Rhizoma Ligustici Chuanxiong Radix Paeoniae Alba Radix Rehmannia Praeparata	10 6 10 15	Tonifying blood and regulating menstruation	Deficiency of blood; menstrual disorders; uterine bleeding	
Blood Tonifying Decoction of Angelicae	Radix Astragali Praeparata Radix Angelicae Sinensis	30 6	Reinforcing vital energy to generate blood	Illness caused by overexertion; deficiency of blood; weakened vital energy and fever	

VITAL-ENERGY REINFORCING AND BLOOD-TONIFYING PRESCRIPTIONS

Prescription	Composition	Amount (grams)	Action(s)	Indication(s)	Remarks
Decoction of Eight Precious Ingredients	*Radix Ginseng*	6	Reinforcing vital energy and tonifying blood	Deficiency of vital energy and blood (e.g., asthenia after illness, various chronic diseases, menstrual disorders, uterine bleeding, protracted boils or furuncles)	This decoction is a combination of Decoction of Four Noble Ingredients and Decoction of Four Herbs; *Radix Zingiberis* and *Fructus Ziziphi Jujubae* are adjurants
	Rhizoma Atractylodis Macrocephalae	9			
	Poria	10			
	Radix Angelicae Sinensis	10			
	Rhizoma Ligustici Chuanxiong	6			
	Radix Paeoniae	10			
	Radix Rehmanniae Praeparata	9			
	Radix Glycyrrhizae Praeparata	6			
	Radix Zingiberis Recens	6			
	Fructus Ziziphi Jujubae	3 dates			

Prescription	Composition	Amount (grams)	Action(s)	Indication(s)	Remarks
Decoction of Glycyrrhizae Praeparata	Radix Glycyrrhizae Praeparata	12	Reinforcing vital energy and nourishing the blood; replenishing vital essence to restore pulse	Insufficiency of vital energy and blood marked by irregular and intermittent pulse and palpitation; coronary heart disease; various forms of myocarditis; rheumatic heart disease	Decoction administered with melted *Colla Corii Asini*
	Radix Ginseng	6			
	Radix Rehmannia	30			
	Ramulus Cinnamomi	10			
	Colla Corii Asini	6			
	Radix Ophiopogonis	10			
	Semen Cannabis	20			
	Radix Zingiberis Recens	10			
	Fructus Ziziphi Jujubae	10 dates			

VITAL-ESSENCE REPLENISHING PRESCRIPTIONS

Prescription	Composition	Amount (grams)	Action(s)	Indication(s)	Remarks
Bolus of Six Ingredients with Rehmannia	Radix Rehmannia Praeparata	240	Replenishing the vital essence of the kidney	Flaring up of pathogenic fire due to consumption of vital essence of the kidney (e.g., pulmonary tuberculosis, diabetes, chronic nephritis, Addison's disease, hyperthyroidism, hypertension, optic neuritis, central retinitis, neurasthenia, nonovulatory functional metrorrhagia)	6–9 g administered 2–3 times daily; for decoction form, amounts of ingredients reduced but proportions kept the same
	Fructus Corni	160			
	Rhizoma Dioscoreae (Chinese yam rhizome)	160			
	Rhizoma Alismatis	90			
	Cortex Moutan Radicis	90			
	Poria alba	90			

Name	Ingredients		Actions	Indications	Administration
Decoction for Adjusting the Flow of Vital Energy by Nourishing the Liver and Kidney	*Radix Glehniae*	10	Nourishing the liver and kidney; regulating the flow of vital energy of the liver	Deficiency of vital essence of the liver and kidney; disturbed flow of vital energy of the liver; hernia; abdominal masses; chronic hepatitis; peptic ulcer; neurosis; hypertension; pleurisy; intercostal neuralgia; chronic orchitis	
	Fructus Meliae Toosendan (Sichuan chinaberry)	5			
	Radix Ophiopogonis	10			
	Radix Angelicae Sinensis	10			
	Radix Rehmannia	30			
	Fructus Lycii	12			
Major Bolus for Tonifying Vital Essence	*Radix Rehmannia Praeparata*	180	Replenishing vital essence to remove pathogenic fire	Flaring up of pathogenic fire due to deficiency of vital essence of the liver and kidney (marked by hectic fever and night sweats, coughing, hemoptysis, hematemesis); hyperthyroidism; renal or bone tuberculosis; diabetes	6–9 every morning and evening; for decoction form amounts of ingredients reduced but proportions kept the same
	Cortex Phellodendri	180			
	Rhizoma Anemarrhenae	180			
	Plastrum Testudinis	180			

VITAL-FUNCTION REINFORCING PRESCRIPTIONS

Prescription	Composition	Amount (grams)	Action(s)	Indication(s)	Remarks
Bolus for Tonifying the Kidney	Radix Rehmannia Rhizoma Dioscoreae Fructus Corni Rhizoma Alismatis Poria Cortex Montan Radicis Ramulus Cinnamomi Radix Aconitiprae-parata	240 120 120 90 90 90 30 30	Invigorating vital function of the kidney	Lowered vital function of the kidney marked by soreness in the lumbar region and knees, cold limbs, difficulty in urination, enuresis, and edema (diabetes, asthmatic cough, hyperaldosteronism, hypothyroidism, neurasthenia, chronic nephritis, chronic bronchial asthma)	6–9 g in bolus form administered twice daily; in decoction form, amounts of ingredients reduced but proportions kept the same
Decoction for Reinforcing Vital Function of the Kidney	Radix Rehmannia Praeparata Rhizoma Dioscoreae Fructus Corni Fructus Lycii Radix Glycyrrhizae Praeparata Cortex Cinnamomi Cortex Eucommiae Radix Aconiti Prae-parata	8–50 6 3 6 5 4 6 7	Invigorating vital function of the kidney; replenishing vital essence of the kidney	As above	
Bolus of Cuscutae	Semen Cuscutae Fructus Schisandrae Concha Ostreae Usta Herba Cistanchis	60 30 60 60	Invigorating vital function of the kidney and arresting discharge	Lowered vital function of the kidney, marked by sluggishness and intolerance of cold, dizziness, soreness in the	6–9 g per dose with salty soup

Prescription	Ingredients	Amount	Action	Indications	Remarks
	Radix Aconiti Praeparata	30		lumbar region, weakness of the legs, continuous dripping of urine (neurasthenia; hypogonadism)	
	Endothelium Corneum Gigeriae Galli	15			
	Cornu Cervi Pantotrichum	30			
	Ootheca Mantidis	30			
	Fructus Alpiniae oxyphyllae (galangal fruit)	30			
	Radix Linderae	30			
	Rhizoma Dioscoreae	30			
Bolus for Seminal Consolidation	Actinolitum (actinolite)	in equal portions	Invigorating vital function of the kidney; consolidating semen	Frequent spontaneous emission due to lowered vital function of the kidney; sexual neurasthenia; hypogonadism	Fine powder mixed with wine to form pills; 6–9 g per dose with salty soup
	Herba Cistanchis				
	Cornu Cervi Pantotrichum				
	Halloysitum Rubrum				
	Radix Morindae Officinalis				
	Semen Allium Tuberosum (seed of fragrant-flowered garlic)				
	Poria Alba				
	Cornu Cervi Degelatinatum				
	Os Draconis Usta (dragon's bone)				
	Radix Aconiti Praeparata				

Prescription	Composition	Amount (grams)	Action(s)	Indication(s)	Remarks
Bolus for Supporting Impregnation	Radix Rehmannia Praeparata	240	Invigorating vital function of the kidney	Seminal deficiency due to decline of the fire of the Vital Gate; impotence; infertility; sexual dysfunction	Add Ginseng 60 g, Cornu Cervi Panlotricbum 60 g to improve effect; 6–9 g per dose
	Rhizoma Atractylodis Macrocephalae	240			
	Radix Angelicae Sinensis	180			
	Fructus Lycii	180			
	Cortex Eucommiae	120			
	Rhizoma Curculiginis	120			
	Radix Morindae Officinalis	120			
	Fructus Corni	120			
	Herba Epimedii	120			
	Herba Cistanchis	120			
	Semen Allium Tuberosum	120			
	Fructus Cnidii	60			
	Radix Aconiti Praeparata	60			
	Cortex Cinnamomi	60			

Astringent Prescriptions

These prescriptions are composed chiefly of astringents and hemostatics. They are used to arrest discharges and thus to treat such conditions as excessive perspiration, persistent diarrhea, spermatorrhea, and urinary incontinence, which result in consumption of vital energy, blood, and fluids.

PRESCRIPTIONS TO ARREST ABNORMAL SWEATING AND STRENGTHEN SUPERFICIAL RESISTANCE

Prescription	Composition	Amount (grams)	Action(s)	Indication(s)	Remarks
Pulvis Ostreae	*Concha Ostreae Usta* *Radix Astragali Recens* *Radix Ephedrae*	30 30 30	Arresting sweating and strengthening superficial resistance	Spontaneous sweating due to debility and lowered superficial resistance	Coarse powder, 9 g per dose, decocted with *Fructus Tritici Levis* 30 g
Decoction of Angelica Sinensis and Six Other Yellow Ingredients	*Radix Rehmannia* *Radix Angelicae Sinensis* *Radix Rehmannia Praeparata* *Radix Scutellariae* *Cortex Phellodendri* *Radix Astragali* *Rhizoma Coptidis* *Radix Astragali*	1 part each 2 parts	Replenishing vital essence and clearing away pathogenic heat; strengthening superficial resistance and arresting sweating	Fever and night sweats due to deficiency of vital energy	Coarse powder 15 g per dose; for decoction form amounts of ingredients as ordered
Jade-Screen Powder	*Radix Astragali Recens* *Rhizoma Actratylodis Macrocephalae* *Radix Ledebouriellae*	180 60 60	Reinforcing vital energy and strengthening superficial resistance to arrest spontaneous sweating	Spontaneous sweating due to lowered superficial resistance	6–9 g per dose; for decoction form amounts of ingredients reduced but proportions kept the same

PRESCRIPTIONS FOR SPERMATORRHEA AND INCONTINENCE OF URINE

Prescription	Composition	Amount (grams)	Action(s)	Indication(s)	Remarks
Pulvis Mantis	Ootheca Mantidis	30	Tonifying the heart and kidney to arrest spermatorrhea and incontinence of urine	Frequent urination, enuresis, spermatorrhea due to deficiency of vital energy of the heart and kidney; neurasthenia	6 g per dose; for decoction form amounts of ingredients reduced but proportions kept the same
	Radix Polygalae (polygala root)	30			
	Rhizoma Acori Graminei	30			
	Os Draconis	30			
	Radix Ginseng	30			
	Rhizoma Poria	30			
	Radix Angelicae Sinensis	30			
	Plastrum Testudinis	30			
Golden Bolus for Seminal Consolidation	Semen Astragali Complanati Praeparata	20	Strengthening kidney function to arrest spermatorrhea	Spermatorrhea due to lowered vital function of the kidney	Powder mixed with paste of lotus powder to form pills, 9 g administered per dose with weak salty soup; for decoction form, lotus seeds added and amounts of ingredients reduced but proportions kept the same
	Semen Euryales	20			
	Stamen Nelumbinis (hindu lotus stamen)	20			
	Os Draconis	20			
	Concha Ostreae	10			

DIARRHEA-CHECKING AND PROLAPSE-PREVENTING PRESCRIPTIONS

Prescription	Composition	Amount (grams)	Action(s)	Indication(s)	Remarks
Powder for Nourishing Viscera	Radix Paeoniae Alba	48	Strengthening the vital function of the stomach and spleen to arrest diarrhea	Chronic dysentery or fecal incontinence due to coldness and lowered function of the spleen and kidney; chronic colitis	6 g of powder per dose; for decoction form, amounts of ingredients reduced but proportions kept the same
	Radix Angelicae Sinensis	18			
	Radix Ginseng	18			
	Cortex Cinnamomi	18			
	Rhizoma Atractylodis Macrocephalae Praeparata	18			
	Semen Myristicae	15			
	Radix Glycyrrhizae Praeparata	24			
	Radix Aucklandiae	42			
	Fructus Chebulae	36			
	Pericarpium Papaveris (poppy shell)	108			

Prescription	Composition	Amount (grams)	Action(s)	Indication(s)	Remarks
Bolus of Four Magical Herbs	Semen Myristicae Fructus Psoraleae Fructus Schisandrae Fructus Evodiae	60 120 60 30	Invigorating the vital function of the kidney and spleen to arrest diarrhea	Diarrhea in the early morning, chronic enteritis, chronic colitis, intestinal tuberculosis due to lowered functioning of the spleen and kidney	Prepared with 100 cooked and crushed jujubes and 240 g of ginger soup, 9–12 g per dose; for decoction form, amounts of ingredients reduced but proportions kept the same

PRESCRIPTIONS FOR UTERINE BLEEDING AND MORBID LEUKORRHEA

Prescription	Composition	Amount (grams)	Action(s)	Indication(s)	Remarks
Decoction for Strengthening the Chong Channels	Rhizoma Atractylodis Macrocephalae Praeparata Radix Astragali Os Draconis Usta Concha Ostrae Usta Fructus Corni	30 18 24 24 24	Replenishing vital energy of the spleen and strengthening the Chong Channel to stop bleeding	Uterine bleeding (e.g., menorrhagia, excessive bleeding after childbirth); peptic ulcer due to deficiency of vital energy of the spleen	

Prescription	Ingredients		Function	Indication
	Radix Paeoniae Alba	12		Excessive leukorrhea
	Os Sepiae (cuttlefish bone)	12		
	Radix Rubiae (madder root)	9		
	Petiolus Trachycarpi carbonistans (burnt petiole of windmill-palm)	6		
	Galla Chinensis	1.5		
Decoction for Treating Leukorrhea	Rhizoma Atractylodis Macrocephalae Praeparata	30	Restoring vital function of the spleen; removing pathogenic dampness to relieve morbid leukorrhea	
	Rhizoma Dioscoreae Praeparata	30		
	Radix Ginseng	6		
	Radix Paeoniae Alba	15		
	Semen Plantaginis	9		
	Rhizoma Atractylodis	9		
	Radix Glycyrrhizae	3		
	Pericarpium Citri Reticulatae	2		
	Spike Schizonepetae Praeparata	2		
	Radix Bupleuri	2		

Sedative Prescriptions

These prescriptions, which contain sedatives and tonics, are used in treating nervous restlessness.

Prescription	Composition	Amount (grams)	Action(s)	Indication(s)	Remarks
Sedative Cinnabar Bolus	*Cinnabar* (cinnabar)	15	Calming the nerves; clearing pathogenic heat and nourishing blood	Flaring up of pathogenic fire of the heart due to insufficiency of vital essence of the heart and marked by neurasthenia, insomnia, amnesia, or mental depression	6–9 g per bolus; taken at bedtime; for decoction form, amounts of ingredients reduced but proportions kept the same
	Rhizoma Coptidis	18			
	Radix Glycyrrhizae Praeparata	16			
	Radix Rehmanniae	8			
	Radix Angelica Sinensis	8			
Decoction of Ziziphi Spinosae	*Semen Ziziphi Spinosae Praeparata* (seed of wild jujube)	18	Nourishing the blood and calming the nerves; clearing pathogenic heat to relieve restlessness	Restlessness and insomnia due to insufficient blood in the liver, which gives rise to endogenous pathogenic heat and in turn to disturbance of the nerves	
	Radix Glycyrrhizae	3			
	Rhizoma Anemarrhenae	6			
	Poria	6			
	Rhizoma Ligustici Chuanxiong	3			
Royal Pills for Mind Easing	*Radix Rehmannia*	120	Replenishing vital essence to ease the mind; regulating vital function of the heart and kidney	Insomnia, palpitation, amnesia, nocturnal emission, cardiopathy, neurasthenia, hyperthyroidism due to lowered functioning of the kidney and	Pills coated with cinnabar, 9 g per dose; for decoction form, amounts of in-
	Fructus Schisandrae	30			
	Radix Angelicae Sinensis	30			
	Radix Asparagi	30			

				gredients reduced but proportions kept the same
	Radix Ophiopogonis	30		insufficient vital essence and blood
	Semen Ziziphi Spinosae	30		
	Radix Ginseng	15		
	Radix Salviae Millorrhizae	15		
	Radix Scrophulariae	15		
	Poria	15		
	Semen Biotae (oriental arborvitae seed)	30		
	Radix Polygalae	15		
	Radix Platycodi	15		
Decoction of Glycyrrhizae, Wheat, and Jujube	Radix Glycyrrhizae	9	Nourishing the heart and calming the nerves; regulating function of the middle burner	Symptom-complex of visceral disturbance due to *yin* deficiency caused by overanxiety (marked by mental dysfunction, fidgeting, restless sleep); psychosis; hysteria; neurasthenia; menopause syndromes; cardiopathy; sinus tachycardia; cardiac neurosis
	Fructus Tritici (wheat)	9		
	Fructus Ziziphi Jujubae	10 dates		

Aromatic and Stimulative Prescriptions

These prescriptions, composed mainly of aromatic stimulants, are used to treat loss of consciousness.

Prescription	Composition	Amount (grams)	Action(s)	Indication(s)	Remarks
Bezoar Resurrection Bolus	Calculus Bovis	30	Clearing away heat toxins; restoring consciousness and treating complicated conditions caused by phlegm	Invasion of the pericardium by pathological factors in infectious febrile disease; coma due to blockage of the heart by phlegm-heat; apoplexy; infantile convulsions due to phlegm-heat; encephalitis B; epidemic meningitis; toxic dysentery; uremia; cerebrovascular disease; toxic hepatitis; hepatic coma	3 g per bolus; 1 bolus per dose
	Radix Curcumae	30			
	Cornu Rhinoceri	30			
	Radix Astragali	30			
	Rhizoma Coptidis	30			
	Realgar (red orpiment)	30			
	Fructus Gardeniae	30			
	Cinnabar	30			
	Borneolum	7.5			
	Moschus	7.5			
	Margarita (pearl)	7.5			
	gold foil	for coating			
Storax Bolus	Rhizoma Atractilodis Macrocephalae	60	Restoring consciousness and promoting the normal flow of vital energy	Apoplectic coma (cerebrovascular disease); sudden loss of consciousness; angina pectoris	1 bolus (3 g) per dose; lower dosage for children
	Radix Aristolochiae (dutchmanspipe root)	60			
	Cinnabar	60			
	Cornu Rhinoceri	60			
	Rhizoma Cyperi	60			
	Fructus Chebulae	60			
	Lignum Santali Alba (sandalwood)	60			
	Benzoinum (benzoin)	60			

Lignum Aquilariae Resinatum (eaglewood)	60
Moschus	60
Flos Caryophylli	60
Fructus Piperis Longi (long pepper fruit)	60
Dryobalanops Aromatica (common borneo camphor)	30
Olium Styrax Liquidus (oil of styrax)	30
Reina Olibani	30

Carminative Prescriptions

These prescriptions are composed of herbs that normalize the flow of vital energy and regulate the functional activities of the viscera. They are used in treating stagnancy of vital energy.

VITAL-ENERGY REGULATION PRESCRIPTIONS

Prescription	Composition	Amount (grams)	Action(s)	Indication(s)	Remarks
Pills of Alpiniae and Cyperus	*Rhizoma Alpiniae Officinarum* (lesser galangal rhizome) *Rhizoma Cyperi Praeparata*	equal amounts	Invigorating the function of the stomach and spleen; promoting the normal flow of vital energy to kill pain	Accumulation of pathogenic cold in the stomach due to stagnancy of vital energy in the liver	6 g per dose; for decoction form, amounts of ingredients reduced but proportions kept the same
Pulvis Meliae	*Fructus Meliae Toosendan* *Rhizoma Corydalis* (corydalis tuber)	30 30	Soothing a depressed liver and eliminating pathogenic heat; promoting the normal flow of vital energy to alleviate pain	Pain in the hypochondriac region; excessive menstrual bleeding; hernial pain due to stagnancy of vital energy of the liver; gastroduodenal ulcer; chronic gastritis; hepatitis; cholecystitis	9 g per dose; for decoction form, amounts of ingredients reduced but proportions kept the same
Decoction of Pinellia and Magnoliae	*Rhizoma Pinellia* *Cortex Magnoliae Officinalis* *Poria* *Rhizoma Zingiberis Recens* *Folium Perillae*	9 9 12 15 6	Promoting the normal flow of vital energy; relieving and resolving phlegm	Globus hystericus; hysteria; gastroenteric neurosis; esophagospasm; chronic laryngitis; tracheitis due to stagnation of vital energy and phlegm	
Decoction of Trichosanthis, Allium, and Spiritus	*Fructus Trichosanthis* (Mongolian snakegourd fruit)	12	Relieving obstruction and dispelling masses; promoting the normal flow of vi-	Chest pain, including angina pectoris; costal pain due to stagnation of vital energy and phlegm	

	Ingredients		Action	Indication	Remarks
	Bulbus Allii Ma-crostemi (onion bulb)	9	tal energy to remove phlegm		For decoction form, amounts of ingredients reduced but proportions kept the same
	white wine				
Pills of Tangerine Seed	*Semen Citri Reticulatae* (tangerine seed)	30	Promoting the normal flow of vital energy to alleviate pain; dispelling masses	Swollen testis due to the invasion of pathogenic cold-dampness into the Liver Channel; hydrocele; orchitis; epididymitis	
	Sargassum	30			
	Thallus Laminariae seu Eckloniae	30			
	Fructus Meliae Toosendan Prae-parata	30			
	Semen Persicae	30			
	Cortex Magnoliae Officinalis	15			
	Caulis Akebiae	15			
	Fructus Aurantium Immaturus Prae-parata	15			
	Rhizoma Corydalis Praeparata	15			
	Cortex Cinnamomi	15			
	Radix Aucklandiae	15			

Prescriptions to Put Down Adverse Upward Flow of Vital Energy

Prescription	Composition	Amount (grams)	Action(s)	Indication(s)	Remarks
Decoction of Perillae to Bring Down Vital Energy	Fructus Perillae (purple perilla fruit)	9	Keeping vital energy going downward to relieve asthma; resolving cold-phlegm	Shortness of breath and asthmatic cough; bronchial asthma; chronic bronchitis; emphysema; cardiac asthma	Decocted with two slices of fresh ginger, a jujube, and a small amount of peppermint
	Rhizoma Pinelliae	9			
	Radix Peucedani (peucedanum root)	6			
	Cortex Magnoliae Officinalis	6			
	Cortex Cinnamomi	2			
	Radix Angelicae Sinensis	6			
	Radix Glycyrrhizae	4			
Antiasthmatic Decoction	Semen Ginkgo (gingko-nut)	9	Ventilating the lung to bring down the adverse upward flow of vital energy and relieve asthma	Asthma caused by internal accumulation of phlegm-heat; chronic bronchitis; bronchial asthma	
	Herba Glycyrrhizae	9			
	Fructus Perillae	6			
	Radix Glycyrrhizae	3			
	Flos Farfarae	9			
	Semen Armeniacae Amarum	5			
	Cortex Mori Radicis	9			
	Radix Scutellariae	5			
	Rhizoma Pinelliae	9			
Decoction of Pericarpium	Pericarpium Citri Reticulatae	9	Eliminating pathogenic heat from the	Hiccups and vomiting due to adverse upward flow of vital	

Citri and Caulis Bambusae in Taenis	Caulis Bambusae in Taenis (bamboo shavings)	9	stomach and promoting the normal flow of vital energy; bringing down adverse upward flow of vital energy to relieve vomiting	energy caused by lowered function of the stomach; morning sickness; vomiting due to incomplete obstruction of the pylorus; incessant hiccups after abdominal operation
	Fructus Ziziphi Jujubae	5 dates		
	Radix Glycyrrhizae	6		
	Rhizoma Zingeberis Recens	9		
	Radix Ginseng	3		
Decoction of Caryophylli and Calyx Kaki	Flos Caryophylli	6	Promoting the normal flow of vital energy and relieving hiccups	Hiccups and vomiting due to lowered function of the stomach; neural hiccups; hiccups after abdominal operation; spasm of the diaphragm
	Calyx Kaki (receptacle of a persimmon)	6		
	Radix Ginseng	3		
	Rhizoma Zingiberis Recens	6		

Blood-Regulating Prescriptions

These prescriptions contain herbs for promoting blood circulation, eradicating blood stasis, and producing hemostasis. They are used to treat various blood disturbances.

PRESCRIPTIONS FOR PROMOTING THE CIRCULATION OF BLOOD AND ERADICATING BLOOD STASIS

Prescription	Composition	Amount (grams)	Action(s)	Indication(s)	Remarks
Blood Regulation Decoction of Semen Persicae	Semen Persicae Radix et Rhizoma Rhei Ramulus Cinnamomi Radix Glycyrrhizae Natrii Sulfas	12 12 6 6 6	Eradicating blood stasis	Absence of menstruation or excessive menstrual bleeding due to blood stagnation in the lower burner; acute pelvic inflammation; retention of the placenta; inflammation of the uterine appendages; intestinal obstruction	
Decoction for Recovery by Activating Blood Circulation	Radix Bupleuri Radix Trichosanthis Radix Angelicae Sinensis Radix Glycyrrhizae Flos Carthami Squama Manitis Radix et Rhizoma Rhei Semen Persicae	15 9 9 6 6 6 30 9	Removing blood stasis by activating blood circulation; restoring the normal flow of vital energy of the liver	Intolerable pain in the costal region due to blood stasis caused by trauma; intercostal neuralgia; costal chrondritis due to blood stasis	
Decoction for Removing Blood Stasis from the Chest	Semen Persicae Flos Carthmi Radix Angelicae Sinensis Radix Rehmannia Rhizoma Ligustici Chuanxiong	12 9 9 9 5	Removing blood stasis by activating blood circulation; relieving pain by regulating the flow of vital energy	Chest pain, absence of menstruation, or excessive menstrual bleeding due to blood stasis in the chest or abdomen; coronary arteriosclerotic angina pectoris; rheumatic heart disease; contusions of	

Prescription	Ingredients	Dose	Action	Indications	Remarks
	Radix Paeoniae Rubra	6		the chest; chest pain due to costal chondritis	
	Radix Achyranthis Bidentatae	9			
	Radix Blatycodi	5			
	Radix Bupleuri	3			
	Fructus Aurantii (bitter orange)	6			
	Radix Glycyrrhizae	3			
Decoction for Recuperating from Hemiplegia by Reinforcing Vital Energy	Radix Astragali	60	Activating blood circulation and unblocking vessels by reinforcing vital energy	Hemiplegia; facial paralysis; paraplegia; monoparesis; other sequelae of cerebrovascular disease or poliomyelitis	
	Tail of Radix Angelicae Sinensis	6			
	Radix Paeoniae Rubra	6			
	Lumbricus	3			
	Rhizoma Ligusti Chuanxiong	3			
	Semen Persicae	3			
	Flos Carthami	3			
Powder for Removing Blood Stasis	Faeces Trogopterorum	in equal portions	Removing blood stasis by activating blood circulation; dispersing masses to alleviate pain	Pain due to blood stasis (e.g., sudden pain in the cardiac region or abdomen, dysmenorrhea, retention of lochia); angina pectoris; extrauterine gestation due to blood stasis	6 g per dose; take with wine or vinegar; for decoction form, amounts of ingredients reduced but proportions kept the same
	Pollen Typhae Praeparata				
Decoction of Salviae	Radix Salviae Miltiorrhizae	30	Promoting normal flow of vital energy to remove blood stasis	Stomachache; chronic gastritis; gastroduodenal ulcer; gastroneurosis; angina pectoris due to stagnancy of vital energy and blood stasis; pain due to chronic pancreatitis	
	Lignum Santali	5			
	Fructus Amomi	5			

Prescription	Composition	Amount (grams)	Action(s)	Indication(s)	Remarks
Coronary Heart Disease Prescription II	Rhizoma Ligustici Chuanxiong	15	Activating blood circulation to remove blood stasis; promoting normal flow of vital energy to kill pain	Coronary arteriosclerotic heart disease or angina pectoris due to blood stasis	
	Radix Paeoniae Rubra	15			
	Flos Carthami	15			
	Lignum Dalbergiae Odoriferae (dalbergia)	15			
	Radix Salviae Miltiorrhizae	30			
Channel-Warming Decoction	Fructus Evodiae	9	Warming the Chong and Ren Channels to dispel pathogenic cold; nourishing blood to remove blood stasis	Menstrual disorders, dysmenorrhea, uterine bleeding due to blood stasis and stagnant pathogenic cold in the Chong and Ren Channels; chronic pelvic inflammation	
	Radix Angelicae Sinensis	9			
	Radix Paeoniae	9			
	Radix Ginseng	6			
	Rhizoma Ligustici Chanxiong	6			
	Ramulus Cinnamomi	6			
	Colla Corii Asini	9			
	Cortex Montan Radicis	6			
	Radix Zingiberis Recens	6			
	Radix Glycyrrhizae	6			
	Radix Ophiopogonis	9			
	Rhizoma Pinelliae	9			
Decoction for Removing Stag-	Radix Angelicae Sinensis	24	Activating blood circulation to remove	Retention of lochia; coldness and pain in the lower abdo-	Decocted with water; add mil-

nant Blood and Promoting Hemogenesis	Rhizoma Ligustici Chuanxiong	9	blood stasis; warming the channels to kill pain	men with a cold sensation due to blood stasis	let wine when the decoction is nearly done
	Radix Zingiberis	2			
	Semen Persicae	6			
	Radix Glycyrrhizae	2			
Prescription for Extrauterine Gestation I	Radix Salviae Miltiorrhizae	15	Activating blood circulation and removing blood stasis; dispersing masses; alleviating pain	Onset of rupture of ectopic pregnancy	
	Radix Paeoniae Rubra	15			
	Semen Persicae	9			
Prescription for Extrauterine Gestation II	Radix Salviae Miltiorrhizae	15	Dispersing masses by activating blood circulation and removing blood stasis; alleviating pain	Inflammations following rupture of ectopic pregnancy; chronic pelvic inflammation or perimetrosalpingitis; adnexitis, pelvic connective tissue inflammations	
	Radix Paeoniae Rubra	15			
	Semen Persicae	9			
	Rhizoma Sparganii	1.5–6			
	Rhizoma Zedoariae	1.5–6			

Hemostatic Prescriptions

Prescription	Composition	Amount (grams)	Action(s)	Indication(s)	Remarks
Powder of Ten Burnt Herbs	*Herba seu Radix Cirsii Japonici Herba Cephalamneploris Folium Nelumbinis Cacumen Biotae Rhizoma Imperatae Radix Rubiae Fructus Gardeniae Radix et Rhizoma Rhei Cortex Montan Radicis Cortex Trachycarpi*	in equal portions	Removing heat from the blood and stopping bleeding	Hematemesis or hemoptysis due to excessive heat in the blood	Powder of the burnt herbs is mixed with either lotus root or radish juice; 9 g per dose, administered twice daily; for decoction form, amounts of ingredients reduced but proportions kept the same
Pills of Four Fresh Herbs	*Folium Nelumbinis Recens Folium Artemisiae Argyi Recens Folium Biotae Recens Radix Rehmannia*	in equal amounts	Removing pathogenic heat from the blood and stopping bleeding	Hematemesis or epistaxis due to intense heat in the blood; hemoptysis due to pulmonary tuberculosis or bronchiectasis; hematemesis due to gastric ulcer	9 g per dose
Recipe for Coughing Blood	*Indigo Naturalis* (natural indigo) *Semen Trichosanthis* (seed of Mongolian snakegourd) *Fructus Gardeniae*	6 9 9	Clearing away pathogenic heat and resolving phlegm; arresting cough and bleeding	Coughing up bloody sputum because of affection of the lung by pathogenic fire in the liver; hemoptysis in bronchiectasis and pulmonary tuberculosis	

			Action	Indication	Dosage
Pulvis Sophorae	Fructus Chebulae	6			
	Pumex (pumice)	9			
	Flos Sophorae Prae-parata	in equal amounts	Clearing pathogenic heat from the intestines to stop bleeding; dispelling pathogenic wind to promote the normal flow of vital energy	Stools containing fresh blood; bleeding due to hemorrhoids	6 g per dose, taken with water or thin rice gruel
	Cacumen Biotae				
	Spike of Schizonepeta				
	Fructus Aurantii				
Decoction of Cephalanoploris	Radix Rehmannia	24	Eliminating pathogenic heat from the blood to stop bleeding; promoting urination	Hematuria due to intense heat in the urinary bladder; acute urinary tract infection; stones in the urinary system	
	Herba Cephalano-plosis	15			
	Fructus Gardeniae	9			
	Talcum	12			
	Caulis Akebia	6			
	Pollon Typhae Prae-parata	9			
	Herba Lopatheri	6			
	Nodus Nelumbinis Rhizomatis (node of lotus rhizome)	9			
	Radix Angelicae Sinensis	6			
	Radix Glycyrrhizae Praeparata	6			

Digestant Prescriptions

Prescription	Composition	Amount (grams)	Action(s)	Indication(s)	Remarks
Stomach Beneficial Bolus	Fructus Crataegi	180	Restoring the normal function of the stomach to remove stagnated food	Retention of undigested food (marked by distension and fullness in the stomach and abdomen, belching with fetid odor, acid regurgitation, anorexia, nausea, and vomiting)	6–9 g per dose; for decoction form, amounts of ingredients reduced but proportions kept the same
	Massa Fermentate Medicinalis (medicated leaven)	60			
	Rhizoma Pinelliae	60			
	Poria	60			
	Pericarium Citri Reticulatae	30			
	Fructus Forsythiae	30			
	Semen Raphani	30			
Bolus for Reinforcing the Spleen	Rhizoma Atractylodis Macrocephalae	75	Invigorating the vital function of the spleen to remove stagnated food	Dyspepsia with pathogenic internal heat due to lowered functioning of the spleen and stomach; fullness in the abdomen; anorexia and indigestion; loose bowels	6–9 g per dose; for decoction form, amounts of ingredients reduced but proportions kept the same
	Radix Auklandiae	22.5			
	Rhizoma Coptidis	22.5			
	Radix Glycyrrhizae	22.5			
	Poria	60			
	Radix Ginseng	45			
	Massa Fermentata Medicinallis Praeparata	30			
	Pericarpium Citri Reticulatae	30			
	Fructus Amomi (longillgular fruit)	30			

Prescription	Ingredients		Actions	Indications	Administration
	Fructus Hordei Germinatus Praeparata	30			
	Fructus Crataegi	30			
	Rhizoma Dioscoreae	30			
	Semen Myristicae (nutmeg)	30			
Pills of Aucklandiae and Arecae	*Radix Auklandiae*	30	Promoting normal flow of vital energy to remove undigested food and purge pathogenic heat	Stagnancy of vital energy due to pathogenic damp-heat produced by retained undigested food (marked by distension and pain in the stomach and abdomen, constipation, dysentery, tenesmus, sticky yellow tongue coating, and full pulse)	Fine powder mixed with water to form small pills; 6 g taken twice or thrice daily with ginger juice
	Semen Arecae	30			
	Pericarpium Citri Reticulatae Viride	30			
	Pericarpium Citri Reticulatae	30			
	Rhizoma Zedoariae	30			
	Rhizoma Coptidis	30			
	Cortex Phellodendri	90			
	Radix et Rhizoma Rhei	90			
	Rhizoma Cyperi Praeparata	120			
	Semen Pharbitidis	120			

Desiccating Prescriptions

These prescriptions, which produce diuresis and desiccation, are used to treat diseases caused by pathogenic dampness.

FRAGRANT PRESCRIPTIONS FOR RESOLVING DAMPNESS

Prescription	Composition	Amount (grams)	Action(s)	Indication(s)	Remarks
Powder for Regulating the Function of the Stomach	Pericarpium Citri Reticulatae	1,560	Removing pathogenic dampness and activating the function of the spleen; promoting the normal flow of vital energy to regulate the function of the stomach	Distension and fullness of the abdomen and stomach, anorexia, nausea, vomiting, belching, acid regurgitation, and general weakness due to stagnancy of vital energy and pathogenic dampness retained in the spleen; chronic gastritis; gastrointestinal neurosis	6–9 g administered mixed with jujube and ginger soup; for decoction form, amounts of ingredients reduced but proportions kept the same
	Cortex Magnoliae Officinalis	1,560			
	Rhizoma Atractylodis Praeparata	2,400			
	Radix Glycyrrhizae Praeparata	900			
Powder of Agastachis for Dispelling Turbidity	Herba Agastachis	90	Removing pathogenic dampness to relieve superficial afflictions; regulating vital energy flow of the spleen and stomach	Pathogenic dampness retained in the spleen and stomach due to exogenous affection by wind and cold; functional disorders of the spleen and stomach caused by summer-heat and dampness; acute gastroenteritis	6–9 g mixed with ginger and jujube soup; for decoction form, amounts of ingredients reduced but proportions kept the same
	Folium Perillae	30			
	Radix Angelicae Dahuricae	30			
	Pericarpium Arecae	30			
	Poria	30			
	Rhizoma Atractylodis Macrocephalae	60			
	Massa Pinelliae Fermentata	60			
	Pericarpium Citri Reticulatae	60			
	Cortex Magnoliae Officinalis	60			
	Radix Platycodi	60			
	Radix Glycyrrhizae Praeparata	75			

FEBRIFUGAL AND DESICCATING PRESCRIPTIONS

Prescription	Composition	Amount (grams)	Action(s)	Indication(s)	Remarks
Decoction of Artemisiae	*Herba Artemisiae Scopariae*	30	Clearing away pathogenic damp-heat	Icteric hepatitis, cholecystitis, gallstones, leptospirosis due to pathogenic damp-heat	
	Fructus Gardeniae	15			
	Radix et Rhizoma Rhei	10			
Decoction of Three Kinds of Seeds	*Semen Armaniacae Ararum*	15	Clearing away pathogenic damp-heat to smooth the normal flow of vital energy	Incipient infectious febrile disease marked by headache, aversion to cold, stuffiness of the chest, hectic fever, pale tongue coating, absence of thirst, weak-floating pulse; typhoid fever; gastroenteritis, pyelonephritis, undulant fever due to pathogenic dampness	
	Talcum	18			
	Medulla Tetrapanacis (stem pith of the rice-paper plant)	6			
	Semen Cardamomi Rotundi	6			
	Herba Lophatheri	6			
	Cortex Magnoliae Officinalis	6			
	Semen Coicis	18			
	Rhizoma Pinelliae	15			
Powder of Two Wonderful Ingredients	*Cortex Phellodenarie Praeparata*	in equal amounts	Clearing away pathogenic damp-heat	Feebleness of the lower limbs, swollen and painful knees due to downward pathogenic damp-heat; morbid leukorrhea due to pathogenic damp-heat; suppurative infection on the surface of the lower part of the body	6–9 g per dose; for decoction form, amounts of ingredients reduced but proportions kept the same
	Rhizoma Atractylodis Praeparata				

Prescription	Composition	Amount (grams)	Action(s)	Indication(s)	Remarks
Decoction for Arthralgia	Radix Stephaniae Tetrandrae	15	Clearing away pathogenic damp-heat to smooth the flow of vital energy in the channels	Arthralgia due to pathogenic damp-heat (marked by joint pain, concentrated urine, sticky yellow tongue coating); rheumatic arthritis; swollen and painful joints	
	Semen Armeniacae Amarum	15			
	Talcum	15			
	Fructus Forsythiae	9			
	Fructus Gardenia	9			
	Semen Coicis	15			
	Rhizoma Pinelliae	9			
	Excrementum Bombycis (silkworm droppings)	9			
	Pericarpium Semen Phaseoli	9			

DIURETIC PRESCRIPTIONS

Prescription	Composition	Amount (grams)	Action(s)	Indication(s)	Remarks
Powder of Five Ingredients Including Poria	Polyporus Umbellatus	9	Eliminating pathogenic dampness through diuresis	Edema, difficulty in urination, or diarrhea; edema due to chronic nephritis	
	Rhizoma Alismatis	15			
	Rhizoma Atractylodis Macrocephalae	9			
	Poria	9			
	Ramulus Cinnamomi	6			

Decoction of Peels of Five Herbs	Exocarpium Zingeberis Recens (ginger peel) Cortex Mori Radicis Pericarpium Citri Reticulatae Pericarpium Arecae Pericarpium Poria	in equal amounts	Relieving edema through diuresis; regulating the flow of vital energy; strengthening the function of the spleen	Edema caused by exuberant dampness due to lowered function of the spleen; edema due to nephritis	Coarse powder 9 g per dose
Decoction of Stephanie and Astragali	Radix Stephaniae Tetranurae Radix Astragali Rhizoma Atractylodis Macrocephalae Radix Glycyrrhizae	12 15 9 6	Promoting the normal flow of vital energy and dispelling pathogenic wind; strengthening the function of the spleen and eliminating retained water	Edema due to pathogenic wind or dampness; edema due to chronic nephritis or cardiopathy	Decocted with 4 slices of fresh ginger and 4 dates

DIURETIC PRESCRIPTIONS OF WARM NATURE

Prescription	Composition	Amount (grams)	Action(s)	Indication(s)	Remarks
Spleen-Strengthening Decoction	Cortex Magnoliae Officinalis	6	Invigorating the vital function of the spleen; promoting the normal flow of vital energy to remove retained water	Edema that is generalized or more severe in the lower half of the body; chronic nephritis; cardiac edema due to lowered vital function	Decocted with 5 slices of fresh ginger and a date
	Rhizoma Atractylodis Macrocephalae	6			
	Fructus Amomi Tsaoko (amomum tsaoko fruit)	6			
	Pericarpium Arecae	6			
	Radix Aconiti Praeparata	6			
	Poria	6			
	Rhizoma Zingeberis Praeparata	3			
	Radix Glycyrrhizae Praeparata	3			
	Fructus Chaenomelis	6			
	Radix Aucklandia	6			
Decoction of Poria, Cinnamomi, Atractylodis, and Glycyrrhizae	Poria	12	Strengthening the functioning of the spleen to eliminate pathogenic dampness, fluid, and phlegm	Chronic bronchitis, bronchial asthma due to deficiency of vital energy of the spleen; edema due to cardiopathy; chronic nephritis due to lowered vital function	
	Ramulus Cinnamomi	9			
	Rhizoma Atractylodis Macrocephalae	6			
	Radix Glycyrrhizae Praeparata	6			

Prescription	Composition	Amount (grams)	Action(s)	Indication(s)	Remarks
Dioscoreae Decoction to Eliminate Damp-Turbidity	*Fructus Alpinia Oxyphylla* *Rhizoma Dioscoreae Hypoglaucae* (yam rhizome) *Rhizoma Acori Graminei* *Radix Linderae*	9 12 9 9	Activating the function of the kidney to eliminate pathogenic dampness		Strangury, chyluria, frequent urination; chronic prostatitis due to deficiency in the kidney and dampness

WIND-DAMPNESS ELIMINATING PRESCRIPTIONS

Prescription	Composition	Amount (grams)	Action(s)	Indication(s)	Remarks
Notopterygium Decoction for Eliminating Dampness	*Rhizoma seu Radix Notopterygii* (notopterygium root) *Radix Angelicae Pubescentis* *Rhizoma Ligustici* *Radix Ledebonriellae* *Radix Glycyrrhizae Praeparata* *Rhizoma Ligustici Chuanxiong* *Fructus Vitex* (vitex fruit)	6 6 4 4 4 4 2	Relieving rheumatic conditions	Generalized aching or severe headache due to pathogenic wind-dampness; common cold; rheumatic arthritis; tension headache	

Prescription	Composition	Amount (grams)	Action(s)	Indication(s)	Remarks
Decoction of Angelicae Pubescentis and Loranthi	Radix Angelicae Pubescentis	9	Dispelling pathogenic wind-dampness to relieve arthralgia; replenishing the liver and kidney and tonifying vital energy and blood	Insufficiency of vital energy and blood due to prolonged arthralgia caused by pathogenic wind and damp-cold; chronic rheumatic arthritis; rheumatic sciatica	
	Ramulus Loranthi	18			
	Cortex Eucommiae	9			
	Radix Achyranthis Bidentatae	9			
	Herba Asari	3			
	Radix Gentianae Macrophyllae	9			
	Poria	12			
	Cortex Cinnamomi	1.5			
	Radix Ledebouriellae	9			
	Rhizoma Ligustici Chuanxiong	6			
	Radix Ginseng	12			
	Radix Glycyrrhizae Praeparata	6			
	Radix Angelicae Sinensis	12			
	Radix Paeoniae	9			
	Radix Rehmannia	15			

Phlegm-Expelling Prescriptions

PHLEGM-DAMPNESS DISSIPATING PRESCRIPTIONS

Prescription	Composition	Amount (grams)	Action(s)	Indication(s)	Remarks
Decoction of Orange Peel and Pinelliae	Rhizoma Pinelliae	9	Removing pathogenic dampness and phlegm; regulating the flow of vital energy and the functioning of the spleen and stomach	Coughing due to pathogenic dampness and phlegm; distension in the chest and costal region; nausea and vomiting	Decocted with slices of fresh ginger and a black plum (*Fructus Mume*)
	Exocarpium Citri Grandis (tangerine peel)	9			
	Poria	6			
	Radix Glycyrrhizae Praeparata	3			

PHLEGM-HEAT DISSIPATING PRESCRIPTIONS

Prescription	Composition	Amount (grams)	Action(s)	Indication(s)	Remarks
Pills for Clearing Away Heat and Phlegm	Semen Trichosanthis	30	Clearing pathogenic heat and resolving phlegm; directing air downward to stop coughing	Coughing with yellow sticky sputum that is difficult to bring up; pneumonia; chronic bronchitis with expectoration of yellow sticky phlegm due to intense heat	6–9 g per dose; for decoction form, amounts of ingredients reduced but proportions kept the same
	Pericarpium Citri Reticulatae	30			
	Radix Scutellariae	30			
	Semen Armeniacae Amarum	30			
	Fructus Aurantii Immaturus	30			
	Poria	30			
	Arisaeme cum Bile	45			
	Rhizoma Pinelliae	45			

Prescription	Composition	Amount (grams)	Action(s)	Indication(s)	Remarks
Phlegm Eliminating Pills of Chloriteschist	*Radix et Rhizoma Rhei* *Radix Scutellariae* *Lignum Aquilariae Resinatum* *Chloriteschist*	240 240 15 30	Eliminating pathogenic fire and resolving phlegm	Insanity, coma, or asthmatic cough with sticky phlegm due to pathogenic fire; dizziness, constipation	6–9 g administered twice daily with warm water
Scrofula Bolus	*Radix Scrophulariae* *Concha Ostreae Usta* *Bulbus Fritillariae Thunbergii*	10 10 10	Clearing away pathogenic heat and resolving phlegm; softening and dispelling masses	Goiter; hyperthyroidism; thyroiditis; uncomplicated acute lymphadenitis	9 g per dose, twice daily

PHLEGM-DRYNESS ELIMINATING PRESCRIPTIONS

Prescription	Composition	Amount (grams)	Action(s)	Indication(s)	Remarks
Decoction of Fritillariae and Trichosanthis	*Bulbus Fritillariae Thunbergii* *Fructus Trichosanthis* *Radix Trichosanthis* *Poria* *Exocarpium Citri Grandis* *Radix Platycodi*	5 3 2 2 2 2	Moistening the lung and clearing away pathogenic heat; regulating the normal flow of vital energy and resolving phlegm	Difficulty in expectorating sputum, dry and sore throat, asthma and dyspnea due to adverse flow of vital energy	

COLD-PHLEGM ELIMINATING PRESCRIPTIONS

Prescription	Composition	Amount (grams)	Action(s)	Indication(s)	Remarks
Decoction of Three Kinds of Seeds for the Benefit of the Parents	*Semen Sinapis Albae*	6	Reversing the upward adverse flow of vital energy and improving digestion; removing phlegm and retained fluid	Asthmatic coughing, profuse sputum and anorexia, sensation of fullness in the chest and stomach	
	Fructus Perillae (fruit of purple perilla)	9			
	Semen Rephani	9			

WIND-PHLEGM EXPELLING PRESCRIPTIONS

Prescription	Composition	Amount (grams)	Action(s)	Indication(s)	Remarks
Antitussive Powder	*Radix Platycodi Praeparata*	960	Dispelling pathogenic wind and ventilating the lung; stopping cough and resolving phlegm	Coughing due to attack of the lung by pathogenic wind; various other kinds of coughing	6–9 g administered per dose; for decoction form, amounts of ingredients reduced but proportions kept the same
	Herba Schizonepetae	960			
	Radix Asteris	960			
	Radix Stemonae	960			
	Rhizoma Cynanchi Glaucescens	960			
	Radix Glycyrrhizae Praeparata	360			
	Pericarpium Citri Reticulatae	480			

Prescription	Composition	Amount (grams)	Action(s)	Indication(s)	Remarks
Decoction of Pinelliae, Atractylodes, and Gastrodiae	Rhizoma Pinelliae Rhizoma Gastrodiae Poria Exocarpium Citri Grandis Rhizoma Atractylodis Macrocephalae Radix Glycyrrhizae	9 6 6 6 9 2	Subduing endogenous wind and resolving phlegm	Giddiness and headache; otogenic or nervous vertigo	Decocted with 1 slice of ginger and 2 dates

Wind-Subduing Prescriptions

These prescriptions contain wind-dispelling herbs pungent in flavor for eliminating exogenous pathogenic wind, or herbs for subduing endogenous wind by nourishing vital essence and checking exuberant vital function.

PRESCRIPTIONS FOR DISPELLING EXOGENOUS WIND

Prescription	Composition	Amount (grams)	Action(s)	Indication(s)	Remarks
Wind-Eliminating Powder	Herba Schizonepetae Radix Ledebouriellae Radix Angelicae Sinensis	3 3 3	Dispelling pathogenic wind and heat; eliminating dampness and arresting itching	Eczema; urticaria; allergic dermatitis; ricefield dermatitis; drug rash; tinea	

		Action	Indication	Dosage
Radix Rehmanniae	3			
Radix Sophorae Flavescentis	3			
Rhizoma Atractylodis	3			
Periostracum Cicadae (cicada slough)	3			
Semen Sesami (black sesame)	3			
Fructus Aretii	3			
Rhizoma Anemarrhenae	3			
Gypsum Fibrosum	3			
Radix Glycyrrhizae	2			
Caulis Akebiae	2			
Mixture of Chuanxiong with Tea		Dispelling pathogenic wind to kill pain	Headache due to affection by exogenous wind, including migraine and pain in the top of the head; tension headache	6 g mixed with green tea, administered twice a day; for decoction form, amounts of ingredients reduced but proportions kept the same
Rhizoma Ligustici Chuanxiong	120			
Herba Schizonepetae	120			
Radix Angelicae Dahuricae	60			
Rhizoma seu Radix Notopterygii	60			
Radix Glycyrrhizae	60			
Herba Asari	30			
Radix Ledebouriellae	45			
Herba Menthae	240			

Prescription	Composition	Amount (grams)	Action(s)	Indication(s)	Remarks
Powder for Correcting Facial Deviation	*Rhizoma Typhonii* (typhonium tuber) *Bombyx Batrticatus* Scorpio (scorpion)	in equal amounts	Dispelling pathogenic wind and resolving phlegm; promoting the normal flow of vital energy in the channels to relieve spasm	Facial paralysis or muscular tics of the face due to apoplexy; trigeminal neuralgia due to obstruction of the channels by pathogenic wind	3 g per dose mixed with warm wine, administered twice a day; for decoction form, amounts of ingredients reduced but proportions kept the same
Mild Pills for Activating Blood Flow in Channels	*Radix Aconiti Praeparata* *Radix Aconiti Kusnezoffii Praeparata* (wild aconite root) *Lambricus* *Rhizoma Arisaematis Praeparata* *Resina Olibani* *Resina Myrrhae*	180 180 180 180 66 66	Activating the normal flow of vital energy in the channels; eliminating pathogenic wind and dampness; resolving phlegm and blood stasis	Numbness of the limbs due to apoplexy resulting from block of the channels and collaterals by blood stasis and dampness; arthralgia; contracture of the limbs; difficulty in movement; hemiplegia	6 g taken once or twice daily with old wine or warm water

PRESCRIPTIONS FOR SUBDUING ENDOGENOUS WIND

Prescription	Composition	Amount (grams)	Action(s)	Indication(s)	Remarks
Decoction for Checking Hyperactivity of the Liver and Subduing Endogenous Wind	Radix Achyranthis Bidentatae	30	Checking hyperactivity of the liver and subduing endogenous wind	Giddiness or motion impairment, Bell's palsy, unconsciousness due to hypertension; pheochromocytoma; premenstrual tension due to hyperfunction of the liver	
	Haematitum	30			
	Os Draconis	15			
	Concha Ostreae	15			
	Plastrum Testudinis	15			
	Radix Paeoniae	15			
	Radix Scrophulariae	15			
	Radix Asparagi	15			
	Fructus Meliae Toosendan	6			
	Fructus Hordei Germinatus	6			
	Herba Artemisiae Scopariae	6			
	Radix Glycyrrhizae	4			
Big Pearls for Stopping Wind	Radix Paeonia Alba	18	Nourishing vital essence and subduing endogenous wind	Unconsciousness and spasms of the limbs due to stirring up of endogenous wind; encephalitis B and the advanced stages of febrile diseases	Decoction is mixed with the yolks after the dregs are discarded
	Colla Corii Asini	9			
	Plastrum Testudinis	12			
	Radix Rehmanniae	18			
	Fructus Cannabis	6			
	Fructus Schisandrae	6			
	Concha Ostreae	12			
	Radix Ophiopogonis	18			
	Radix Glycyrrhizae	12			
	Praeparata raw egg yolk	2 yolks			
	Carapax Tronycis	12			

Prescription	Composition	Amount (grams)	Action(s)	Indication(s)	Remarks
Decoction of Rehmannia	Radix Rehmanniae	90	Nourishing vital essence of the kidney; invigorating vital function of the kidney; resolving phlegm and inducing resuscitation	Sudden loss of voice, inability to walk; syringomyelia	Ingredients ground into powder, 9 g per dose decocted with two slices of ginger, two peppermint leaves, and two dates
	Radix Morindae Officinalis	30			
	Fructus Corni	30			
	Herba Dendrobii	30			
	Herba Cistanchis	30			
	Fructus Schisandrae	15			
	Radix Aconiti Praeparata	30			
	Cortex Cinnamomi	30			
	Poria Alba	30			
	Radix Ophiopogonis	30			
	Rhizoma Acorus Graminei	30			
	Radix Polygalae	30			

Dryness-Eliminating Prescriptions

These prescriptions contain herbs warm or cool in property and bitter, pungent, or sweet in flavor. They are used to remove pathogenic dryness.

Prescription	Composition	Amount (grams)	Action(s)	Indication(s)	Remarks
Powder of Bitter Armeniacae and Perillae	Folium Perillae	9	Dispelling pathogenic cold-dryness; ventilating the lung and resolving phlegm	Chronic bronchitis, bronchiectasis, emphysema due to affliction with pathogenic cold-dryness	Amounts of ingredients adjusted according to patient's condition
	Semen Armeniacae Amarum	5			
	Rhizoma Zingeberis	9			
	Radix Platycodi	9			

Prescription	Ingredients	Amount	Action	Indication
	Poria	9		
	Rhizoma Pinelliae	9		
	Radix Glycyrrhizae	6		
	Radix Peucedani	9		
	Pericarpium Citri Reticulatae	9		
	Fructus Aurantii			
	Fructus Ziziphi Jujubae	3 dates		
Decoction for Restoring Lung Function by Clearing Pathogenic Heat	*Folium Mori*	9	Eliminating pathogenic dryness from the lung	Impairment of the lung by pathogenic dryness, marked by headache, fever, unproductive cough, asthma
	Calcined Gypsum Fibrosum	15		
	Radix Glycyrrhizae	3		
	Fructus Cannabis	3		
	Radix Ginseng	2		
	Colla Corii Asini	3		
	Radix Ophiopogonis	4		
	Semen Armeniacae Amarum	2		
	Folium Eriobotryae	6		
Decoction to Replenish Vital Essence and Remove Pathogenic Factors From the Lung	*Radix Rehmanniae*	9	Replenishing vital essence of the lung and removing pathogenic factors from the lung	Diphtheria, tonsillitis, laryngopharyngitis, nasopharyngeal cancer due to deficiency of vital essence
	Radix Ophiopogonia	6		
	Radix Glycyrrhizae	2		
	Radix Scrophulariae	6		
	Bulbus Fritillariae Cirrhosae	6		
	Cortex Moutan	3		
	Herba Menthae	2		
	Radix Paeoniae Alba Praeparata	3		

Prescription	Composition	Amount (grams)	Action(s)	Indication(s)	Remarks
Decoction of Lilii for Strengthening the Lung	Radix Rehmannia	6	Nourishing vital essence and clearing pathogenic heat from the lung; removing dryness from the lung and resolving phlegm	Dry-pain of the throat, asthmatic cough, bloody sputum, feverish sensation of the palms, soles, and heart region; pulmonary tuberculosis; tracheitis; bronchiectasis due to deficiency of vital essence of the lung and kidney	
	Radix Rehmannia Praeparata	9			
	Radix Ophiopogonis	5			
	Bulbus Lilii (lily bulb)	2			
	Radix Paeoniae	2			
	Radix Angelicae Sinensis	2			
	Bulbus Fritillariae Cirrhosiae	2			
	Radix Scrophulariae	2			
	Radix Platycodi	2			
	Radix Glycyrrhizae	2			
Decoction of Ophiopogonis	Radix Ophiopogonis	35	Activating vital function of the stomach to generate fluid and reverse the adverse upward flow of vital energy	Lung cancer; pleurisy due to deficiency of vital essence of the lung and stomach; asthma, shortness of breath; tuberculosis; chronic bronchitis	
	Rhizoma Pinelliae	5			
	Radix Ginseng	5			
	Radix Glycyrrhizae Praeparata	3			
	Semen Oryzae Nongglutinosae	5			
	Fructus Ziziphi Jujubae	4 dates			

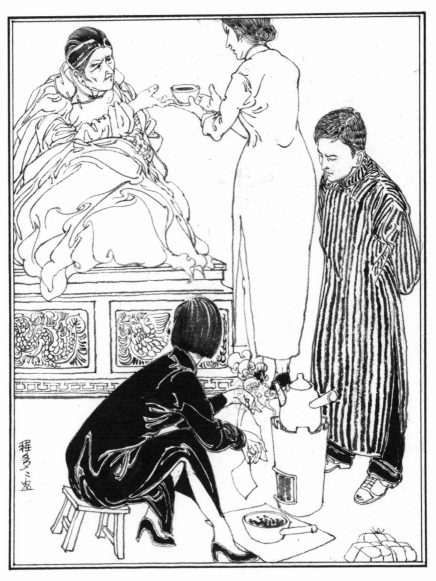

Family member preparing an herbal decoction for mother, who is ill.

CHAPTER FOUR

———◆———

Treatment of
Some Common Conditions

TRADITIONAL CHINESE MEDICINE emphasizes the careful observation and analysis of pathologic conditions. Only when the patient's disease state is understood according to the theories described in volume 1 can appropriate treatment be prescribed. This chapter describes how various common conditions are treated in keeping with this principle. The conditions discussed are the following: the common cold, fever due to internal injury, pneumonia, pleurisy, acute gastroenteritis, diarrhea, primary hypertension, coronary atherosclerotic heart disease, cerebrovascular accident, nephritis, low back pain, seminal emission, impotence, insomnia, and syncope.

THE COMMON COLD

The cold is a common affection by exogenous pathogenic factors. It is manifested by nasal obstruction, rhinorrhea, sneezing, headache, chills, fever, cough, and sore throat. Common colds occur throughout the year, especially in winter and spring. A severe case is called "a bad cold attacked by pathogenic wind or cold." "A prevalent bad cold" denotes an especially severe cold.

What traditional Chinese medicine calls the common cold encompasses a wide range of disorders in Western medicine: upper respiratory infection due to bacteria or viruses, acute tonsillitis, and the early stages of many infectious diseases. Influenza falls within the category of prevalent bad cold and can be treated accordingly.

Etiology

"The common cold is caused by exogenous pathogenic factors. But when invasion of the channels by strong pathogenic factors succeeds, a bad cold occurs" ("Treatise on the Common Cold," *Jingyue's Complete Works*).

The onset of the common cold is often closely related to abnormal weather. For instance, if it is cold in spring instead of warm, cool in summer instead of hot, hot in autumn instead of cool, or warm in winter instead of cold, pathogenic wind, cold, summer heat, or dampness will attack and cause common cold or prevalent bad cold. Invasion by pathogenic factors can also occur when an irregular lifestyle or overexertion lowers defensive vital function of the superficial portion of the body. The lung is associated with the skin surface; it has its specific body opening in the nose. When pathogenic wind or cold attacks the body through the skin and nose, the lung is the site first attacked. The lung fails to keep inspired air flowing downward; thus symptoms such as coughing, asthma, oliguria, and edema may occur.

Essentials of Diagnosis and Treatment

The common cold is due to pathogenic wind or cold or to contagious infection. Manifestations of functional disturbance in the superficial defensive system occur in the common cold. Severe generalized manifestations are present in the prevalent bad cold.

Differentiation of the disorders—for example, whether they are of exterior-cold or exterior-heat, or of exterior-deficiency or exterior-excessiveness—is based on assessment of aversion to cold, fever, perspiration, pulse, and tongue coating. The seasons, climatic changes, and affection by different pathogenic factors should also be considered.

Because the illness is a superficial disorder, the therapeutic approach is to dispel pathogenic factors from the exterior of the body by diaphoresis. In patients of weak constitution or advanced age, it is necessary to strengthen body resistance in addition to dispelling the invading pathogenic factors.

Treatment According to Differentiation of Symptom-Complexes

COMMON COLD DUE TO PATHOGENIC WIND-COLD. Manifestations: Chills, no or moderate fever, absence of sweat, nasal obstruction, watery nasal discharge, sneezing, headache, aching joints, tickling sensation in the throat, cough with expectoration of scanty sputum, thin pale tongue coating, floating or tight pulse.

Principle of treatment: Dispelling pathogenic cold from the exterior of the body and restoring the normal function of the lung with medicinal herbs pungent in flavor and warm in property.

Prescription: Antiphlogistic Decoction of Schizonepeta and Ledebouriella, with Modifications.

Herba Schizonepetae	6	grams
Radix Ledebouriellae	6	"
Rhizoma seu Radix Notopterygii	9	"
Radix Peucedani	9	"
Fructus Aurantii	9	"
Radix Platycodi	9	"
Semen Armeniacae Amarum	9	"
Rhizoma Ligustici Chuanxiong	6	"
Radix Glycyrrhizae	6	"

Modifications include: For cases with severe chills, absence of sweating, and floating tight pulse, add 9 grams *Ramulus Cinnamomi,* or substitute Ephedra Decoction:

Herba Ephedrae	6	grams
Ramulus Cinnamomi	9	"
Semen Armeniacae Amarum	9	"
Folium Perillae	6	"
Radix Puerariae	9	"
Radix Glycyrrhizae	6	"

For cases with severe headache, add 9 grams *Rhizoma Ligustici Chuanxiong* and 6 grams *Radix Angelicae Dahuricae.*

For cases with nasal obstruction, add 9 grams *Flos Magnoliae* (magnolia flower).

For cases with heaviness of the head, fatigue, feeling of oppression in the chest, nausea, anorexia, lack of taste sensation, and slimy white tongue coating, add 9 grams *Cortex Magnoliae Officinalis,* 9 grams *Pericarpium Citri Reticulatae,* 9 grams *Rhizoma Atractylodis,* and 9 grams *Rhizoma Pinelliae.*

COMMON COLD DUE TO PATHOGENIC WIND-HEAT. Manifestations: High fever, slight intolerance of wind and cold, sweating, headache, nasal obstruction, thick nasal discharge, dry and sore throat, cough with expectoration of scanty sticky sputum, thin yellow tongue coating, floating and rapid pulse.

Principle of treatment: Dispelling pathogenic heat from the exterior of the body and the lung.

Prescription: Decoction of Lonicera and Forsythia, with Modifications.

Flos Lonicerae	15 grams
Fructus Forsythiae	15 "
Fructus Arctii	6 "
Herba Menthae (added when decoction is nearly done)	6 "
Radix Isatidis	15 "
Radix Scrophulariae	9 "
Radix Platycodi	9 "
Herba Schizonepetae	6 "
Herba Lophatheri	3 "
Radix Glycyrrhizae	6 "

Modifications include: For cases with severe cough and expectoration of purulent sputum, omit *Herba Schizonepetae,* and add 9 grams *Bulbus Fritillariae,* 9 grams *Radix Peucedani,* and 9 grams *Semen Armeniacae Amarum.*

For cases with sore, swollen throat or tonsillitis, add 30 grams *Flos Lonicerae,* 9 grams *Rhizoma Belamcandae* (blackberry lily) and 9 grams *Radix Sophorae Subprostratae.*

For severe cases due to pathogenic wind-heat, marked by high fever, headache, dry nose, thirst and reddened tongue with yellow coating, add 9 grams *Radix Puerariae,* 9 grams *Radix Scutellariae,* 30 grams *Gypsum Fibrosum,* 9 grams *Rhizoma Anemarrhenae,* and 12 grams *Radix Trichosanthis.*

For cases with pathogenic dampness, heaviness of the head, fatigue, feeling of oppression in the chest, and slimy yellow tongue coating, add 12 grams *Herba Agastachis,* and 12 grams *Herba Eupatorii.*

Seasonal Common Cold

COMMON COLD DUE TO PATHOGENIC SUMMER-HEAT AND DAMP-NESS. Manifestations: Protracted high fever, chills, sweating, lassitude, fatigue, thirst, concentrated urine, reddened tongue with slimy yellow coating, soft and rapid pulse.

Principle of treatment: Dispelling pathogenic summer-heat and dampness from the exterior of the body.

Prescription: Renewed Decoction of Elsholtzia, with Modifications.

Herba Agastachis	9	grams
Flos Lonicerae	15	"
Herba Elsholtziae seu Moslae	9	"
Cortex Magnoliae Officinal	4	"
Flos Dolichoris	12	"
Talcum	15	"
Flos Chrysanthemi	9	"
Herba Eupatorii	9	"

Modifications include: For cases with exuberant summer-heat, add 9 grams *Radix Scutellariae,* 6 grams *Rhizoma Coptidis,* and 6 grams *Fructus Gardeniae.*

For cases with exuberant dampness, add 9 grams *Poria,* 6 grams *Rhizoma Pinelliae,* 9 grams *Pericarpium Citri Reticulatae,* and 12 grams *Rhizoma Atractylodis.*

COMMON COLD DUE TO EXUBERANT PATHOGENIC DAMPNESS DURING THE LONG SUMMER PERIOD (JUNE). Manifestations: Moderate fever, chills, absence of sweating, extreme heaviness of the head and joints, cough with expectoration of purulent sputum, feeling of oppression in the chest, nausea, vomiting, anorexia, lack of taste sensation, loose stools, slimy white tongue coating, soft and slow pulse.

Principle of treatment: Dispelling pathogenic dampness from the exterior of the body.

Prescription: Notoptergyium Decoction for Eliminating Dampness.

Rhizoma seu Radix Notopterygii	9 grams
Radix Angelicae Pulescentis	9 "
Rhizoma Ligustici	9 "
Radix Ledebouriellae	6 "
Rhizoma Ligustici Chuanxiong	9 "
Fructus Vitex	9 "
Herba Agastachis	9 "
Herba Eupatorii	9 "
Rhizoma Atractylodis	9 "
Radix Glycyrrhizae	6 "

Modifications: For cases with nausea, vomiting, feeling of oppression in the chest, abdominal distension, and loose stools, add 9 grams *Pericarpium Citri Reticulatae,* 6 grams *Rhizoma Pinnelliae,* 6 grams *Cortex Magnoliae Officinal,* 12 grams *Semen Coicis,* and 9 grams *Semen Myristicae* or substitute Powder of Agastache for Dispelling Turbidity.

COMMON COLD DUE TO PATHOGENIC DRYNESS IN AUTUMN. Manifestations: Fever, chills, headache, dry unproductive cough, dry mouth and nose, thirst, reddened tongue with thin coating and scanty saliva, floating and rapid pulse.

Principle of treatment: Dispelling pathogenic wind and dryness to soothe the disturbed lung and generate saliva.

Prescription: Decoction of Mori and Armeniacae, with Modifications.

Folium Mori	9 grams
Semen Armeniacae Amerum	9 "
Radix Platycodi	9 "
Radix Glehniae	12 "
Radix Ophiopogonis	12 "
Bulbus Fritillariae	9 "
Fructus Gardeniae	9 "

Modifications include: For cases with dry, itchy throat, add 9 grams *Fructus Arctii.*

For cases with expectoration of purulent sputum, add 15 grams *Fructus Trichosanthis* and 15 grams *Fructus Aristolochiae* (birthwort fruit).

For cases with epistaxis, add 15 grams *Rhizoma Imperatae* and 9 grams *Radix Rehmannia.*

COMMON COLD DUE TO WEAK CONSTITUTION

COMMON COLD DUE TO DEFICIENCY OF VITAL ENERGY AND AFFECTION BY PATHOGENIC WIND-COLD. Manifestations: Chills, fever, headache, nasal obstruction, cough with expectoration of white sputum, lassitude, shortness of breath, apathy, pale tongue with white coating, floating and forceless pulse.

Principle of treatment: Reinforcing vital energy to dispel pathogenic factors from the exterior of the body.

Prescription: Decoction of Codonopsis and Perillae, with Modifications.

Radix Codonopsis Pilosulae	9 grams
Folium Perillae	6 "
Radix Puerariae	9 "
Radix Peucedani	9 "
Rhizoma Pinelliae	9 "
Poria	9 "
Exocarpium Citri Grandis	9 "
Radix Platycodi	9 "
Fructus Aurantii	9 "
Rhizoma Zingiberis Recens	3 slices
Fructus Ziziphi Jujubae	3 dates

Modifications: For cases with severe deficiency of vital energy, substitute Decoction for Reinforcing Vital Energy and Strengthening the Spleen and Stomach with Modifications.

For cases with spontaneous sweating, substitute Jade Screen Powder: *Radix Astragali, Rhizoma Atractylodis Macrocephalae,* and *Radix Ledebouriellae.*

RECURRENT COMMON COLD DUE TO LOWERED VITAL FUNCTION. Manifestations: Moderate fever, severe chills, generalized aching, headache, presence or absence of sweating, pallor, apathy, cold limbs, flabby tongue with white coating, deep and forceless pulse.

Principle of treatment: Reinforcing vital function and vital energy to dispel pathogenic factors from the exterior of the body.

Prescription: Rehabilitation Powder, with Modifications.

Radix Ginseng	3 grams
Radix Astragali	15　"
Ramulus Cinnamomi	6　"
Radix Paeoniae Alba	9　"
Radix Glycyrrhizae	3　"
Radix Aconiti Praeparata	3　"
Herba Asari	3　"
Rhizoma seu Radix Notopterygii (notopterygium root)	6　"
Radix Ledebouriellae	6　"
Rhizoma Ligustici Chuanxiong	6　"
Rhizoma Zingiberis Recens	3 slices
Fructus Ziziphi Jujubae	3 dates

Modifications include: For cases with severe chills, add 6 grams *Herba Schizonepetae* and 3 grams *Folium Perillae.*

COMMON COLD DUE TO DEFICIENCY OF BLOOD. This condition results from want of blood after an illness, loss of blood, or lack of proper care after childbirth, together with affliction by exogenous pathogenic factors.

Manifestations: Headache, fever, slight chills, absence of sweating, haggard look, pale lips and nails, palpitation, dizziness, pale tongue with white coating, and thready or floating forceless pulse.

Principle of treatment: Nourishing the blood to dispel pathogenic factors from the exterior of the body.

Prescription: Decoction of Caulis Allii and Seven Other Herbs, with Modifications.

Radix Rehmannia	15 grams
Radix Ophiopogonis	9　"
Radix Puerariae	6　"
Semen Sojae Praeparatum	6　"
Caulis Allii Fistulosum	3 inches

Modifications include: For cases with severe chills, add 6 grams *Folium Perillae* and 6 grams *Herba Schizonepetae.*

For cases with high fever, add 9 grams *Flos Lonicerae,* 9 grams *Fructus Forsythiae,* and 6 grams *Radix Scutellariea.*

COMMON COLD DUE TO DEFICIENCY OF VITAL ESSENCE. Manifestations: Headache, fever, slight intolerance of wind and cold, presence or absence of sweating, dizziness, restlessness, thirst, hot sensation in the palms and soles, dry cough, thready and rapid pulse.

Principle of treatment: Replenishing vital essence to dispel pathogenic factors from the exterior of the body.

Prescription: Decoction of Polygonatum Odoratum, with Modifications.

Rhizoma Polygonati Odorati	9 grams
Radix Platydedi	6 "
Radix Cynanchi Atrati	6 "
Semen Sojae Praeparatum (fermented soya beans)	6 "
Herba Menthae	6 "
Radix Glycyrrhizae	3 "
Caulis Allii Fistulosum	2 inches
Fructus Ziziphi Jujubae	3 dates

Modifications include: For severe cases, add 6 grams *Herba Schizonepetae* and 6 grams *Radix Ledebouriellae.*

For cases with unproductive cough, add 6 grams *Pericarpium Trichosanthis* and 3 grams *Fructus Arctii.*

For cases with thirst, add 6 grams *Herba Lophatheri* and 9 grams *Radix Trichosanthis.*

Other Common Methods of Preventing and Treating Common Colds

PROVEN RECIPES [1]

Decoction given to prevent influenza:

Folium Isatidis	30 grams
Radix Isatidis	30 "
Rhizoma Cyrtomii (cyrtomium rhizome)	30 "

1. Proven recipes are folk remedies; they are simple and effective, and are commonly used in the incipient stage of a disease or to prevent a disease. Classic prescriptions, on the other hand, are prescriptions that have been used effectively through the years and subsequently have been recorded in the classics.

Decoction given to treat common cold:

Radix Isatidis	9 grams
Herba Houttuyniae	15 "

Decoction to treat common cold or cold brought on by drenching:

Caulis Allii Fistulosum	5 sticks
Rhizoma Zingiberis Recens	3 slices

Decocted with brown sugar.
Decoction given to prevent common cold in summer:

Herba Agastachis	15 grams
Flos Chrysanthemi Indici	30 "
Folium Nelumbinis	30 "

To prevent influenza, put 150 grams *Rhizoma Cyrtomii* wrapped in gauze in the bottom of drinking-water container as a beverage for persons at risk.

ACUPUNCTURE TREATMENT

Main points: Fengchi (GB 20), Hegu (LI 4), Lieque (Lu 7), Dazhui (Du 14).
Points according to manifestations:

Nasal obstruction—Yingxiang (LI 20)
Headache—Fengchi (GB 20), Taiyang (Extra 2)
High fever—Quchi (LI 11)
Cough—Tiantu (Ren 22), Feishu (UB 13)
Sore throat—Shaoshang (Lu 11), prick to bloodlet
Anorexia—Zusanli (St 36)

Reducing method with strong stimulation is applied until sweating is induced.

EAR ACUPUNCUTRE THERAPY. Internal Nose, Forehead, Occiput, Adrenal, Subcortex

---

CASE HISTORY
Male, age 40, first visit on March 5, 1971.

History

The patient was in good health until three days before being seen in the clinic. His complaints included fever, intolerance of cold, absence of sweating, aching limb joints, nasal obstruction, coarse breathing, restlessness, sore throat, cough with expectoration of purulent sputum, shortness of breath, and concentrated urine.

Diagnosis and Treatment

On examination, a yellow tongue coating and floating and rapid pulse were found. It was concluded that the disease was due to retention of pathogenic heat in the lung plus exogenous affection by pathogenic wind-cold, resulting in symptoms of exogenous cold and endogenous heat.

It was thus considered advisable to dispel wind-cold and clear heat from the lung. Therefore, Decoction of Ephedra, Armeniacae, Gypsum, and Glycyrrhizae, with Modifications, was prescribed:

Herba Ephedrae	6	grams
Gypsum Fibrosum	30	"
Semen Armeniacae Amarum	9	"
Radix Glycyrrhizae	4.5	"
Radix Ledebouriellae	9	"
Cortex Mori	9	"
Radix Scutellariae	9	"

After three doses, the fever disappeared through sweating. Then two doses of the same decoction with *Fructus Gardeniae* added were administered.

When the patient came to the clinic on March 12, the symptoms were nearly gone, and treatment was stopped.

—From Pan Yangzhi, *A Collection of Case Histories of Traditional Chinese Medicine* (Gansu People's Publishing House, 1981), pp. 182–83.

Two or three of the above points are selected for each treatment; needles are retained for 30 minutes.

FEVER DUE TO INTERNAL INJURY

This condition is caused by consumption of *yin, yang,* vital energy, and/or blood, or by an imbalance thereof. The fever usually is moderate, but sometimes it is high. This category also includes a sensation of heat felt in the chest, palms, and soles although body temperature is normal. It encompasses any moderate fever caused by tumor, blood disorders, connective tissue disorders, endocrine disorders, tuberculosis, or other chronic infectious disease.

Etiology

Such fever can be caused by the following:

- In patients with deficiency symptoms, impairment of vital energy and vital essence by febrile disease.
- Impairment of vital essence by overdose of herbs warm in property, leading to disharmony of *yin* and *yang* and thus to internal growth of pathogenic fire.
- Massive hemorrhage, deficiency of blood in the liver and heart, or consumption of essence and blood due to failure of the spleen to generate blood.
- Overexertion, improper diet, or sinking of vital energy of the stomach and spleen.
- Stagnancy of vital energy of the liver due to emotional strain.
- Blood stasis due to stagnancy of vital energy or to trauma.
- Lowered vital function in patients with deficiency symptoms, or lowered vital function of the kidney, leading to superficial pseudo-heat manifestations.

Essentials of Diagnosis and Treatment

It is most important to distinguish fever due to internal injury from that due to exogenous affection. The differences are listed below:

	Fever Due to Internal Injury	*Fever Due to Exogenous Affection*
Disease history	Slow onset and protracted course	Sudden onset and short course
Nature of fever	Moderate fever or a heat sensation; chills relieved by keeping warm	High fever; chills not relieved by keeping warm
Manifestations	Dizziness, lassitude, spontaneous and night sweats, forceless pulse	Headache, nasal obstruction, floating pulse

Treatment of fever due to internal injury should be in keeping with the cause. It is inadvisable to administer only diaphoretics or herbs cool in nature. Such agents may impede the vital function of the spleen or injure vital essence, and thus they may worsen the condition.

Treatment According to Differentiation of Symptom-Complexes

FEVER DUE TO DEFICIENCY OF VITAL ESSENCE. Manifestations: Moderate fever or afternoon fever, night sweats, heat sensation in the chest, palms, and soles, malar flush, insomnia, excessive dreaming during sleep, restlessness, dry mouth, dizziness, weakness of the back and knees, reddened tongue without coating or with scanty coating, thready and rapid pulse.

Principle of treatment: Replenishing vital essence to eliminate pathogenic heat.

Prescription: Decoction for Removing Heat from the Bones, with Modifications.

Carapax Trionycis	9	grams
Rhizoma Anemarrhenae	9	"
Radix Rehmannia	6	"
Radix Scrophulariae	9	"
Radix Polygoni Multiflori	15	"
Cortex Lycii Radicis	9	"
Radix Stellariae	9	"
Herba Artemiziae Chinghao	9	"
Radix Gentianae Macrophyllae	9	"
Rhizoma Picrorrhizae	6	"

Modifications include: For cases with marked dryness of the mouth, add 12 grams *Bulbus Lilii* and 9 grams *Radix Ophiopogonis.*

For cases with severe insomnia, add 15 grams *Semen Ziziphi Spinosae,* 9 grams *Semen Biotae,* and 9 grams *Caulis Polygoni Multiflori.*

For cases with prominent night sweats, add 15 grams *Concha Ostreae* and 30 grams *Fructus Tritici Levis.*

For cases with restlessness, dry mouth, reddened tongue, and malar flush due to flaring up of fire, substitute Major Bolus for Tonifying Vital Essence, which consists of 2 grams *Cortex Phellodendri,* 2 grams *Rhizoma Anemarrhenae,* 3 grams *Radix Rehmanniae Praeparata,* and 3 grams *Plastrum Testudinis*. Or Substitute Rehmanniae Bolus of Anemarrhenae and Phellodendri, which consists of 4.5 grams *Radix Rehmannia Praeparata*, 3 grams *Fructus Corni*, 3 grams *Rhizoma Dioscoreae*, 3 grams *Poria*, 3 grams *Cortex Moutan Radicis*, 3 grams *Rhizoma Anemarrhenae*, and 3 grams *Cortex Phellodendri*.

FEVER DUE TO DEFICIENCY OF BLOOD. Manifestations: Protracted moderate fever, pale or livid complexion, emaciation, dizziness, palpitation, lassitude, spontaneous or night sweats, insomnia, amnesia, scanty menstruation or excessive menstrual bleeding, pale tongue with white coating, deep and rapid pulse.

Principle of treatment: Tonifying the blood and reinforcing vital energy to relieve fever.

Prescription: Decoction of Four Herbs, with Modifications.

Radix Angelicae Sinensis	9 grams
Radix Rehmannia Praeparata	18 "
Radix Paeoniae Alba	9 "
Radix Codonopsis Pilosula	15 "
Colla Corri Asini (mixed in with the decoction)	9 "
Carapax Trionycis	15 "

FEVER DUE TO DEFICIENCY OF VITAL ENERGY. Manifestations: Onset of moderate or high fever after over-exertion, dizziness, lassitude, spontaneous sweating, shortness of breath, apathy, anorexia, loose stools, pale tongue, thready weak or empty rapid pulse.

Principle of treatment: Reinforcing vital energy to strengthen superficial resistance and eliminate pathogenic heat.

Prescription: Decoction for Reinforcing Vital Energy and Strengthening the Spleen and Stomach.

Radix Astragali	12 grams
Radix Codonopsis Pilosula	12 "
Rhizoma Atractylodis Macrocephalae Praeparata	9 "
Radix Angelica Sinensis	9 "
Rhizoma Cimicifugae	3 "
Radix Bupleuri	6 "
Radix Ophiopogonis	9 "
Fructus Schisandrae (Chinese magnoliavine fruit)	6 "
Radix Glycyrrhizae Praeparata	6 "

Modifications include: For cases with frequent spontaneous sweating, add 15 grams *Concha Ostreae Usta* and 15 grams *Os Draconis Usta*.

For cases with alternating fever and chills, sweating, and intolerance of wind, add 6 grams *Ramulus Cinnamomi* and 9 grams *Radix Paeoniae Alba*.

For cases with feeling of oppression in the chest and slimy white tongue coating due to pathogenic dampness, add 9 grams *Rhizoma Atractylodis,* 9 grams *Poria,* and 6 grams *Cortex Magnoliae Officinalis.*

For cases with moderate fever and thirst due to summer heat, omit *Radix Astragali, Radix Angelica Sinensis,* and *Radix Bupleuri* and add 3 grams *Rhizoma Coptidis,* 9 grams *Caulis Nelumbinis,* and 30 grams *Exocarpium Citrulli* (watermelon peel).

FEVER DUE TO DEFICIENCY OF VITAL ENERGY AND VITAL ESSENCE. Manifestations: Protracted moderate fever after subsidence of high fever, lassitude, dry mouth, dry unproductive cough, reddened tongue with scanty coating, thready and rapid pulse.

Principle of treatment: Reinforcing vital energy and replenishing vital essence to relieve fever.

Prescription: Decoction of Lophatheri and Gypsum, with Modifications.

Radix Glehniae	12 grams
Radix Ophiopogonis	12 "
Radix Codonopsis Pilosulae	9 "
Fructus Schisandrae	9 "
Cortex Mori Radicis	9 "
Gypsum Fibrosum	12 "
Radix Cynanchi Atrati	9 "
Rhizoma Pinelliae	6 "
Herba Lophatheri (bamboo leaf)	3 "
Caulis Bambusae in Taenium	9 "

Modifications include: For cases with dry unproductive cough, add 6 grams *Semen Armeniacae Amarum* and 12 grams *Folium Eriobotryae.*

FEVER DUE TO LOWERED VITAL FUNCATION. Manifestations: Fever, malar flush, chills, cold limbs, dyspnea, palpitation, headache, somnolence, aching in the low back and knees, oliguria, swollen feet, pale flabby moist tongue with teethprints along the borders and white coating, deep threaty weak or floating forceless pulse.

Principle of treatment: Invigorating the function of the kidney to dispel pathogenic cold.

Prescription: Decoction for Reinforcing Vital Function of the Kidney, with Modifications.

Radix Rehmannia Praeparata	18 grams
Fructus Corni	9 "
Semen Cuscutae	9 "
Radix Angelica Sinensis	9 "
Radix Glycyrrhizae Praeparata	6 "
Cortex Cinnamomi	1.5 "

FEVER DUE TO STAGNANCY OF VITAL ENERGY. Manifestations: Heat sensation due to emotional strain, restlessness, irritability or depression, distension of the hypochondria, frequent sighing, bitter taste in the mouth, menstrual disorders, dysmenorrhea, reddened tongue with light yellow coating, taut and rapid pulse.

Principle of treatment: Restoring smooth flow of vital energy of the liver to eliminate pathogenic heat.

Prescription: Ease Decoction with Moutan and Gardeniae.

Radix Bupleuri	9 grams
Radix Paeoniae Alba	9 "
Radix Angelica Sinensis	9 "
Cortex Moutan Radicis	9 "
Herba Menthae	6 "
Radix Scutellariae	6 "
Poria	9 "
Rhizoma Atractylodis Macrocephalae	9 "
Radix Cynanchi Atrati (swallow wort root)	6 "
Fructus Gardeniae	6 "
Folium Mori	6 "

Modifications include: For cases with prominent heat sensation, dry mouth, and constipation, omit *Rhizoma Atractylodis Macrocephalae* and *Poria,* and add 9 grams *Radix Scutellariae.*

For cases with pain in the hypochondria, add 9 grams *Fructus Meliae Toosendan* and 9 grams *Radix Curcumae.*

For cases with fever and lower abdominal pain during menstruation, omit *Radix Scutellariae* and add 9 grams *Pollen Typhae* and 9 grams *Faeces Trogopterorum*.

FEVER DUE TO BLOOD STASIS. Manifestations: Moderate fever that is more severe at night or sometimes high fever, dry mouth, fixed pain in the limbs or masses in the limbs, livid complexion, purple lips, thready and choppy pulse.

Principle of treatment: Invigorating the flow of blood to remove stasis and pathogenic heat.

Prescription: Decoction for Removing Blood Stasis from the Chest, with Modifications.

Radix Angelica Sinensis	9	grams
Radix Rehmannia	6	"
Radix Paeoniae Rubra	6	"
Rhizoma Ligustici Chuanxiong	6	"
Semen Persicae	6	"
Flos Carthami	6	"
Radix Achyranthis Bidentatae (bidentate achyranthes root)	9	"
Radix Bupleuri	6	"
Fructus Aurantii	6	"
Cortex Moutan Radicis	6	"
Eupolyphaga seu Steleophaga (ground beetle)	6	"
Radix et Rhizoma Rhei	3	"

Other Common Methods of Treating Fever Due to Internal Injury

ACUPUNCTURE TREATMENT FOR FEVER

Main points: Dazhui (Du 14), Quchi (LI 11), and Fuliu (K 7). Points according to manifestations:

Afternoon fever—Yuji (Lu 10)
High fever—Shixuan (Ex 30), prick to bloodlet
Stuffiness in the chest—Neiguan (P 6)
Anorexia—Zusanli (St 36) and Pishu (UB 20)

CASE HISTORY

Female, age 40, first visit on June 17, 1973.

History

Complaints included afternoon fever (37.7°–37.8° C), numbness of the legs at night, and lassitude.

Diagnosis and Treatment

On examination, a thready and rapid pulse and slightly reddened tongue without coating were found. It was concluded that the condition was due to deficiency of vital essence and to endogenous intense heat. The patient was prescribed a decoction of the following ingredients:

Radix Rehmannia	24 grams	
Fructus Corni	12	"
Rhizoma Dioscoreae	12	"
Cortex Moutan Radicis	12	"
Rhizoma Alismatis	9	"
Poria	9	"
Radix Bupleuri	9	"
Fructus Schizandrae	6	"
Radix Paeoniae Alba	9	"
Cortex Cinnamomi	6	"

This decoction is used to replenish vital energy and dispel intense heat in order to relieve moderate fever.

The patient paid a second visit on June 26. The moderate fever had subsided after seven doses. The patient was advised to take ten doses more to improve her health.

—From *A Collection of Case Records* by Dr.
Yue Meizhong, compiled by Academy of
Traditional Chinese Medicine (People's
Medical Publishing House, 1978), p. 100.

Uniform reducing and reinforcing method is applied for moderate fever, and reducing method for high fever.

EAR-ACUPUNCTURE THERAPY. Ear-Shenmen, Sympathetic Nerve, Lung, Subcortex.

One or two points are selected for each treatment, and needles are embedded for three to five days.

PNEUMONIA

Pneumonia (including lobar pneumonia, bronchopneumonia, and atypical pneumonia) is inflammation of the lung caused by bacterial or viral infection. Clinically, fever, chills, coughing, shortness of breath, and chest pain are commonly present. In traditional Chinese medicine, forms of pneumonia are known as "acute febrile disease caused by pathogenic wind," "invasion of the lung by pathogenic heat," and "asthmatic breathing due to lung trouble."

Etiology

Pneumonia is due to blockage of the lung by phlegm-heat; it occurs when excessive heat in the lung, in conjunction with invasion of pathogenic wind, impedes normal flow of vital energy of the lung. If the pathogenic factors remain in the *qi* (secondary defensive) system, the *ying* (nutrient) system may become involved. In severe cases, pathogenic factors dominate, and there is a decline of body resistance—a critical condition that may result in prostration due to depletion of *yang*. Deficiencies of vital energy and vital essence are often found in the late stage of the disease.

Essentials of Diagnosis and Treatment

In diagnosis, the stage of invasion by pathogenic wind (i.e., invasion of the *wei, qi, ying,* or *xue* system) should be determined. Clinically, there are five kinds of symptom-complexes: invasion of the lung by pathogenic wind; blockage of the lung by phlegm-heat; penetration of pathogenic heat into the pericardium; prostration due to exhaustion of *yang* and accumulation of pathogenic heat; and deficiency of vital energy and vital essence.

Because the disease is located in the lung and the causative factor is phlegm-heat, the treatment is focused on removing toxic heat from the lung and resolving phlegm. The development of the disease can be controlled only if large dosages of drugs for eliminating toxic heat are administered, for the disease often evolves rapidly.

Prostration due to exhaustion of *yang* and accumulation of pathogenic heat is a critical condition and demands first the use of emergency treatment to check profuse sweating and rescue the patient by reinforcing vital function and vital energy. Then the condition is treated according to the root cause.

Treatment Based on the Differentiation of Symptom-Complexes

INVASION OF THE LUNG BY PATHOGENIC WIND (usually seen in atypical pneumonia and bronchopneumonia). Manifestations: Fever, intolerance of cold, cough, expectoration of white mucoid or purulent sputum, suffocating or painful sensation in the chest, thirst, reddened tongue border, thin white or light yellow tongue coating, floating and rapid pulse.

Principle of treatment: Dispelling pathogenic factors from the exterior of the body with herbs pungent in flavor and cool in property.

Prescription: Decoction of Lonicera and Forsythia, with Modifications.

Flos Lonicerae	15 grams
Fructus Forsythiae	15 "
Herba Lophatheri	6 "
Herba Schizonepetae	6 "
Herba Menthae	6 "
Radix Peucedani	6 "
Semen Armeniacae Amarum	9 "
Semen Sojae Praeparatum	9 "
Cortex Mori Radicis	12 "
Pericarpium Trichosanthis (peel of snakegourd fruit)	12 "
Radix Scutellariae	9 "

Modifications include: For cases with dull pain in the hypochondrium, add 9 grams *Radix Paeonia Rubra* and 9 grams *Radix Curcumae*.

For cases with extreme heat and restlessness, add 9 grams *Fructus Gardeniae Praeparata*.

For cases with purulent sputum or dry cough, add 9 grams *Radix Platycodi* and 9 grams *Bulbus Tritillariae*.

BLOCKAGE OF THE LUNG BY PHLEGM-HEAT (usually seen in bronchopneumonia and lobar pneumonia). Manifestations: Fever with or without chills, flushed face, profuse or scanty sweating, extreme thirst, chest pain exacerbated by coughing, expectoration of purulent, rust-colored, or blood-flecked sputum, flaring of the nostrils, shortness of breath, concentrated urine, reddened, dry tongue with yellow coating, gigantic pulse or slippery and rapid pulse.

Principle of treatment: Removing toxic heat, clearing the lung, and eliminating phlegm.

Prescription: Decoction of Ephedra, Armeniacae, Gypsum, and Glycyrrhizae in Combination with Phragmitis Decoction Worth a Thousand Pieces of Gold, with Modifications.

Herba Ephedrae	6	grams
Semen Armeniacae Amerum	9	"
Gypsum Fibrosum (decocted first)	60	"
Flos Lonicerae	15	"
Fructus Forsythiae	15	"
Radix Scutellariae	9	"
Herba Houttuyniae	15	"
Rhizoma Phragmitis	30	"
Semen Benincasae	12	"
Semen Persicae	6	"
Semen Coicis	15	"
Concretio Silicea Bambusae	9	"

Modifications include: For cases with profuse sputum and shortness of breath, add 9 grams *Semen Lepidii seu Descurainiae* and 9 grams *Cortex Mori Radicis.*

For cases with bloody sputum, add 9 grams *Cacumen Biotae* and 30 grams *Rhizoma Imperatae.*

For cases with sharp chest pain, add 9 grams *Radix Paeoniae Rubra,* 15 grams *Fructus Trichosanthis,* and 9 grams *Radix Curcumae.*

For cases with abdominal distension and constipation, omit *Herba Ephedrae* and add 15 grams *Fructus Trichosanthis* and 6 grams *Natrii Sulfas Exsiccatus* (taken with the decoction).

For cases with profuse sweating and thirst, omit *Herba Ephedrae* and add 15 grams *Radix Glehniae,* 9 grams *Rhizoma Anemarrhenae,* and 12 grams *Radix Trichosanthis.*

Penetration of pathogenic heat into the pericardium (usually found in the acute stage of septic pneumonia). Manifestations: Protracted high fever that is worse at night, cough, shortness of breath, sensation of oppression in the chest, irritability, delirium, loss of consciousness, convulsions, stiff neck, flaring of the nostrils, wheezing, chest pain, expectoration of blood-flecked sputum, dry mouth and lips, reddened tongue with brown coating, deep, taut, thready, and rapid pulse.

Principle of treatment: Dispelling pathogenic heat from the nutrient system, removing toxic heat, and resuscitating the patient.

Prescription: Nutrient System Clearing Decoction, with Modifications.

Radix Rehmannia	15	grams
Radix Scrophulariae	15	"
Fructus Forsythiae	9	"
Rhizoma Acori Graminei	9	"
Flos Lonicerae	15	"
Cortex Moutan Radicis	9	"
Rhizoma Coptidis	3	"
Radix Curcumae	3	"
Semen Armenicae Amerum	9	"
Herba Houttuyniae	24	"
Cornu Rhinoceri	3	"

Modifications include: For cases with coma, administer one Bezoar Bolus for Clearing Heart-Fire twice daily.

For cases with irritability and spasms of the limbs, add 15 grams *Ramulus Uncariae cum Uncis,* 30 grams *Concha Haliotidis,* and 6 grams *Lumbrious,* and take 1.5 grams Purple Snowy Powder with the decoction.

For cases with wheezing, shortness of breath, and flaring of the nostrils, add 9 grams *Bulbus Fritillariae* (fritillary bulb), 15 grams *Pulvis Concha Meretricis* (wrapped in a piece of gauze), and 9 grams *Concretio Silicea Bambusae.*

For cases with delirium, administer a *Bezoar Resurrection Bolus.*

PROSTRATION DUE TO DEPLETION OF YANG AND ACCUMULATION OF PATHOGENIC HEAT (usually seen in acute septic pneumonia associated with heart failure). Manifestations: High fever and cold limbs (or sudden subsidence of fever, profuse sweating, and cold limbs), pallid countenance, cyanosis, restlessness, loss of consciousness, purpura at the tongue border, deep and thready pulse.

Principle of treatment: Restoring vital function from collapse and reinforcing vital energy.

Prescription: Decoction for Prostration with Cold Limbs in Combination with Ginseng.

Radix Ginseng	9 grams	
Radix Ophiopogonis	9	"
Fructus Schisandrae	6	"
Radix Aconiti Praeparata	12	"
Rhizoma Zingiberis	9	"
Concha Ostreae Usta	12	"
Os Draconis Ustum	12	"
Radix Glycyrrhizae Praeparata	6	"

DEFICIENCY OF VITAL ENERGY AND VITAL ESSENCE ASSOCIATED WITH REMAINING PHLEGM AND PATHOGENIC HEAT (usually seen in the convalescent stage of pneumonia).

Manifestations: Dry unproductive cough, moderate fever, afternoon fever, feverish sensation in the palms and soles, lassitude, restlessness, anorexia, profuse sweating, dry mouth, deep reddened tongue with scanty coating or shedding of some fur in the middle, deep and rapid pulse.

Principle of treatment: Reinforcing vital energy and replenishing vital essence, moistening the lung, and eliminating phlegm.

Prescription: Decoction of Lophatheri and Gypsum, with Modifications.

Radix Glehniae	12 grams	
Radix Ophiopogonis	12	"
Bulbus Fritillariae	9	"
Poria	9	"
Radix Codonopsis Pilosulae	9	"
Gypsum Fibrosum	30	"
Semen Armenicae Amerum	9	"
Herba Lophatheri	9	"
Radix Rehmannia	12	"
Radix Trichosanthis	15	"

Modifications include: For cases with malar flush and restlessness, add 3 grams *Fructus Gardeniae Praeparata* and 9 grams *Semen Sojae Praeparatum*.

CASE HISTORY
Male, age 17, admitted March 1, 1964.

History

The patient had had a cough for one week. On the morning of admission to the hospital, he experienced sudden onset of chills and fever, sweating, chest pain, and cough with expectoration of yellowish sputum.

Diagnosis and Treatment

On examination, the patient's face was found to be flushed, his temperature was 39.8°C, and there were diminished breath sounds in the lower right lung. The white cell count was 19,000/mm^3, with 90% neutrophils. Chest x-ray showed patchy shadowing in the lower right lung. The patient had a thin tongue coating and floating, rapid pulse. The diagnosis was invasion of the lung by pathogenic wind and excessive heat in the vital energy system, and it was considered advisable to dispel excessive heat from the vital energy system to clear away sputum. The patient was admitted to the hospital, and the following prescription was given:

Periostracum Cicadae	3 grams	
Fructus Forsythiae	12	"
Rhizoma Anemarrhenae	15	"
Semen Oryzae Nonglutinosae	30	"
Radix Glycyrrhizae	3	"
Gypsum Fibrosum	60	"
Bulbus Fritillariae	9	"

One-half of the above decoction was taken every six hours. In addition, 10 ml of Cough-Relieving Syrup was administered three times daily.

Second examination: April 3.

The patient's temperature was 37.1°C. Rust-colored sputum was expectorated. Upon percussion, a dull resonance was heard in the lower right chest. Sonorous breathing and moist rales were present. The white blood cell count was 10,100/mm^3, with 78% neutrophils. A thin tongue coating and slippery pulse were present. The treatment described above was continued.

Third examination: April 4.

There were no signs of symptoms other than unproductive cough. Chest x-ray showed that the patchy shadowing had been absorbed. A thin tongue coating and slippery pulse were present. It was thought that pathogenic factors remained, and it was considered advisable to remove the disturbance and sputum from the lung. A decoction of the following ingredients was given:

Folium Mori Radicis	9 grams	
Periostracum Cicadae	3	"
Fructus Forsythiae	9	"
Retinervus Citri Fructus (tangerine pith)	4.5	"
Exocarpium Citri Grandis	4.5	"
Semen Armeniacae Amarum	9	"
Cortex Mori Radicis	9	"
Pericarpium Fructus Trichosanthis	12	"
Radix Glycyrrhizae Praeparata	3	"

Fourth examination: April 6.
Mucoid, yellowish sputum was produced by coughing. A thin tongue coating and slippery pulse were present. It was thought that sputum, heat, and functional disturbance of the lung remained. A decoction of the following ingredients was given:

Radix Glehniae	9	grams
Cortex Mori Radicis	9	"
Exocarpium Citri Grandis	4.5	"
Semen Armeniacae Amarum	9	"
Fructus Trichosanthis	12	"
Radix Glycyrrhizae Praeparata	3	"

Fifth examination: April 8.
The white blood cell count had returned to normal. Chest x-ray showed that the lesion in the lower right lung had nearly disappeared. A moderate cough remained. The patient was discharged from the hospital.

—From *Selected Case Records,* compiled by Longhua Hospital (Affiliated with Shanghai College of Traditional Chinese Medicine) (Shanghai People's Publishing House, 1977), pp. 11–12.

For cases with sweating on exertion or slight shortness of breath, add 3 grams *Fructus Schisandrae* and 12 grams *Semen Juglandis* (walnut meat).

For persistent moderate fever, administer Decoction for Removing Heat from the Bones with Modifications.

Radix Stellariae	9	grams
Rhizoma Picrorrhizae	9	"
Carapax Trionycis	18	"
Cortex Lycii Radicis	12	"
Herba Artemisiae Chinghao	4.5	"
Rhizoma Anemarrhenae	9	"
Radix Ophiopogonis	9	"

Other Common Methods of Treating Pneumonia

PROVEN RECIPES

Decoction given for lobar pneumonia:

Herba Houttuyniae	30 grams
Herba Scutellariae Barbatae	30 "
Herba Commelinae (dayflower herb)	30 "

Decoction given for lobar pneumonia:

| Herba Houttuyniae | 30 grams |
| Radix Platycodi | 15 " |

Decoction given for lobar pneumonia:

| Herba Andrographitis (fresh creat) | 30 grams |

Decoction given for bronchopneumonia:

Herba Houttuyniae	30 grams
Herba Taraxaci	15 "
Semen Armeniacae Amarum	9 "
Cortex Mori Radicis	9 "

ACUPUNCTURE TREATMENT

Main Points: Hegu (LI 4), Feishu (UB 13), Lieque (Lu 7), Shaoshang (Lu 11) (prick to bloodlet), Shangyang (LI 1) (prick to bloodlet). Reducing method is usually applied.
Points according to manifestations:

Fever—Quchi (LI 11)
High fever—Chize (Lu 5) or Shixuan (Extra 30) (prick to bloodlet)
Profuse sputum—Fenglong (St 40)
Chest pain—Neiguan (P 6), Shanzhong (Ren 17)

EAR-ACUPUNCTURE THERAPY. Lung, Trachea, Ear-Asthma, Sympathetic Nerve, Ear-Shenmen.
Two or three points are selected for each treatment, and needles are retained for 15 minutes or embedded for three to five days.

PLEURISY

Pleurisy is inflammation of the pleura. It results either from spread of lung infections (such as tuberculosis) or from complications of chest diseases. The chief clinical manifestations include chest pain exacerbated by coughing, fever, and pleural effusion. In traditional Chinese medicine, pleurisy is known as "water distension in the chest" and "pain in the hypochondria."

Etiology

Pleurisy is caused by protracted deficiency of vital energy of the lung and invasion of the lung by pathogenic factors. At the incipient stage, the pathogenic changes are located neither in the exterior nor in the interior but in between. The body resistance and pathogenic factors confront each other sharply; thus, fever and chills are present. Once the pathogenic factors invade the lung, cough and shortness of breath occur because of impaired circulation of vital energy of the lung. When dispersal of body fluid is impeded because of stagnancy of vital energy of the lung, water is retained in the chest and chest pain appears. At the late stage, water retention produces collection of pathogenic heat, which in turn lowers vital function; thus, vital essence is injured.

Essential of Diagnosis and Treatment

In the incipient stage of pleurisy, when the pathogenic changes are located between the exterior and interior, the main symptoms are fever and chills. When the pleura becomes edematous and congested, pain and sensation of oppression in the chest as well as dyspnea are noted. In the ensuing stage of stagnancy of vital energy, night sweats, a suffocating sensation, and general weakness are evident. Late stage pleurisy, in which vital essence is deficient, is marked by an unproductive cough and hectic fever.

Treatment should be based on the differentiation of symptom-complexes. Because pleural effusion is the chief problem, it is important to eliminate fluid retention with hydrogogues.

Treatment Based on the Differentiation of Symptom-Complexes

AFFECTION LOCATED BETWEEN THE EXTERIOR AND INTERIOR (usually seen in the incipient stage of pleurisy). Manifestations: Fever, chills, perspiration, cough, distending chest pain exacerbated by respiration and motion, shortness of breath, dry throat, retching, thin white or yellow tongue coating, taut and rapid pulse.

Principle of treatment: Eliminating pathogenic factors through the regulating effect of herbs.

Prescription: Decoction of Bupleuri, Aurantii, and Pinelliae, with Modifications.

Radix Bupleuri	9	grams
Radix Scutellariae	9	"
Rhizoma Pinelliae Praeparata	9	"
Radix Paeoniae Rubra	9	"
Fructus Trichosanthis	9	"
Fructus Aurantii	9	"
Radix Platycodi	6	"
Semen Benincasae	9	"
Semen Sinapis Albae	9	"

Modifications include: For cases with high fever, profuse sweating, cough, and dyspnea, omit *Radix Bupleuri* and add 6 grams *Herba Ephedrae,* 60 grams *Gypsum,* 9 grams *Semen Armeniacae Amarum,* and 3 grams *Radix Glycyrrhizae.*

For cases with sensation of oppression in the chest, cough, and shortness of breath, add 9 grams *Semen Lepidii seu Descurainiae* and 15 grams *Cortex Mori Radicis.*

For cases with sharp pain in the chest and costal region, add 9 grams *Semen Persicae* and 9 grams *Radix Curcumae.*

WATER RETENTION IN THE CHEST (usually seen in pleural effusion). Manifestations: Cough, distending pain in the chest, shortness of breath, difficulty breathing when lying flat, pain on respiration and motion, thin white tongue coating, taut and slippery pulse.

Principle of treatment: Eliminating water retention and promoting normal flow of vital energy.

Prescription: Pills for Controlling Phlegm-Fluid.

Radix Euphorbiae Kansui (soaked in decoction of *Radix*   1 portion
    Glycyrrhizae for one day, and charred after coating
    with flour)
Radix Euphorbiae Pekinensis   1   "
Semen Sinapis Albae   1   "

The pills should be taken with jujube decoction before breakfast; the daily dose should start at 1.8–2.4 g and gradually increase to 2.7–4.5 g. They should be taken for three to five days, discontinued for two to three days, and then taken for three to five more days. Moderate abdominal pain and diarrhea may occur. If severe diarrhea occurs, the drug should be discontinued and a bowl of rice water taken.

Meanwhile, other medicinal herbs should be administered. They include *Rhizoma Cyperi, Flos Inulae, Fructus Perillae, Lignum Aquilariae Resinatum, Radix Curcumae,* and *Fructus Aurantii.*

STAGNANCY OF VITAL ENERGY (usually found in the late stage of pleurisy, associated with pleural thickening). Manifestations: Pain in the chest and hypochondria. suffocating feeling, dyspnea, cough that is worse on cloudy days, thin tongue coating, taut pulse.

Principle of treatment: Promoting the flow of vital energy.

Prescription: Decoction of Cyperi and Inulae, with Modifications.

Rhizoma Cyperi Praeparata	9	grams
Flos Inulae	6	"
Fructus Perillae	9	"
Lignum Dalbergiae Odoriferae	3	"
Radix Curcumae	9	"
Radix Bupleuri	4.5	"
Radix Paeoniae Rubra	9	"
Fructus Aurantii	4.5	"
Rhizoma Corydalis	9	"

Modifications include: For cases with severe cough, add 9 grams *Semen Armeniacae Amarum,* 9 grams *Pericarpium Trichosanthis,* and 9 grams *Folium Eriobotryae.*

For cases with persistent chest pain, add 9 grams *Semen Persicae,* 6 grams *Flos Carthemi,* 9 grams *Radix Angelicae Sinensis,* and 3 grams *Resina Myrrhae.*

DEFICIENCY OF VITAL ESSENCE AND INTERNAL COLLECTION OF PATHOGENIC HEAT (usually seen in late pleurisy accompanied by active pulmonary tuberculosis). Manifestations: Cough, expectoration of scanty mucoid sputum or dry unproductive cough, dry mouth and throat, emaciation, distending pain in the chest and hypochondria, afternoon fever, restlessness, feverish sensation in the palms and soles, malar flush, night sweats, reddened tongue with scanty coating, thready and rapid pulse.

Principle of treatment: Replenishing vital essence to remove pathogenic heat.

Prescription: Decoction of Adenophorae and Ophiopogonis, with Modifications.

Radix Adenophorae Strictae (straight lady bell root)	12 grams
Rhizoma Polygonati Odorati	15 "
Radix Ophiopogonis	9 "
Radix Paeoniae Alba	9 "
Cortex Lycii Radicis	9 "
Cortex Mori Radicis	9 "
Retinervus Citri Fructus	3 "
Bulbus Fritillariae	4.5 "
Radix Stellariae	6 "

Modifications include: For cases with pallor, lassitude, and shortness of breath, add 15 grams *Radix Codonopsis Pilosulae,* 15 grams *Radix Astragali,* and 6 grams *Fructus Schisandrae.*

For cases with remaining effusion in the chest, add 30 grams *Concha Ostreae Usta* and 9 grams *Rhizoma Alismatis.*

For cases with pain in the chest and hypochondria, add 9 grams *Pericarpium Trichosanthis,* 6 grams *Fructus Aurantii,* 9 grams *Radix Curcumae,* and 9 grams *Retinervus Luffae Fructus* (pith loofah).

Other Common Methods of Treating Pleurisy

PROVEN RECIPES

Decoction given 3–4 times daily for pleurisy caused by spread of infection from pulmonary tuberculosis: *Herba Xanthii* (cocklebur), 120–150 grams.

For pleurisy caused by spread of infection from pulmonary tuberculosis: *Herba Ajugae Decumbens* (bugle) (decocted with lean meat), 30–60 grams.

ACUPUNCTURE TREATMENT

Main points: Zhigou (SJ 6), Qimen (Liv 14), Yanglingquan (GB 34). Reducing method is usually applied.

Points according to manifestations: Suffocating feeling in the chest—Neiguan (P 6), or cupping on the pain area.

EAR-ACUPUNCTURE THERAPY. Sympathetic Nerve, Ear-Shenmen, Heart, Chest, Lung.

Two or three points are selected for each treatment, and needles are retained for 15 minutes or embedded for three to five days.

ACUTE GASTROENTERITIS

Acute gastroenteritis is common in the summer and autumn. The chief clinical manifestations are vomiting, diarrhea, and abdominal pain. In traditional Chinese medicine, acute gastroenteritis is known as "injury from diet" and "vomiting and diarrhea."

Etiology

Acute gastroenteritis is usually caused by contaminated food and drink, by ingestion of too much raw, cold, or greasy food, or by food poisoning. In addition, it can be caused by invasion of the body by pathogenic summer heat and dampness, leading to disturbance of digestion and transport by the gastrointestinal system and impeding normal flow of vital energy. In severe cases, exhaustion of body fluid through continuous vomiting and diarrhea can lead to collapse.

Essentials of Diagnosis and Treatment

It is important to differentiate acute gastroenteritis from dysentery and cholera. In dysentery, the stools contain blood and mucus, and tenesmus is present. Cholera is manifested first by drastic vomiting and diarrhea without abdominal pain; dehydration soon occurs. The main manifestations, however, of acute gastroenteritis are drastic vomiting and watery diarrhea, with abdominal cramps.

Various symptom-complexes are seen in acute gastroenteritis. They include vomiting and diarrhea due to pathogenic damp-cold or damp-heat, injury of body fluid by vomiting and diarrhea, and injury of vital function by vomiting and diarrhea.

It is inadvisable to administer antiemetics and antidiarrheals at the incipient stage of the disease. Symptoms should be observed, causes determined, and the appropriate treatment method adopted.

Treatment Based on Differentiation of Symptom-Complexes

VOMITING AND DIARRHEA DUE TO PATHOGENIC DAMP-COLD. Manifestations: Watery vomiting, watery diarrhea, suffocating feeling in the epigastric region, distending pain in the abdomen, absence of thirst (or preference for hot drink), chills and fever, headache, generalized aching, thin white or slimy tongue coating, soft pulse.

Principle of treatment: Dissolving turbidity with aromatics and strengthening digestion by warming the stomach and spleen to remove dampness.

Prescription: Decoction of Agastachis for Dispelling Turbidity, with Modifications.

Herba Agastachis	9	grams
Herba Eupatorii	9	"
Folium Perilliae	6	"
Rhizoma Atractylodis	9	"
Cortex Magnoliae Officinalis	9	"
Radix Aucklandiae	6	"
Semen Cardamomi Rotundi	3	"
Pericarpium Citri Reticulatae	9	"
Rhizoma Pinelliae Praeparata	9	"
Massa Fermentata Medicinalis	9	"
Poria	9	"
Rhizoma Zingiberis	3	"

Modifications include: For cases with a suffocating feeling in the epigastric region, add 9 grams *Fructus Aurantii Immaturus* and 9 grams *Fructus Crataegi*.

For cases with persistent vomiting and diarrhea and abdominal cramps, add 3 grams *Cortex Cinnamomi* and 6 grams *Radix Aconiti Praeparata*.

For cases with drastic diarrhea, add 9 grams *Radix Codonopsis Pilosulae*, 6 grams *Radix Puerariae*, 12 grams *Rhizoma Dioscoreae*, and 12 grams *Semen Dolichoris Albae*.

VOMITING AND DIARRHEA DUE TO PATHOGENIC DAMP-HEAT. Manifestations: Distending pain in the epigastric region, sour fermented vomitus, belching of foul gas, fever, thirst, restlessness, sharp abdominal pain aggravated by pressure, watery foul-smelling stools (sometimes with scanty mucus or blood), burning sensation of the anus after defecation, concentrated urine, reddened tongue with yellow coating, slippery and rapid pulse.

Principle of treatment: Eliminating pathogenic damp-heat and dissolving turbidity with aromatics.

Prescription: Decoction of Puerariae, Scutellariae, and Coptidis with Modifications.

Radix Puerariae	12 grams	
Radix Scutellariae Praeparata	9	"
Rhizoma Coptidis	6	"
Folium Nelumbinis	9	"
Herba Agastachis	9	"
Herba Eupatorii	9	"
Radix Aucklandiae	6	"
Herba Lophatheri	6	"
Pulvis Talci	15	"
Radix Glycyrrhizae	3	"

Modifications include: For cases with retention of undigested food, add 15 grams *Massa Fermentata Medicinalis* and 9 grams *Fructus Crataegi*.

For cases with profuse sweating and oliguria, add 15 grams *Radix Rehmannia* and 12 grams *Radix Trichosanthis*.

For cases with mucoid and bloody stools and burning sensation of the anus, add 9 grams *Radix Pulsatillae*.

For cases with abdominal pain aggravated by pressure, add 6 grams *Radix et Rhizoma Rhei* and 6 grams Fructus Aurantii Immaturus.

For cases with marked nausea, add 9 grams *Caulis Bambusae in Taenia* and 6 grams *Rhizoma Pinelliae Praeparata.*

INJURY OF BODY FLUID BY VOMITING AND DIARRHEA (usually seen in acute gastroenteritis with dehydration.) Manifestations: Fever, irritability, restlessness, lassitude, thirst, profuse sweating, apathy, concentrated urine, sunken eyes, leg cramps, reddened prickly tongue with dry dark coating, deep, rapid and thready pulse.

Principle of treatment: Removing pathogenic heat and reinforcing vital energy to replenish body fluid.

Prescription: Decoction for Invigorating Pulse-Beat, with Modifications.

Radix Codonopsis Pilosulae	12	grams
Radix Glehniae	12	"
Herba Dendrobii	12	"
Rhizoma Polygonati Odorati	12	"
Radix Ophiopogonis	9	"
Radix Rehmannia	30	"
Fructus Schisandrae	6	"
Pulvis Talci	15	"
Herba Lophatheri	6	"
Radix Glycyrrhizae	3	"

Modifications include: For cases with profuse sweating, add 9 grams *Radix Paeoniae Alba* and 15 grams *Fructus Tritici Levis.*

For cases with leg cramps or leg pains, add 12 grams *Fructus Chaenomelis* and 9 grams *Excrementum Bombycis.*

For cases with persistent diarrhea, add 15 grams *Radix Puerariae Praeparata* and 9 grams *Fructus Chebulae Praeparata.*

INJURY OF VITAL FUNCTION DUE TO VOMITING AND DIARRHEA (usually seen in gastroenteritis complicated by peripheral circulatory failure). Manifestations: Intolerance of cold due to drastic vomiting and diarrhea, lassitude, apathy, pallor, cold sweat, cold limbs, decreased body temperature, dimming consciousness, pale tongue with white coating, deep, thready, and forceless pulse.

Principle of treatment: Restoring vital function from collapse and reinforcing vital function.

Prescription: Decoction for Promoting Blood Circulation and Relieving Cold Limbs, with Modifications.

Radix Codonopsis Pilosulae	15 grams
or	
Radix Ginseng	6 "
Radix Astragali	12 "
Rhizoma Atractylodis Macrocephalae	9 "
Rhizoma Zingiberis	6 "
Radix Aconiti Praeparata	9 "
Ramulus Cinnamomi	6 "
Fructus Schisandrae	3 "
Radix Glycyrrhizae Praeparata	9 "

Modifications include: For cases with cold sweat, add 12 grams *Os Draconis Usta* and 12 grams *Concha Ostreae Usta*.

Other Common Methods of Treating Acute Gastroenteritis

PROVEN RECIPES

1. *Bulbus Allii* (garlic)   3 cloves
   vinegar   100 ml

Administer vinegar with mashed garlic.

2. *Herba Portulacae*, 60 grams. Decoction given for vomiting and diarrhea due to pathogenic damp-heat.

3. *Rhizoma Zingiberis*   15 grams
   Brown sugar   12 "

Decoction given for vomiting and diarrhea due to pathogenic damp-cold.

4. *Pulvis Alumen* (alum powder), 3 grams. Taken with water twice daily.

CASE HISTORY
Male, age 63, first visit on August 2, 1964.

History

The day before the first visit, the patient had suddenly developed watery diarrhea without abdominal pain; he had had 20 loose stools. He also had vomiting, lassitude, cold limbs, abdominal distension, borborygmi, leg cramps, pale slimy tongue coating, and soft, thready, and deep pulse.

The herbs given were as follows:

Rhizoma Coptidis	3 grams
Radix Scutellariae	6 "
Rhizoma Zingiberis	9 "
Radix Glycyrrhizae Praeparata	4.5 "
Poria	9 "
Excrementum Bombycis	12 "

Second visit: August 4.

The vomiting and diarrhea had stopped, and the leg cramps were no longer present. But cold limbs, lassitude, abdominal distension, anorexia, thin white tongue coating, and soft, slow pulse remained. Therefore *Excrementum Bombycis* and *Rhizoma Zingiberis* were omitted from the above prescription and the amount of *Poria* was doubled.

Third visit: August 6.

There had been no loose stools, but poor appetite, lassitude, and soft, slow pulse remained. It seemed that normal functioning of the spleen and stomach had not returned after the vomiting and diarrhea. Therefore herbs to strengthen the function of the spleen and stomach were given; the prescription was as follows:

Rhizoma Atractylodis Macrocephalae	9 grams
Fructus Aurantii Immaturus	4.5 "
Radix Aucklandiae Praeparata	3 "
Fructus Amomi	3 "
Pericarpium Citri Reticulatae	4.5 "
Poria	12 "
Semen Coicis Praeparata	12 "
Radix Glycyrrhizae Praeparata	3 "
Fructus Oryzae Germinatus	9 "

Fourth visit: August 9.

All signs and symptoms except a slightly cold sensation of the skin and limbs had disappeared. Pills of Scutellariae and Allii, *Radix Scutellariae, Bulbus Allii,* were given, 15 grams daily, for convalescence.

—From *Selected Case Records,* compiled by Longhua Hospital (Affiliated with Shanghai College of Traditional Chinese Medicine) (Shanghai People's Publishing House, 1977), p. 35.

ACUPUNCTURE TREATMENT

Main points: Neiguan (P 6), Zhongwan (Ren 12), Zusanli (St 36), Hegu (LI 4), Dachangshu (UB 25).
Points according to manifestations:

Abdominal pain—Qihai (Ren 6), Tianshu (St 25)
Fever—Quchi (LI 11)
Profuse sweating and cold limbs—Shenque (Ren 8) (moxibustion is applied)

Generally, the reducing method is applied in cases due to heat. Even reinforcing and reducing methods are applied together with moxibustion for cases due to cold; one or two treatments are given per day.

EAR-ACUPUNCTURE THERAPY. Large Intestine, Small Intestine, Stomach, Spleen.
One or two points are selected for each treatment, and needles are embedded for three to five days.

DIARRHEA

Diarrhea refers to fecal discharges of increased frequency and liquidity, accompanied by neither pus, blood, nor tenesmus. It commonly occurs in acute and chronic enteritis, irritable bowel syndrome, colitis, gastrointestinal neurosis, and functional disturbances of digestion and absorption.

Etiology

Diarrhea can result from the following:

- Exogenous pathogenic factors (cold, dampness, summer heat) causing dysfunction of the spleen in transporting and distributing nutrients and water.
- Impairment of the spleen and stomach by improper diet, by ex-

cessive intake of greasy, sweet, cold, raw, or contaminated matter, or by retention of undigested food.
- Dysfunction of the spleen caused by emotional strain leading to stagnation of the liver's vital energy, which adversely attacks the spleen.
- Dysfunction of the spleen caused by protracted illness leading to lowered vital function of the kidney, which fails to strengthen the spleen.

Essentials of Diagnosis and Treatment

Diagnosis of diarrhea should be based on its nature, i.e., whether it is of pathogenic cold or heat, or of excessiveness or deficiency. In general, diarrhea due to pathogenic cold is manifested by loose stools and dyspepsia; that due to pathogenic heat by foul-smelling stools and a burning sensation in the anus; that due to deficiency of vital energy by abdominal pain relieved on pressure and by preference for warmth; that due to excessiveness by sharp abdominal pain aggravated by pressure and relieved by defecation.

Chronic diarrhea may also be of different kinds. That due to dysfunction of both the spleen and kidney is characterized by diarrhea occurring before dawn daily; that due to deficiency of vital energy of the spleen, by a feeling of fullness and lack of desire for food.

The primary method of treating diarrhea is to strengthen the function of the spleen and kidney and remove dampness through urination. It is inadvisable to administer antidiarrheals in incipient diarrhea; they should be used only in the second or late stages of the illness. Patients with diarrhea should avoid cold, raw, and greasy food.

Treatment According to Differentiation of Symptom-Complexes

Acute Diarrhea

Diarrhea due to retention of cold. Manifestations: Watery diarrhea with abdominal pain and borborygmus, aversion to cold accompanied by fever, headache, absence of sweat, aching limbs, slimy white tongue coating, soft pulse.

Principle of treatment: Dispelling pathogenic cold from the exterior of the body and removing dampness.

Prescription: Powder of Agastachis for Dispelling Turbidity, with Modifications.

Herba Agastachis	9	grams
Folium Perillae	9	"
Cortex Magnoliae Officinalis	6	"
Radix Angelicae Dahuricae	9	"
Pericarpium Arecae	9	"
Rhizoma Pinelliae Praeparata	9	"
Pericarpium Citri Reticulatae	9	"
Radix Platycodi	9	"
Poria	12	"
Rhizoma Atractylodis Macrocephalae	9	"
Radix Glycyrrhizae Praeparata	6	"

Modifications include: For cases with strong superficial affection, add 6 grams *Herba Schizonepetae* and 6 grams *Radix Ledebouriellae*.

For cases with feeling of oppression in the epigastric region and lassitude due to pathogenic dampness, add 9 grams *Rhizoma Atractylodis,* 9 grams *Rhizoma Alismatis,* 6 grams *Semen Cardamomi Rotundi,* and 9 grams *Semen Coicis.*

DIARRHEA DUE TO DAMP-HEAT OR SUMMER-HEAT. Manifestations: Diarrhea with loose and dark yellow fetid stools, burning sensation in the anus, thirst, concentrated urine, slimy yellow tongue coating, soft, slippery, and rapid pulse.

Principle of treatment: Clearing away pathogenic damp-heat to stop diarrhea.

Prescription: Decoction of Puerariae, Scutellariae, and Coptidis, with Modifications.

Radix Puerariae	9	grams
Radix Scutellariae	9	"
Rhizoma Coptidis	6	"
Flos Lonicerae	15	"
Poria	12	"
Caulis Akebiae	6	"
Rhizoma Atractylodis	12	"

Talcum   15 grams
Radix Glycyrrhizae   6   "

Modifications include: For cases with retention of undigested food, add 9 grams *Massa Fermentata Medicinalis,* 9 grams *Fructus Hordei Germinatus,* and 9 grams *Fructus Crataegi.*

For cases with sharp abdominal pain, add 12 grams *Radix Paeoniae Alba Praeparata* and 6 grams *Radix Aucklandiae.*

For cases due to summer-heat, add 12 grams *Herba Agastachis,* 9 grams *Herba Elsholtziae seu Moslae,* 6 grams *Pericarpium Dolichoris Albae* (hyacinth dolichos peel), and 6 grams *Folium Nelumbinis.*

DIARRHEA DUE TO UNDIGESTED FOOD. Manifestations: Abdominal pain relieved by defecation, borborygmus, diarrhea with fetid stools, oppressed feeling in the stomach and abdomen, belching, acid regurgitation, thick slimy tongue coating, slippery pulse.

Principle of treatment: Promoting digestion to stop diarrhea.

Prescription: Stomach Beneficial Decoction, with Modifications.

Pericarpium Citri Reticulatae	9 grams
Rhizoma Pinelliae Praeparata	9 "
Poria	12 "
Fructus Forsythiae	9 "
Fructus Crataegi	9 "
Massa Fermentata Medicinalis	9 "
Fructus Hordei Germinatus	9 "
Semen Raphani Praeparata	15 "
Semen Arecae Praeparata	9 "
Rhizoma Atractylodis Macrocephalae Praeparata	9 "

Modifications include: For cases with pronounced retention of undigested food, pain and feeling of oppression in the abdomen, add 6 grams *Radix et Rhizoma Rhei,* 6 grams *Fructus Aurantii Immaturus,* and 9 grams *Semen Arecae Praeparata.*

For cases with sharp abdominal pain, add 12 grams *Radix Paeoniae Alba Praeparata* and 6 grams *Radix Aucklandiae.*

CHRONIC DIARRHEA

DIARRHEA DUE TO DISHARMONY OF THE SPLEEN AND LIVER. Manifestations: Diarrhea with abdominal pain due to emotional strain, feeling of oppression in the chest and hypochondrium, belching, anorexia, reddened tongue with thin coating, taut pulse.

Principle of treatment: Strengthening the function of the spleen, subduing the liver, and regulating the flow of vital energy.

Prescription: Decoction of Atractylodis Macrocephalae and Paeoniae in Combination with Powder for Cold Limbs, with Modifications.

Rhizoma Atractylodis Macrocephalae	12 grams	
Rhizoma Dioscorea	12	"
Radix Paeoniae Alba Praeparata	12	"
Pericarpium Citri Reticulatae	9	"
Radix Ledebouriellae	6	"
Radix Bupleuri	6	"
Fructus Aurantii Praeparata	6	"
Radix Glycyrrhizae Praeparata	6	"

Modifications include: For cases with persistent diarrhea, add 9 grams *Fructus Schisandrae* and 6 grams *Fructus Mume.*

For cases with anorexia and lassitude, add 12 grams *Radix Codonopsis Pilosulae,* 9 grams *Massa Fermentata Medicinalis,* and 9 grams *Fructus Crataegi.*

DIARRHEA DUE TO DEFICIENCY OF THE SPLEEN. Manifestations: Persistent loose stools containing undigested food, frequent defecation after intake of greasy food, anorexia, feeling of oppression in the epigastric region, livid complexion, lassitude, pale tongue with white coating, thready and weak pulse.

Principle of treatment: Reinforcing vital energy of the spleen to stop diarrhea.

Prescription: Decoction of Codonopsis, Poria, and Atractylodis, with Modifications:

Radix Codonopsis Pilosulae	12 grams	
Poria	12	"
Rhizoma Atractylodis Macrocephalae	9	"
Rhizoma Dioscorea	15	"
Semen Dolichoris Albae	15	"
Pericarpium Citri Reticulatae	6	"
Semen Nelumbinis	9	"
Fructus Amomi	6	"
Semen Coicis	15	"
Radix Glycyrrhizae Praeparata	6	"

Modifications include: For cases with anorexia, add 9 grams *Fructus Crataegi,* 9 grams *Massa Fermentata Medicinalis,* and 9 grams *Fructus Hordei Germinatus.*

For cases with watery diarrhea, intolerance of cold, cold limbs, and borborygmus, add 6 grams *Radix Aconiti Praeparata* and 6 grams *Rhizoma Zingiberis Praeparata.*

For cases with persistent anal prolapse due to sinking of vital energy, substitute Decoction for Reinforcing Vital Energy and Strengthening the Spleen and Stomach.

DIARRHEA DUE TO DEFICIENCY OF THE KIDNEY. Manifestations: Diarrhea in the early morning, abdominal pain relieved by defecation, intolerance of cold, cold limbs, weakness of the low back and knees, pale tongue with white coating, deep and thready pulse.

Principle of treatment: Strengthening the function of the kidney and spleen.

Prescription: Decoction of Four Magical Herbs, with Modifications.

Fructus Psoraleae	12 grams
Semen Myristicae	9 "
Fructus Evodiae	6 "
Fructus Schisandrae	6 "
Radix Codonopsis Pilosulae	9 "
Radix Aconiti Praeparata	6 "
Fructus Chebulae	9 "

Modifications include: For chronic diarrhea in the aged, add 12 grams *Radix Astragali* and 9 grams *Rhizoma Atractylodis Macrocephalae Praeparata.*

For chronic diarrhea with anal prolapse, add 15 grams *Hallorysitum Rubrum* and 15 grams *Limonitum* (limonite).

For cases with loose stools, add 3 grams *Cortex Cinnamomi* and 12 grams *Semen Caesalpiniae* (caesalpinia).

Other Common Methods of Treating Diarrhea

PROVEN RECIPES

Decoction used in treating diarrhea due to hypofunction of the spleen: *Pericarpium Granati* (one entire peel) and some brown sugar or 1.5 grams *Pulvis Galla Chinensis.*
Decoction given for diarrhea due to cold-dampness:

Semen Plantaginis	30–60 grams	
Herba Agastachis	9	"
Rhizoma Zingiberis Recens	9	"

ACUPUNCTURE TREATMENT

Main points: Group 1: Changqiang (Du 1), Yinlingquan (Sp 9)
Group 2: Tianshu (St 25), Zusanli (St 36), Zhengxie (2.5 *cun* below the umbilicus).
Reducing method is applied for diarrhea due to pathogenic heat; uniform reducing and reinforcing method is applied for diarrhea due to deficiency.

EAR-ACUPUNCTURE THERAPY. Ear–Large Intestine, Small Intestine, Stomach, Spleen.
One or two points are selected for each treatment, and needles are embedded for three to five days.

PRIMARY HYPERTENSION

Primary hypertension is a common cardiovascular disease. It is characterized by a progressive rise in diastolic blood pressure. Manifestations include dizziness, headache, feeling of pressure in the head, tinnitus, and lassitude. Hypertension is also a causative factor in palpitation and hemiplegia. In traditional Chinese medicine, it is linked with "dizziness," "headache," "hyperfunction of the liver," and "flaring up of liver heat."

Etiology

Hypertension is often related to emotional stress, improper diet, and internal injury caused by loss of balance and harmony between vital essence and vital function of the liver and kidney. It also can result from impairment of vital essence due to hyperactivity of the liver, or from deficiency of vital essence of the kidney and exuberance of vital function.

Hypertension due to emotional stress, worry, or persistently having a load on one's mind may induce stagnancy of vital energy of the liver, which may transform into fire and then flare up to the head, thus disturbing the function of the sense organs.

Hypertension may also be caused by improper diet. Overeating of greasy foods and alcohol addiction may damage the function of the spleen and stomach. Water and nutrients within the body cannot be transported properly, and retained substances are transformed into fire, which scorches the body fluid, turning it into phlegm. The phlegm and liver fire flare up to the head, thus blocking the sense organs.

Overwork or aging may also lead to hypertension. In these conditions, vital essence of the kidney wanes, leading to deficiency of liver essence, so that liver fire flares up to the head. In the advanced stage, loss of vital energy may also appear due to deficiency of vital essence.

At the incipient stage of the disease, exuberance of vital function of the liver is often found. Deficiency of vital essence of the liver and kidney develops in the second stage, and deficiency of vital essence and lowered vital function are common in the late stage.

Cerebrovascular accidents (strokes), which sometimes produce hemiplegia, can occur in persistent or severe disease leading to blockage of the Heart Channel by phlegm. Sometimes congestive heart failure occurs because of internal retension of dampness and stagnancy of vital energy and blood resulting from deficiency in the heart and kidney.

Essentials of Diagnosis and Treatment

It is important to determine whether the disease is due to retention of fire and phlegm or to deficiency of vital essence of the liver and kidney and hyperactivity of the liver. In treatment, special attention is given to regulating vital function and vital essence of the liver and kidney. In cases with hyperactivity of the liver, it is essential to eliminate fire and phlegm. In cases with deficiency of vital essence and exuberance of vital function, it is important to replenish vital essence and check hyperactivity.

Treatment Based on Differentiation of Pathological Conditions

FLARING UP OF EXCESSIVE HEAT OF THE LIVER (usually found in hypertensive encephalopathy and hypertensive crisis). Manifestations: Dizziness, distending pain in the head, blurred vision, elevated blood pressure, flushed face, bitter taste in the mouth, irritability, trembling of the hands, slight numbness of the lips, tongue, and limbs, insomnia, reddened tongue tip, yellow tongue coating, taut and rapid pulse.

Principle of treatment: Subduing hyperfunction of the liver and endogenous wind.

Prescription: Decoction of Gentianae to Purge the Liver in Combination with Decoction of Gastrodia and Uncaria, with Modifications.

Rhizoma Gastrodiae	6	grams
Radix Gentianae	9	"
Fructus Gardeniae	9	"
Radix Scutellariae	9	"
Radix Rehmannia	15	"
Flos Chrysanthemi	9	"
Ramulus Uncariae cum Uncis	15	"
Fructus Tribuli	9	"
Herba Siegesbeckiae	9	"
Folium Clerodendri Trichotomi (harlequin glorybower leaf)	12	"
Lumbricus	9	"
Concha Ostrea (decocted first)	30	"
Concha Margaritifera Usta (decocted first)	30	"

Modifications include:For cases with headache and dizziness, add 30 grams *Concha Haliotidis* and take 0.3–0.6 grams *Pulvis Cornu Antelopis* separately.

For cases with constipation, add 6 grams *Radix et Rhizoma Rhei*.

EXCESS PHLEGM AND FIRE (usually found in the incipient or second stage of the disease). Manifestations: Dizziness, distending pain in the head, elevated blood pressure, suffocating feeling in the epigastric region, nausea and vomiting, expectoration of mucoid sputum, bitter taste in the mouth, anorexia, dream-disturbed sleep, pale tongue with reddened tip, slimy yellow tongue coating, taut and slippery pulse.

Principle of treatment: Eliminating fire and phlegm; subduing hyperfunction of the liver and endogenous wind.

Prescription: Coptidis Decoction for Warming the Gallbladder, with Modifications.

Rhizoma Coptidis	3	grams
Radix Scutellariae	9	"
Spica Prunellae	15	"
Arisaema cum Bile	6	"
Pericarpium Citri Reticulatae	6	"
Semen Cassiae	12	"
Rhizoma Pinelliae	9	"
Rhizoma Acori Graminei	9	"
Poria	9	"
Caulis Bambusae in Taenis	6	"
Herba Siegesbeckiae	12	"

Modifications include: For cases with headache and irritability, add 3 grams *Radix Gentianae,* 6 grams *Cortex Moutan Radicis,* 9 grams *Fructus Gardeniae,* 6 grams *Folium Ilex* (broad leaf holly), and 30 grams *Concha Ostreae.*

For cases with insomnia, add 3 grams *Plumula Nelumbinis.*

For cases with profuse phlegm-dampness marked by heaviness of the head, blurred vision, numbness of the limbs, suffocating feeling in the chest, and slimy white tongue coating, omit *Rhizoma Coptidis, Radix Scutellariae,* and *Semen Cassiae* and add 9 grams *Bombyx Batryticatus,* 6 grams *Rhizoma Gastrodiae,* 9 grams *Rhizoma Atractylodis Macrocephalae,* and 9 grams *Rhizoma Alismatis.*

DEFICIENCY OF VITAL ESSENCE OF THE LIVER AND KIDNEY AND HYPERACTIVITY OF THE LIVER (usually seen in the second stage of the disease or in hypertension at menopause). Manifestations: Dizziness, headache, tinnitus, blurred vision, flushed face on exertion or emotional strain, dry mouth, emaciation, weakness of the low back and legs, seminal emission, deep reddened tongue with little coating, thready and taut pulse.

Principle of treatment: Replenishing vital essence and checking hyperactivity; tonifying the liver and kidney.

Prescription: Rehmanniae Decoction of Anemarrhenae and Phellodendri, with Modifications.

Radix Rehmannia	15	grams
Radix Rehmannia Praeparata	9	"
Fructus Corni	9	"
Cortex Moutan Radicis	9	"
Rhizoma Anemarrhenae	6	"
Cortex Phellodendri	6	"
Radix Paeoniae Alba	9	"
Radix Polygoni Multiflori Praeparata	12	"
Ramulus Loranthi	12	"
Fructus Ligustri Lucidi	12	"
Plastrum Testudinis	12	"
Concha Ostreae	18	"
Concha Haliotidis (decocted first)	30	"

Modifications include: For cases with palpitation and insomnia, omit *Radix Paeoniae Alba* and *Ramulus Loranthi* and add 9 grams *Rhizoma Polygonatu Odorati,* 9 grams *Semen Ziziphi Spinosae,* and 9 grams *Semen Biotae* (seed of oriental arborvitae).

For cases with headache, flushed face, restlessness, thirst, and deep reddened tongue, add 30 grams *Spica Prunellae* and 9 grams *Flos Chrysanthemi.*

For cases of hypertension due to climacteric menstrual disorders, add 9 grams *Radix Angelicae Sinensis,* 9 grams *Radix Achyranthis Bidentatae,* and 15 grams *Herba Leonuri.*

For cases with palpitation and propensity to be frightened, add 12 grams *Ramulus Uncariae cum Uncis* and 30 grams *Concha Margaritifera Usta.*

For cases with seminal emission, add 12 grams *Fructus Rosae Laevigatae* and 12 grams *Semen Cuscutae.*

DEFICIENCY OF VITAL ESSENCE AND VITAL FUNCTION (usually seen in the late stage of the disease or in hypertension at menopause).

Manifestations: Dizziness, weakness of the low back and legs, intolerance of cold, cold limbs, puffiness of the face, nocturia, impotence, spermatorrhea, pallor, anorexia, lassitude, flabby pale tongue, deep and thready pulse.

Principle of treatment: Replenishing vital essence and strengthening the function of the kidney.

Prescription: Restoring Kidney Decoction Prescribed by the Golden Chamber in Combination with Two Fairies Decoction, with Modifications.

Herba Epimedii	9	grams
Rhizoma Curculiginis	9	"
Radix Aconiti Praeparata	6	"
Cortex Cinnamomi	24	"
Fructus Corni	9	"
Radix Rehmannia Praeparata	9	"
Plastrum Testudinis	18	"
Cortex Eucommiae	12	"
Ramulus Loranthi	15	"

Modifications include: For cases with palpitation and shortness of breath, add 15 grams *Fluoritum* (fluorite, decocted first), 24 grams *Magnetitum* (decocted first), 9 grams *Radix Codonopsis Pilosulae*, 3 grams *Fructus Schisandrae,* and 6 grams *Radix Glycyrrhizae Praeparata.*

For cases with puffiness of the face and legs, add 9 grams *Radix Astragali,* 9 grams *Rhizoma Atractylodi Macrocephalae,* and 9 grams *Radix Stephaniae Tetrandrae.*

For cases with nocturia, add 12 grams *Fructus Alpiniae Oxyphyllae* and 9 grams *Oötheca Mantidis.*

For cases with seminal emission and spermatorrhea, add 12 grams *Fructus Rosae Laevigatae* and 12 grams *Semen Eurylaes.*

Other Common Methods of Treating Primary Hypertension

PROVEN RECIPES

1. *Herba Cephalanoploris,* 30–60 grams. Decoction given for incipient hypertension.

2. *Folium Clerodendri Trichotomi*, 15–30 grams. Decoction given for hypertension due to deficiency of vital essence and lowered vital function.

3. *Herba Cephalanoploris*   30 grams
   Herba Plantaginis   30   "
   Herba Siegesbeckiae   15   "

Decoction given for hypertension.

4. Pulvis of *Radix Aristolochiae,* 1.5 grams. Taken after each meal (three times daily) for three months.

5. *Fructus Aristochiae* (fresh), 30 grams. Decoction prepared with sugar and taken three times daily.

6. *Herba Apium Graveolens* (celery), 2–3 kg. Cut into pieces, boiled, and kept in a sealed jar until sour; one bowlful taken with 2–4 ounces sugar daily.

7. *Fructus Evodiae.* Powder prepared with vinegar and applied to soles for hypertension.

8. *Semen Ricini* (castor bean). Crushed and applied to Point Yongquan (K 1) on both sides for hypertensive crisis or apoplexy.

9. Two Fairies Decoction

   Radix Curuliginis   12 grams
   Herba Epimedii   12   "
   Radix Angelicae Sinensis   9   "
   Radix Morindae Officinalis   9   "
   Cortex Phellodendri   9   "
   Rhizoma Anemarrhanae   9   "

Decoction given for climacteric hypertension.

10. Other single ingredients good for hypertension include the following: *Herba Ajugae, Semen Cassiae, Ramulus Uncariae Cum Uncis, Semen Celosiae, Radix Scutellariae, Flos Chrysanthemi Indici, Lumbricus, Flos Sophorae, Fructus Leonuri* (motherwort fruit), *Cortex Moutan Radicis, Herba seu Radix Cirsii Japonici, Cortex Eucommiae, Ramulus Loranthi.*

Decoction of two or three ingredients prepared for each treatment.

CASE HISTORY
Male, age 57, first visit on March 19, 1977.

History

The patient's complaints included dizziness, dry mouth, and cough.

Diagnosis and Treatment

On examination, the blood pressure was found to be 190/110 mm Hg. Floating (in *cun* area) and deep (in *guan* area) pulse was observed. Therefore Decoction of Loranthi was prescribed; the ingredients were:

Ramulus Loranthi	24	grams
Radix Achyranthis	24	"
Rhizoma Dioscoreae	24	"
Os Draconis	24	"
Radix Angelicae Sinensis	9	"
Radix Paeoniae Alba	9	"
Radix Rehmannia	12	"
Radix Aristolochiae	18	"
Rhizoma Polygonatu Odorati	15	"

Second visit: March 22.

The above symptoms had been relieved but constipation had developed. Weak and deep pulse was felt, indicating impeded blood circulation. Therefore, the following ingredients were administered:

Radix et Rhizoma Rhei Praeparata cum wine	9	grams
Rhizoma Dioscoreae	9	"
Radix Ledebouriellae	9	"
Radix Angelicae Pubescentis	9	"
Semen Pruni	12	"
Fructus Cannabis	12	"
Radix Angelicae Dahuricae	12	"
Semen Cuscutae	12	"
Radix Achyranthis	18	"
Rhizoma Polygonati Odorati	18	"
Semen Plantaginis	6	"

Third visit: March 27.

All symptoms had nearly disappeared, and the blood pressure had decreased to 140/90 mm Hg. After another two doses of the above prescription, omitting *Radix et Rhizoma Rhei*, were given, the patient fully recovered.

—From Feng Jinming, *A Collection of Case Histories of Traditional Chinese Medicine* (Gansu People's Publishing House, 1981), p. 118.

ACUPUNCTURE TREATMENT

Main points: Taichong (Liv 3), Ganshu (UB 18), Zusanli (St 36), Quchi (LI 11).
Points according to manifestations:

Dizziness—Shenmen (H 7), Yintang (Extra 1)
Palpitation—Neiguan (P 6), Xinshu (UB 15)
Insomnia—Shenmen (H 7), Sanyinjiao (Sp 6)

Reducing method is usually applied and moxibustion administered to Shenshu (UB 23), Taixi (K 3) and Ganshu (UB 18).

EAR-ACUPUNCTURE THERAPY. Groove for Lowering Blood Pressure, Ear-shenmen, Sympathetic Nerve, Kidney, Liver.
One or two points are selected for each treatment, and needles are embedded for three to five days.

CORONARY ATHEROSCLEROTIC HEART DISEASE

Coronary atherosclerotic heart disease is often present by the age of 40. Manifestations include cardiac pain of sudden onset, palpitation, and shortness of breath. Such conditions as angina pectoris, myocardial infarction, hardening of the cardiac muscle, and chronic coronary atherosclerotic disease fall within this category. In traditional Chinese medicine, the disorder is known by such designations as "pectoral pain with stuffiness," "cardiac pain with stuffiness," "true cardiac pain," and "gastralgia with cold limbs."

Etiology

The main cause of the disease is a blockage of the Heart Channel. Such blockage can result from weakened functioning of the kidney in the elderly and feeble, phlegm obstruction due to consumption of too much fat, collection of pathogenic coldness impeding vital function of the heart, stagnancy of vital energy and blood due to emotional strain, and anxiety and overexertion injuring the heart and spleen.

Manifestations of the disease include excess and deficiency symptom-complexes. The former are due to impairment of vital function of the heart by blood stasis and phlegm. The latter are due to functional disturbance of the internal organs, which results in unsteady flow of vital energy and blood of the heart.

Essentials of Diagnosis and Treatment

In diagnosis, it is of primary importance to determine the location and nature of the pain. Generally, cardiac pain is felt in the pectoral region or lower chest. The pain may radiate into the arm or neck, and it has different characteristics in different cases. Often, a dull pain, a sharp sting, or angina is brought about by overexertion, excitement, overeating, cold, or unexpected climatic change. The pain may be relieved by rest.

Different treatments are used for different conditions. For example, a blockage in the Heart Channel, which is considered an excess symptom-complex, is removed by promoting smooth flow of vital energy and blood; in contrast, lowered functioning of the internal organs, which is considered a deficiency symptom-complex, is treated by reinforcing vital energy and blood. Complicated manifestations are usually seen, and treatment should be in accordance with the symptoms and signs.

Treatment Based on Differentiation of Pathological Conditions

IMPEDED CARDIAC VITAL FUNCTION (usually seen in angina pectoris or acute myocardial infarction). Manifestations: Persistent cold-induced pain in the cardiac region, palpitation, shortness of breath, stuffiness in the chest, retrosternal pain and tightness, pallid countenance, lassitude, pale tongue with slimy white coating or purpura, taut, slippery pulse or irregular, intermittent pulse.

Principle of treatment: Strengthening cardiac vital function and killing pain.

Prescription: Decoction of Trichosanthis, Allium, and Pinelliae, with Modifications.

Fructus Trichosanthis	15	grams
Bulbus Allii Macrostemi (onion bulb)	6	"
Rhizoma Pinelliae Praeparata	9	"
Pericarpium Citri Reticulatae	6	"
Fructus Auranthii	6	"
Poria	15	"
Ramulus Cinnamomi	3	"
Cortex Magnoliae Officinalis	6	"

Modifications include: In severe cases, administer a Storax Bolus.

For cases with intolerance of cold, cold limbs, and irregular and intermittent pulse, add 9 grams *Radix Codonopsis Pilosulae,* 9 grams *Rhizoma Atractylodis Macrocephale,* and 9 grams *Radix Aconiti Praeparatae.*

For cases with pain and difficulty breathing when lying flat, administer 15 grams *Rhizoma Pinelliae Praeparatae.*

BLOCKAGE OF THE HEART CHANNEL BY BLOOD STASIS (usually seen in angina pectoris or acute myocardial infarction). Manifestations: Sharp stinging located in the cardiac region and radiating into the left shoulder and arm, distending pain in the hypochondria, palpitation, difficulty breathing, restlessness, cyanosis, dark purple tongue with ecchymosis, taut, thready, and choppy pulse or irregular, intermittent pulse.

Principle of treatment: Invigorating smooth flow of vital energy and blood to kill pain.

Prescription: Decoction of Salviae in Combination with Decoction of Four Herbs with Perisicae and Carthami.

Radix Salviae Miltiorrhizae	15	grams
Lignum Santali	3	"
Pericarpium Citri Reticulatae Viride	6	"
Radix Linderae	6	"
Fructus Amomi	3	"
Radix Angelicae Sinensis	9	"
Rhizoma Ligustici Chuanxiong	6	"
Semen Persicae	9	"

Radix Paeoniae Rubra (red peony)   9 grams
Flos Carthami   6   "

Or Coronary Heart Disease Prescription II (see chapter 3), one dose daily for 4 weeks.

Modifications include: For cases with cyanosis, administer a Storax Bolus or add 9 grams *Pollen Typhae,* 9 grams *Faeces Trogopterorum,* or 1.5 grams *Pulvis Notoginseng.*

For cases with palpitation and irregular, intermittent pulse, add 12 grams *Colla Corii Asini* and 15 grams *Radix Codonopsis Pilosulae.*

BLOCKAGE OF THE HEART CHANNEL BY PHLEGM (usually seen in angina pectoris or acute myocardial infarction). Manifestations: Crushing pain in the cardiac region, lassitude, profuse sputum, coughing, nausea, anorexia, dizziness, pale tongue with thick, slimy coating, taut, slippery pulse or soft, slow pulse.

Principle of treatment: Dissolving turbidity with aromatics; regulating the function of the spleen to resolve phlegm.

Prescriptions: (a) Crushing Pain-Relieving Pills (*Fructus Piperis Longi, Rhizoma Alpiniae Officinarum, Lignum Santali, Borneolum, Herba Asari,* and *Rhizoma Corydalis*) or *Storax Bolus.* (b) Gallbladder-Warming Decoction.

Rhizoma Pinelliae Praeparata	9	grams
Pericarpium Citri Reticulatae	6	"
Fructus Aurantii	6	"
Cortex Magnoliae Officinalis	6	"
Poria	9	"
Caulis Bambusae in Taenis	6	"
Radix Glycyrrhizae	6	"
Rhizoma Atratylodis Macrocephalae	9	"

Modifications include: For cases with stagnation of phlegm-heat, marked by restlessness, fever, reddened tongue, and slippery, rapid pulse, add 3 grams *Rhizoma Coptidis,* 9 grams *Caulis Bambusae in Taenis,* and 6 grams *Arisaema cum Bile.*

For cases with severe blood stasis and sharp pain, add 9 grams *Rhizoma Sparganii,* 9 grams *Rhizoma Zedoariae,* 9 grams *Pollen Typhae,* 9 grams *Faeces Trogopterorum,* and 15 grams *Fructus Crataegi.*

To strengthen the result, herbs such as the following may be added:

Styrax Liquidus (storax), *Fructus Piperis Longi, Lignum Santali, Lignum Aquilariae Resinatum, Radix Aristolochiae.*

DEFICIENCY OF VITAL ENERGY AND VITAL ESSENCE (usually seen in the remission stage of angina pectoris and myocardial infarction). Manifestations: Pain in the cardiac region, shortness of breath, palpitation, spontaneous sweating, thirst, scanty saliva, reddened tongue with little coating, taut, thready pulse or irregular, intermittent pulse.

Principle of treatment: Reinforcing vital energy and replenishing vital essence.

Prescription: Decoction for Invigorating the Pulse-Beat, with Modifications.

Radix Codonopsis Pilosulae	9 grams
Radix Ophiopogonis	9 "
Fructus Schisandrae	6 "
Radix Rehmannia	15 "
Radix Glycyrrhizae Praeparata	9 "
Ramulus Cinnamomi	6 "
Radix Paeoniae Alba	9 "

Modifications include: For cases with prominent precordial pain, add 6 grams *Lignum Aquilariae Resinatum* and 9 grams *Radix Curcumae.*

For cases with dizziness, tinnitus, numbness of the tongue and limbs, restlessness, irritability, and hypertension, add 4.5 grams *Rhizoma Gastodrae,* 12 grams *Ramulus Uncariae cum Uncis,* 15 grams *Concha Haliotidis,* 24 grams *Concha Ostreae,* 6 grams *Folium Mori Radicis,* 9 grams *Cortex Moutan Radicis,* and 6 grams *Fructus Gardeniae.*

For cases with restlessness, palpitation, and insomnia, add 12 grams *Lignum Pini Poriaferum* (the core of poria), 9 grams *Fructus Ziziphi Spinosae Praeparata,* 9 grams *Radix Polygalae,* 15 grams *Cortex Albiziae,* and 6 grams *Folium Mori Radicis.*

WEAKENED FUNCTIONING OF THE HEART AND KIDNEY (usually seen in hardening of the cardiac muscle or after acute myocardial infarction). Manifestations: Suffocating feeling in the chest, intermittent cardiac pain, palpitation, shortness of breath, low back pain, lassitude, intolerance of cold, cold limbs, pallor, cyanosis, pale or dark purple tongue, deep and thready or irregular, intermittent pulse.

Principle of treatment: Strengthening the function of the heart and kidney to promote blood circulation.

Prescription: Decoction for Reinforcing Vital Function of the Kidney, with Modifications.

Radix Rehmannia Praeparata	12 grams
Radix Aconiti Praeparata	6 "
Ramulus Cinnamomi	6 "
Rhizoma Pinelliae Praeparata	6 "
Bulbus Allii Macrostemi	6 "
Colla Cornus Cervi	9 "
Radix Angelicae Sinensis	9 "
Semen Cuscutae	9 "
Radix Codonopsis Pilosulae	9 "
Fructus Corni	9 "

Modifications include: For cases with low back pain, spermatorrhea, seminal emission, and impotence, add 9 grams *Rhizoma Curculiginis* and 9 grams *Herba Epimedii.*

For cases with frequent urination, add 12 grams *Fructus Alpiniae Opsyphyllae* and 6 grams *Oötheca Mantidis.*

For cases with puffiness of the face and legs, add 12 grams *Radix Astragali* and 9 grams *Radix Stephaniae Tetrandrae.* For cases with dyspnea upon exertion and palpitations, add 3 grams *Fructus Schisandrae,* 3 grams *Gecko,* 30 grams *Semen Juglandis,* and 1.5 grams *Lignum Aquilariae Resinatum.*

For cases with insomnia, add 15 grams *Os Draconis,* 15 grams *Concha Ostreae,* 9 grams *Radix Polygalae,* and 15 grams *Semen Ziziphi Spinosae Praeparata.*

GREATLY LOWERED VITAL FUNCTION (usually seen in myocardial infarction complicated by heart failure and shock). Manifestations: Sharp and repeated cardiac pain, palpitation, dyspnea, cyanosis, pallor, cold sweat, cold limbs, coma (in severe cases), purple tongue, deep, thready, and faint pulse or irregular and intermittent pulse.

Principle of treatment: Strengthening vital function for resuscitation; promoting normal circulation of blood to remove stasis.

Prescription: Decoction of Ginseng, Aconiti, Draconis, and Ostreae, with Modifications.

Radix Ginseng Rubra (simmered separately)	15 grams
Radix Aconiti Praeparata	9 "
Os Draconis	15 "
Concha Ostreae	15 "
Radix Glycyrrhizae Praeparata	9 "
Cortex Cinnamomi	3 "
Radix Astragali	15 "
Fructus Schisandrae	6 "
Radix Ophiopogonis	9 "
Storax Bolus	1 bolus

Modifications include: For cases with dyspnea and sensation of oppression in the chest, add 6 grams *Semen Persicae*, 6 grams *Flos Carthami*, 9 grams *Faeces Trogopterorum*, and 9 grams *Pollen Typhae*.

Other Common Methods of Treating Coronary Atherosclerotic Heart Disease

PROVEN RECIPES

1. Storax Bolus: one bolus is taken 1–3 times daily to prevent angina pectoris, or one bolus is taken for attack of angina pectoris.

2. Crushing-Pain-Relieving Pills: 90 grams *Fructus Piperis Longi*, 45 grams *Lignum Santali*, 45 grams *Rhizoma Alpiniae Officinarum*, 30 grams *Rhizoma Corydalis*, 24 grams *Borneolum*, 15 grams *Herba Asari*. The preparations of extract and volatile oil are put in capsules, and 0.3 grams taken 3 times daily to prevent angina pectoris.

3. Pills of Rhinoceros Gallstone (patent medicine) 4.5 grams twice daily.

4. Coronary Heart Disease Pills

Folium Ginkgo (ginkgo leaf)	3 kg
Radix Scrophulariae	2 "
Caulis Spatholobi	1 "
Spica Prunellae	1 "
Fructus Crataegi	1 "
Radix Angelicae Sinensis	1 "
Flos Carthami	0.5 "
Radix Polygoni Multiflori	0.75 "

Rhizoma Polygonati	0.5	kg
Rhizoma Corydalis	0.25	"
Resina Myrrhae	90	"
Resina Draconis (dragon's blood)	30	"

Pills weighing 15 grams are prepared; one pill is taken 2–3 times daily for angina pectoris.

5. Compound Salviae Injection for angina pectoris: Every ml contains 1–2 g each of *Radix Salviae* and *Lignum Dalbergiae Odoriferae.* Two ml is injected intramuscularly twice daily, or diluted with glucose or dextran solution and injected intravenously.

| 6. *Radix Codonopsis Pilosulae* | 9 grams |
| *Rhizoma Polygonati Odorati* | 15 " |

Decoction given for deficiency of vital energy and vital essence in coronary disease.

7. *Radix Ilicis Pubescentis* (hairy holly root), 90–120 grams. Decoction or injection given for attack of angina pectoris.

Decoction: One dose daily.

Injection: 1–2 times daily, 2–4 ml per intramuscular injection.

8. *Succinum*	1 portion
Pulvis Notoginseng	1 "
Resina Draconis	1 "
Lignum Aquilariae Resinatum	1 "

or

| *Rhizoma Sparganii* | 1 " |
| *Rhizoma Zedoariae* | 1 " |

or

Radix Curcumae	60 grams
Rhizoma Corydalis	60 "
Lignum Aquilariae Resinatum	30 "

Powdered; 3 grams administered daily.

ACUPUNCTURE TREATMENT

Main points: Neiguan (P 6), Xinshu (UB 15), Ximen (P 4), Shanzhong (Ren 17).

CASE HISTORY

Male, age 36, admitted on February 2, 1963.

History

The patient had suffered frequent crushing precordial pain for nearly a year. The pain radiated to the left shoulder and nape; it often lasted for half an hour, and sometimes it occurred five or six times per day. Other complaints included sweating, shortness of breath, irritability, palpitation, constipation, concentrated urine, and productive cough.

Diagnosis and Treatment

On examination, a taut, slippery, and slightly rapid pulse was felt. In modern medical terms, the diagnosis was coronary atherosclerotic heart disease with angina pectoris. In traditional Chinese terms, it was thought that the disease was due to blockage of the channels by phlegm caused by lowered vital function of the heart.

It was considered advisable to eliminate phlegm from the channels and promote blood flow to kill pain. Therefore Decoction of Trichosanthis, Allium, and Pinelliae in Combination with Powder for Removing Blood Stasis with Modifications was given; the ingredients were:

Fructus Trichosanthis	9 grams
Bulbus Allii Macrostemi	6 "
Radix Paeoniae Alba	15 "
Bulbus Fritillariae	6 "
Radix Aucklandiae	3 "
Radix Curcumae	9 "
Rhizoma Acori Graminei	6 "
Radix Angelicae Sinensis	9 "
Radix Salviae Miltiorrhizae	9 "
Lumbricus	6 "
Flos Carthami	3 "
Magnetitum	9 "
Radix Polygalae mixed with Cinnabaris	9 "
Semen Ziziphi Spinosae	9 "

In addition, a powder consisting of the following ingredients was prepared.

Pollen Typhae	3 grams
Faeces Trogopterorum	3 "
Resina Olibani	3 "
Succinum	1.5 "
Resina Myrrhae	3 "

The powder was divided into four doses, and two doses were taken daily with the above decoction.

Storax Bolus was also given; one half bolus was administered three times daily.

Half a month later, the patient was markedly better than before. As of February 16, there had been four days on which no attacks of angina pectoris had occurred. After discharge from the hospital, the patient was advised to take the prescription with modifications for another three months; during that time he had no further attacks of angina pectoris. No relapses occurred in the five months after treatment.

—Liu Yanchi, "The Treatment of Coronary Atherosclerotic Heart Disease," *Journal of Traditional Chinese Medicine* (1964), no. 6, pp. 12–13.

Secondary points: Quchi (LI 11), Zusanli (St 36), Dushu (UB 16), Jueyinshu (UB 14).

Two main points and one secondary point are selected for each treatment, and needles are retained for 20 to 40 minutes. One or two treatments are applied per day. Needles should be inserted toward the vertebrae from the Back-*shu* points; needle sensation should spread to the chest for better results.

EAR-ACUPUNCTURE THERAPY. Heart, Ear-Shenmen, Subcortex, Sympathetic Nerve, Endocrine, Small Intestine.

One or two points are selected for each treatment, and needles are embedded for three to five days.

CEREBROVASCULAR ACCIDENTS

Cerebrovascular accidents (strokes) are those conditions in which acute pathologic changes in the cerebral vessels produce neurologic impairment due to local disturbance in blood supply. Manifestations can include coma, semiconsciousness, hemiplegia, and facial paresis. The disease is divided into two classes: hemorrhage and ischemia (lack of blood). The former includes cerebral hemorrhage and subarachnoid hemorrhage. The latter includes cerebral angiospasm, cerebral thrombosis, and cerebral embolism. In traditional Chinese medicine, cerebrovascular accident is known as "stricken by wind" (apoplexy), which is further divided into "hollow visceral apoplexy" (marked by sudden fainting and hemiplegia) and "channel apoplexy" (marked by hemiplegia without coma).

Etiology

The occurrence of the disease is closely related to such factors as old age, debility, emotional disturbance, irregular diet, and obesity. When one passes middle age, deficiency of vital essence of the liver and kidney and hyperactivity of vital function usually occur. The retained pathogenic heat of the heart and liver turns vital essence into phlegm or phlegm-dampness. Phlegm-fire produced internally because of obesity, addiction to alcohol, or excessive intake of greasy food goes upward. As a result phlegm-fire disturbs the equilibrium of *yin* and *yang,* and the circulation of vital energy and blood is deranged. Then blood follows the upward trend of vital energy and rushes to the brain, producing coma. If the body resistance fails in the struggle against pathogenic factors, collapse occurs owing to depletion of vital essence and vital function; the condition is known as "hollow visceral apoplexy." If pathogenic wind of the liver adversely attacks the channels together with phlegm and impedes smooth flow of vital energy and blood, facial paresis and hemiplegia occur; this condition is called "channel apoplexy."

Essentials of Diagnosis and Treatment

First, the location of the disease must be determined. If the channels are affected, the case is moderate, and it is advisable to remove phlegm from the channels and to check the liver and subdue its wind. If the internal organs are affected, the case is severe and it is advisable to remove phlegm in order to resuscitate the patient or to strengthen vital function to prevent collapse.

It is also important to tell whether the case is an emergency. As a rule, in emergency cases, treat the acute symptoms first; when these are relieved, treat the fundamental cause. If there is a preponderance of pathogenic wind, fire, or phlegm, it is necessary to eliminate these pathogenic factors. If there is a deficiency of vital essence, vital energy, and blood, it is necessary to replenish vital essence and nourish blood. As for the sequelae (such as hemiplegia, speech defect, and facial paresis), it is advisable to reinforce vital energy, nourish blood, and remove blood stasis from the vessels; meanwhile acupuncture treatment is applied.

Treatment Based on Differentiation of Pathological Conditions

BLOCKAGE OF THE CHANNELS BY PATHOGENIC WIND-PHLEGM (a manifestation of channel apoplexy; usually found in cerebral thrombosis, cerebral embolism, cerebral angiospasm, and sequelae of cerebrovascular accidents). Manifestations: unilateral facial paresis, hemiplegia, numbness of the face and limbs, contractures and stiffnesses of the hand and foot, dizziness, heavy sensation of the head, profuse sputum, rigidity of the tongue, impairment or loss of speech, thin white or slimy white tongue coating, taut-slippery or taut-thready pulse.

Principle of treatment: Eliminating phlegm from the channels; subduing wind of the liver.

Prescription: Decoction for Expelling Phlegm combined with Powder for Correcting Facial Deviation, with Modifications.

Rhizoma Pinelliae Praeparata	9	grams
Arisaema cum Bile	6	"
Caulis Bambusae in Taenis	9	"
Poria	9	"
Pericarpium Citri Reticulatae (tangerine pith)	9	"
Fructus Aurantii Immaturus	6	"
Rhizoma Gastrodiae	4.5	"
Ramulus Uncariae cum Uncis	12	"
Bombyx Batryticatus	9	"
Fructus Tribuli	12	"
Rhizoma Typhonii Praeparata	3	"
Lumbricus	9	"

Modifications include: For cases with marked deviation of the mouth and eyes (facial paresis), add 6 grams *Scorpio.*

For cases with contractures of the hand and foot, cramps, and pain, add 12 grams *Herba Siegesbeckiae* and 12 grams *Folium Clerodendri Trichotomi.*

For cases with headache and dizziness, add 30 grams *Concha Margaritifera Usta*, 15 grams *Concha Ostreae*, 15 grams *Spica Prunellae*, and 12 grams *Radix Paeoniae Alba.*

For cases with dull facial expression, add 9 grams *Radix Polygalae* and 9 grams *Rhizoma Acori Graminei.*

RETENSION OF PHLEGM AND FIRE (a manifestation of hollow visceral apoplexy; usually seen in cerebral embolism and cerebral angiospasm). Manifestations: Sudden loss of consciousness, spasm of jaw muscles, clenched fists, convulsions, flushed face, feverish sensation, delirium, hyperpnea with rattling in the throat, severe headache, vomiting, constipation, concentrated urine, reddened tongue with slimy yellowish coating, taut and slippery pulse.

Principle of treatment: Clearing away pathogenic heat to subdue wind; eliminating phlegm for resuscitation.

Prescription: Decoction of Cornu Antelopis and Uncariae, with Modifications.

Pulvis Cornu Antelopis (mix with the decoction)	1.5 grams
Ramulus Uncariae cum Uncis	15 "
Rhizoma Coptidis	3 "
Concha Margaritifera Usta	30 "
Radix Curcumae	6 "
Radix Gentianae	9 "
Rhizoma Acori Graminei	9 "
Arisaema cum Bile	6 "
Concretio Silicea Bambusae	9 "

In addition, one Priceless Treasure Pill or one Bezoar Bolus for Clearing Away Heart Fire is administered twice daily.

Modifications include: For cases with constipation, add 9 grams *Radix et Rhizoma Rhei* and 6 grams *Natrii Salfas Exsiccatus.*

For cases with severe headache, add 3 grams *Rhizoma seu Radix Notopterygii,* 6 grams *Rhizoma Ligustici Chuanxiong,* and 9 grams *Fructus Gardeniae praeparata.*

For cases with dry mouth and reddened tongue, add 9 grams *Radix Glehniae,* 9 grams *Herba Dendrobii,* 9 grams *Radix Ophiopogonis,* and 9 grams *Radix Trichosanthis.*

For cases with convulsions, rigidity of the tongue, and spasm of jaw muscles, add 30 grams *Concha Haliotidis,* 4.5 grams *Scorpio,* and 9 grams *Lumbricus.*

RETENTION OF COLD-PHLEGM (usually seen in cerebral embolism and cerebral angiospasm). Manifestations: Sudden onset of convulsions and coma, speech defect, headache, dizziness, nausea, vomiting, hemiplegia, pallor, cyanosis, flabby tongue with purpura on its border, deep, taut, and slippery pulse.

Principle of treatment: Dispelling pathogenic wind and eliminating phlegm; pacifying the liver and relieving convulsions.

Prescription: Decoction for Longevity and Normal Speech Ability, with Modifications.

Pulvis Cornu Antelopis	1.5	grams
Ramulus Cinnamomi	3	"
Fructus Aconiti Praeparata	3	"
Rhizoma seu Radix Notopterygii	4.5	"
Radix Ledebouriellae	4.5	"
Rhizoma Gastrodiae	9	"
Semen Ziziphi Spinosae	12	"
Rhizoma Pinelliae Praeparata	6	"
Succus Bambusae (bamboo juice)	30	"

Modifications include: For cases with pectoral stuffiness, shortness of breath, and cyanosis, add one Storax Bolus, twice daily.

For cases with profuse sputum, add 4.5 grams *Arisaema cum Bilis* (arisaema with bile) and 4.5 grams *Rhizoma Acori Graminei.*

For cases with cramps of limbs, add 4.5 grams *Scorpio* and 9 grams *Bombyx Batryticatus.*

PROSTRATION DUE TO DEPLETION OF VITAL FUNCTION AND VITAL ESSENCE (a manifestation of hollow visceral apoplexy; usually found in cerebral hemorrhage and subarachnoid hemorrhage). Manifestations: Closed eyes, open mouth, shortness of breath, coma, pallor, slightly flushed face, sweating, cold limbs, urinary incontinence, thready, rapid or deep, hidden pulse.

Principle of treatment: Reinforcing vital function and replenishing vital essence to rescue the patient.

Prescription: Decoction of Ginseng and Aconiti, with Modifications.

Radix Ginseng (simmered separately)	9	grams
Fructus Aconiti Praeparata	9	"
Radix Ophiopogonis	9	"
Fructus Schisandrae	6	"
Os Draconis Ustum (decocted first)	15	"
Concha Ostreae (decocted first)	15	"

Modifications include: For cases with profuse sweating, add 15 grams *Radix Astragali* and 9 grams *Radix Paeoniae Alba.*

For cases with deficiency of vital essence and flushed cheeks, add 15 grams *Radix Rehmannia,* 6 grams *Fructus Corni,* and 9 grams *Herba Dendrobii.*

For cases with deficiency of vital energy and pallor, add 3 grams *Cortex Cinnamomi.*

DEFICIENCY OF BLOOD AND BLOOD STASIS (usually seen in seque-lae of channel apoplexy or cerebrovascular accident). Manifestations: Hemiplegia, speech defect, numbness of the hand and foot, flaccid muscles, apathy, dull expression, livid complexion or pallor, pale tongue with white coating or with purpura on its border, deep, thready, and choppy pulse.

Principle of treatment: Reinforcing vital energy and nourishing blood; promoting normal blood flow to remove stasis.

Prescription: Decoction for Recuperating from Hemiplegia by Reinforcing Vital Energy, with Modifications.

Radix Astragali	30	grams
Rhizoma Ligustici Chuanxiong	9	"
Radix Angelicae Sinensis	9	"
Radix Paeoniae Rubra	9	"
Lumbricus	15	"
Semen Persicae	9	"
Flos Carthami	6	"
Radix Achyranthis Bidentatae	9	"
Radix Salviae Miltiorrhizae	9	"

Modifications include: For cases with numbness, cramps, pain, and heaviness of the limbs, add 6 grams *Squama Manitis Praeparata,* 9 grams *Herba Siegesbeckiae,* 9 grams *Bombyx Batryticatus,* 4.5 grams *Scorpio,* and 3 grams *Arisaema cum Bilis.*

For cases with numbness and cold limbs, add 6 grams *Ramulus Cinnamomi* and 6 grams *Radix Aconiti Praeparata.*

For dull expression, add 9 grams *Redix Curcumae* and 6 grams *Rhizoma Acori Graminei.*

DEFICIENCY OF VITAL ESSENCE OF THE LIVER (usually found in sequelae of cerebrovascular accident). Manifestations: Speech defect, hemiparesis or hemiplegia, numbness of the limbs, uncontrolled drooling, dizziness, flushed face, dull expression, reddened tongue, thready pulse.

CASE HISTORY
Female, age 66, first visit on August 7, 1972.

History

One week before seeing the doctor, the patient had suddenly lost consciousness and then developed right-sided hemiplegia, speech defect, profuse sputum, uncontrolled drooling, lassitude, and anorexia.

Diagnosis and Treatment

On examination, a white tongue coating and taut and slippery pulse were found. It was thought that the disease was due to retention of phlegm and stagnation of vital energy, causing blockage of the channels. The ingredients given were as follows:

Concha Margaritifera Usta	30	grams
Flos Chrysanthemi	9	"
Gypsum Fibrosum	18	"
Ramulus Loranthi	24	"
Radix Achyranthis Bidentatae	9	"
Rhizoma Acori Graminei	9	"
Semen Armeniacae Amarum	9	"
Exocarpium Citri Grandis	9	"
Radix Salviae Miltiorrhizae	15	"
Flos Carthemi	9	"
Caulis Spatholobi	30	"
Ramulus Mori (mulberry branch)	30	"
Retinervus Luffae Fructus	12	"
Fructus Hordei Germinatus	15	"
Fructus Oryzae Germinatus	15	"

One dose daily was given for seven days.

Second visit: August 14.

The patient could walk with a stick, but the movement of her right arm was impaired. A white tongue coating and taut, slippery pulse were present.

The above prescription was given again except that *Flos Charysanthemi* was deleted and 9 grams *Resina Olibani*, 9 grams *Resina Myrrhae*, and 9 grams *Lumbricus* were added.

Third visit: August 21.

The motion impairment had decreased, but the patient felt weak and had no appetite. The pulse condition and tongue picture were the same as before. The above prescription was continued except that *Gypsum* and *Ramulus Loranthi* were deleted and 12 grams *Radix Astragali*, 12 grams *Radix Codonopsis Pilosulae*, and 6 grams *Fructus Amomi* were added.

Fourth visit: August 28.

The motion impairment of the right arm and the speech defect had nearly disappeared. The following ingredients were prescribed for convalescence:

Radix Astragali	24	grams
Radix Codonopsis Pilosulae	12	"
Radix Angelicae Sinensis	12	"
Radix Salviae Miltiorrhizae	15	"

Ramulus Mori	30	grams
Caulis Spatholobi	30	"
Lignum Sappan (sappan caesalpinia)	6	"
Ramulus Cinammonia	9	"
Lumbricus	9	"
Herba Epimedii	15	"
Squama Manitis	9	"
Retinervus Luffae Fructus	12	"
Concha Margaritifera Usta	30	"
Radix Achyranthis Bidentatae	9	"
Resina Olibani	9	"
Resina Myrrhae	9	"

—Wang Hongshi, *Veteran Traditional Doctors' Experiences in Beijing* (Beijing Publishing House, 1980), p. 138.

Principle of treatment: Replenishing vital essence of the liver and kidney to nourish blood.

Prescription: Decoction of Rehmannia, with Modifications.

Radix Rehmannia Praeparata	15	grams
Radix Morindae Officinalis	12	"
Herba Cistanchis	12	"
Herba Dendrobii	12	"
Fructus Corni	9	"
Radix Achyranthis Bidentatae	12	"
Fructus Schisandrae	3	"
Radix Ophiopogonis	9	"
Fructus Aconiti Praeparata	3	"
Cortex Eucommiae	12	"
Ramulus Loranthi	12	"

Modifications include: For cases with dry mouth and reddened tongue, omit *Fructus Aconiti* and add 9 grams *Colla Corii Asini* (melted) and 15 grams *Plastrum Testudinis*.

For cases with muscle spasm, add 9 grams *Colla Corii Asini* (melted) and 9 grams *Radix Paeoniae Alba*.

For cases with constipation, add 12 grams *Fructus Cannabis* and 12 grams *Fructus Leonuri*.

For cases with dull expression, add 9 grams *Rhizoma Acori Graminei* and 9 grams *Radix Polygalae*.

For cases with insomnia, add 12 grams *Semen Biotae* and 12 grams *Semen Ziziphi Spinosae*.

Other Common Methods of Treating Cerebrovascular Accident

PROVEN RECIPES

1. Major Bolus for Activating Blood Flow in Channels: For sequelae of cerebrovascular accident (e.g., hemiplegia), one bolus twice daily.
2. Siegesbeckiae and Clerodendri Pills: for sequelae of cerebrovascular accident and prevention of cerebral hemorrhage, 6–9 grams twice daily.

ACUPUNCTURE TREATMENT

1. Hollow visceral apoplexy.
Main points: Renzhong (Du 26), Yongquan (K 1), Neiguan (P 6), Zusanli (St 36).
Points according to manifestations:

Flushed face, irritability, gigantic and rapid pulse—Shixuan (needling until bleeding)
Headache, muscle spasm—Hegu (LI 4), Taichong (Liv 3)
Profuse sputum—Fenglong (St 40), Tiantu (Ren 22)
Cold limbs, faint pulse—Moxibustion applied to Qihai (Ren 6), Guanyuan (Ren 4), Zusanli (St 36)

2. Channel apoplexy or sequelae of apoplexy.
Main points: For paralysis of the upper limbs, Jianyu (LI 15), Quchi (LI 11), Hegu (LI 4) through Laogong (P 8), Waiguan (SJ 5) through Neiguan (P 6), Baxie (Extra 28). For paralysis of the lower limbs, Huantiao (GB 30), Fengshi (GB 31), Zusanli (St 36), Yanglingquan (GB 34), Jiexi (St 41), Bafeng (Extra 36).
Points according to manifestations:

Deviation of the mouth and eyes (facial paresis) Taiyang (Extra 2), Fengchi (GB 20), Xiaguan (St 7), Jiache (St 6), Yingxiang (LI 20), Dicang (St 4), Hegu (LI 4), Zusanli (St 36)
Speech defect—Lianquan (Ren 23), Yamen (Du 15), Tongli (H 5), Sanyinjiao (Sp 6), Jinjin (Extra 10), Yuye (Extra 10) (prick to bloodlet), Zhaohai (K 6)

Difficulty in swallowing—Yamen (Du 15), Lianquan (Ren 23), Zhaohai (K 6), Tiantu (Ren 22), Sanyinjiao (SP 6)

EAR-ACUPUNCTURE THERAPY. Heart, Kidney, Ear-Shenmen, Subcortex, Brain Point, corresponding points on the affected limbs.

Two or three points are selected for each treatment, and needles
are embedded for three to five days.

NEPHRITIS

Nephritis is inflammation of the kidney, either acute or chronic.
One form of this condition follows infection by hemolytic strepto-
cocci. Clinical manifestations include edema, hypertension, protein-
uria, and sometimes heart failure, hypertensive encephalopathy, and
uremia. In traditional Chinese medicine, nephritis is classified as
"edema of *yang* nature" (i.e., edema due to dysfunction of the lung)
or "edema of *yin* nature" (i.e., edema due to dysfunction of the spleen
and kidney); acute nephritis is usually known as "edema due to affection by pathogenic wind" and chronic nephritis as "generalized
anasarca" or "abdominal fullness."

Etiology

Acute nephritis is caused by exogenous affection by pathogenic
wind or inflamed lesions of the body surface. When the body is
bound up by pathogenic wind, water is retained, the spleen and
stomach malfunction, and water metabolism is impeded. Thus, generalized anasarca and oliguria follow. In some cases, frequency or
urgency of urination occurs because of pathogenic damp-heat entering the urinary bladder. Hematuria occurs when damp-heat collects
in the urinary bladder, turns to pathogenic fire, and injures the vessels. When damp-heat rushes to the head and when vital energy of
the lung and stomach flows upward, dizziness, headache, nausea, and
vomiting appear.

Chronic nephritis develops from acute nephritis. It is induced by
overexertion, common cold, and improper diet; thus, the disease is
related to dysfunction of the spleen, kidney, and liver. Failure of

water transport brings about edema and anorexia due to lowered functioning of the spleen and kidney. Livid complexion, low back pain, and lassitude are caused by insufficient vital essence of the kidney and depletion of essence and blood. Repeated edema due to persistent kidney disorders eventually leads to severe disease, marked by lowered vital function and insufficient vital essence of the *zang-fu* organs.

Essentials of Diagnosis and Treatment

At the incipient stage, the disease is manifested by retention of water and dysfunction in water metabolism. But in protracted cases, lowered vital function and insufficient vital essence are common. Clinically, acute nephritis may be divided into the following symptom-complexes: collection of pathogenic wind-water, accumulation of pathogenic damp-heat, and accumulation of pathogenic dampness in the spleen. Chronic nephritis may be divided into the following symptom-complexes: weakened spleen due to abundant dampness, weak functioning of the spleen and kidney, and deficiency of vital essence and preponderance of vital function. In the late stage of nephritis, there may be uremia, symptom-complexes of which are divided into lowered vital functioning and upward attack of pathogenic dampness, lowered body resistance and excessive heat in the blood system, and depletion of vital essence and vital function.

In acute nephritis, it is important to expel pathogenic factors by diaphoresis and remove dampness through diuresis. If edema is present in chronic nephritis, it is advisable to remove dampness through diuresis by replenishing vital essence. If edema is not prominent but headache and dizziness occur, it is advisable to replenish vital essence of the liver and kidney. After edema disappears, it is necessary to tonify the spleen and kidney. When uremia occurs, treatment methods such as strengthening body resistance to cool blood and subduing wind for resuscitation are employed.

Treatment Based on Differentiation of Pathological Conditions

COLLECTION OF PATHOGENIC WIND-WATER (usually seen at the incipient stage of acute nephritis). Manifestations: Aversion to wind, headache, low back pain, puffiness of the face and limbs, concentrated urine or hematuria, coughing, shortness of breath, pale, reddened tongue with white coating, floating and slippery pulse.

Principle of treatment: Removing pathogenic wind and heat; clearing the lung to promote urination and relieve edema.

Prescription: Decoction of Ephedra, Forsythia, and Phaseoli, with Modifications.

Herba Ephedrae	6	grams
Fructus Forsythiae	15	"
Semen Phaseoli	30	"
Gypsum Fibrosum	30	"
Rhizoma Imperatae	30	"
Folium Perillae	9	"

Modifications include: For cases with cough, add 9 grams *Semen Armeniacae Amarum* and 9 grams *Radix Peucedani*.

For cases with hematuria or dark red urine, add 15 grams *Radix Rehmannia* and 30 grams *Herba Cephalanoploris*.

ACCUMULATION OF PATHOGENIC DAMP-HEAT (usually found in acute nephritis marked by edema, hematuria, and hypertension). Manifestations: Generalized anasarca, scanty urine, hematuria, frequent urination, urgency, headache, dizziness, hypertension, bitter taste and dryness in the mouth, nausea, vomiting, constipation, abdominal distension, slimy yellow tongue coating, taut and slippery pulse.

Principle of treatment: Clearing away heat to cool blood; promoting urination to relieve edema.

Prescription: Decoction of Cephalanoploris, with Modifications.

Herba Cephalanoploris	30	grams
Rhizoma Imperatae	30	"
Pulvis Talci	15	"
Folium Pyrrosiae (pyrrosia leaf)	30	"
Semen Plantaginis (wrapped with gauze)	15	"
Poria	9	"
Rhizoma Alismatis	9	"
Radix Stephaniae Tetrandrae	9	"
Radix Rehmannia	18	"
Nodus Nelumbinis Rhizomatis	15	"
Herba Leonuri	15	"

Modifications include: For cases with dermatopathy (e.g., boils and furuncles), add 12 grams *Flos Lonicerae* and 12 grams *Cortex Dictamni Radicis*.

For cases with urgency and frequency of urination, add 12 grams *Spora Lygodii* (climbing fern).

For cases with headache, dizziness, and hypertension, add 15 grams *Spica Prunellae* and 15 grams *Herba Siegesbeckiae*.

ACCUMULATION OF PATHOGENIC DAMPNESS IN THE SPLEEN (usually found in acute nephritis). Manifestations: Edema (worse below the loins), scanty urine, loose stools, lassitude, anorexia, stuffiness in the chest and abdomen, nausea, vomiting, pale tongue with slippery white or slimy white coating, deep slow or deep thready pulse.

Principle of treatment: Strengthening the function of the spleen; removing dampness through diuresis.

Prescription: Decoction of Five Ingredients Including Poria and Decoction of Peels of Five Herbs, with Modifications.

Poria	30	grams
Polyporus Umbellatus	15	"
Rhizoma Alismatis	15	"
Rhizoma Atractylodis Macrocephalae	15	"
Ramulus Cinnamomi	9	"
Pericarpium Arecae	15	"
Exocarpium Zingiberis	9	"
Cortex Mori Radicis	15	"
Rhizoma Atractylodis	15	"
Exocarpium Benincasae	30	"
Pericarpium Citri Reticulatae	9	"
Rhizoma Alismatis	12	"

WEAKENED SPLEEN DUE TO ABUNDANT DAMPNESS (usually seen in chronic nephritis diffuse glomerular and tubular stage). Manifestations: Recurrent edema (worse below the low back), livid complexion, lassitude, stuffiness in the chest and abdomen, anorexia, loose stools, pale tongue with white or slimy white coating, soft and slow pulse.

Principle of treatment: Invigorating vital function of the spleen and removing dampness through diuresis.

Prescription: Spleen Strengthening Decoction, with Modifications.

Cortex Magnoliae Officinalis	9 grams
Rhizoma Alismatis	9 "
Fructus Aconiti Praeparata	6 "
Rhizoma Atractylodis	9 "
Ramulus Cinnamomi	6 "
Semen Alpiniae Katsumadai	6 "
Cortex Poria	15 "
Radix Astragali	15 "
Semen Plantaginis (wrapped in gauze)	15 "
Rhizoma Atracylodis Macrocephalae	9 "

Modifications include: For cases with prominent edema, add 15 grams *Pericarpium Arecae* and 15 grams *Exocarpium Benincasae.*

WEAKENED FUNCTIONING OF THE SPLEEN AND KIDNEY (usually seen in chronic nephritis, diffuse glomerular and tubular stage). Manifestations: Protracted severe edema (worse below the loins), scanty urine, distended abdomen, pallor, anorexia, fullness sensation after meals, loose stools, aching loins and legs, aversion to cold, cold limbs, flabby tongue with dental indentations along its border, white tongue coating, deep and thready pulse.

Principle of treatment: Invigorating vital function of the spleen and kidney; removing obstruction through diuresis.

Prescription: Restoring Kidney Decoction Prescribed by the Golden Chamber, with Modifications.

Fructus Aconiti Praeparata	9 grams
Cortex Cinnamomi	3 "
Radix Rehmannia Praeparata	15 "
Fructus Corni	9 "
Rhizoma Dioscoreae	15 "
Poria	15 "
Rhizoma Alismatis	9 "
Rhizoma Zingiberis	3 "
Rhizoma Atractylodis Macrocephalae	9 "

Modifications include: For cases with prominent edema, add 9 grams *Radix Achyranthis Bidentatae* and 15 grams *Semen Plantaginis.*

For cases with lassitude, palpitation, and profuse sweating, omit *Rhizoma Alismatis* and *Rhizoma Zingiberis,* halve the amounts of *Cortex Cinnamomi* and *Fructus Aconiti Praeparata,* and add 12 grams *Radix*

Codonopsis Philosulae, 12 grams *Radix Astragali,* and 9 grams *Radix Angelicae Sinensis.*

For cases with dizziness, anemia and purple tongue in females, add 6 grams *Colla Corii Asini,* 12 grams *Radix Astragali,* 9 grams *Radix Angelicae Sinensis,* 9 grams *Herba Leonuri,* and 12 grams *Radix Glycyrrhizae Praeparata.*

DEFICIENCY OF VITAL ESSENCE AND PREPONDERANCE OF VITAL FUNCTION (usually found in chronic nephritis and renal hypertension). Manifestations: Moderate or no edema, dizziness, headache, hypertension, flushed face, tinnitus, blurred vision, aching loins, dry throat, restlessness, insomnia, night sweats, seminal emission, yellowish urine, reddened tongue with scanty coating, thready and taut pulse.

Principle of treatment: Nourishing the liver and kidney, subduing hyperactivity of the liver, and checking exuberance of vital function.

Prescription: Rehmannia Decoction of Lycii and Chrysanthemum, with Modifications.

Radix Polygoni Multiflori Praeparata	15	grams
Radix Rehmannia Praeparata	15	"
Fructus Lycii	12	"
Ramulus Loranthi	15	"
Concha Margaritifera Usta	30	"
Concha Ostreae	30	"
Fructus Tribuli	12	"
Flos Chrysanthemi	9	"
Cortex Moutan Radicis	9	"
Fructus Leonuri	12	"

Modifications include: For cases with prominent dizziness, add 12 grams *Semen Cassiae,* 12 grams *Ramulus Uncariae cum Uncis,* and 9 grams *Spica Prunellae.*

For cases with prominent edema, omit *Radix Rehmannia Praeparata* and *Radix Polygoni Multiflori* and add 12 grams *Cortex Poria.*

For cases with moderate fever and dry throat, add 12 grams *Radix Glehniae,* 12 grams *Radix Cynanchi Atrati,* and 9 grams *Radix Ophiopogonis.*

LOWERED VITAL FUNCTION AND UPWARD ATTACK OF PATHO-
GENIC DAMPNESS (usually seen in the first stage of uremia). Manifestations: Protracted anasarca, dizziness, nausea, vomiting, pallor, lassitude, anorexia, stuffiness in the chest and abdomen, aversion to
cold, somnolence, decreased amount of urine or anuria, loose stools,
flabby tongue with dental indentations along its border, deep, thready,
and slow pulse.

Principle of treatment: Invigorating vital function to remove
dampness; regulating the function of the stomach and spleen to bring
down adverse flow of vital energy.

Prescription: Decoction for Controlling Water, with Modifications.

Radix Aconiti Praeparata	6	grams
Radix Paeoniae Alba	9	"
Rhizoma Atracylodis Macrocephalae	9	"
Rhizoma Pinelliae Praeparata	9	"
Cortex Poria	12	"
Exocarpium Zingiberis	12	"
Radix Codonopsis Pilosulae	12	"
Pericarpium Citri Reticulatae	6	"
Caulis Bambusae in Taenis	9	"

Modifications include: For cases with thick, slimy tongue coating,
constipation, and abdominal distension, add 9 grams *Radix et Rhizoma Rhei* and 6 grams *Fructus Aurantii Immaturus.*

For cases with urinary retention and distension in the lower abdomen, add 12 grams *Semen Plantaginis* and 12 grams *Radix Achyranthis Bidentatae.*

LOWERED BODY RESISTANCE AND EXCESSIVE HEAT IN THE BLOOD
SYSTEM (usually found in uremia). Manifestations: Moderate edema,
emaciation, dizziness, dull expression, delirium, fever, restlessness,
epistaxis, bleeding gums, dry mouth, azotemic breath odor, blurred
vision, constipation, convulsions of the limbs, reddened or prickly
tongue with brown coating, thready and rapid pulse.

Principle of treatment: Clearing away pathogenic heat and cooling
blood; subduing hyperfunction of the liver and endogenous wind and
reinforcing vital energy.

Prescription: Decoction of Rhinoceros Cornu and Rehmannia, with Modifications.

Pulvis Rhinocori (rhinoceros horn powder)   1.5 grams
or
Pulvis Bubali (buffalo horn powder)   30–60   "
Radix Rehmannia   30   "
Cortex Moutan Radicis   9   "
Radix Paeoniae Rubra   9   "
Rhizoma Imperatae   30   "
Herba Dendrobii   15   "
Fructus Gardeniae   9   "
Radix et Rhizoma Rhei (decocted later)   9   "
Radix Scutellariae   12   "
Radix Ginseng   9   "
Rhizoma Acori Graminei   9   "

Modifications include: For cases with epistaxis and bleeding gums, omit *Rhizoma Acori Graminei* and add 15 grams *Herba Ecliptae* (eclipta herb).

For cases with dry mouth and reddened tongue, add 12 grams *Radix Scrophulariae,* 12 grams *Radix Ophiopogonis,* 12 grams *Concha Ostreae,* 12 grams *Plastrum Testudinis,* and 12 grams *Carapax Triony- cis.*

For cases with coma and rattling in the throat, administer a *Bezoar Resurrection Bolus.*

For cases with delirium, restlessness, and cramps of limbs, add 1.5 grams *Purple Snowy Powder.*

DEPLETION OF VITAL ESSENCE AND VITAL FUNCTION (usually seen in the late stage of uremia). Manifestations: Pallor, feeble respiration or shortness of breath, azotemic breath odor, coma or somnolence, profuse sweating, scanty or no urine, pale tongue with little coating, feeble or faint pulse.

Principle of treatment: Reinforcing vital energy to revive patient.

Prescription: Decoction of Ginseng and Aconiti in Combination with Decoction for Invigorating Pulse-Beat, with Modifications.

Radix Ginseng   9 grams
Fructus Schisandrae   9   "

Radix Glycyrrhizae Praeparata	9 grams
Radix Aconiti Praeparata	15 "
Radix Ophiopogonis	15 "
Os Draconis Ustum	15 "
Concha Ostreae Usta	15 "

Modifications include: For cases with profuse sweating, add 15 grams *Radix Astragali,* 9 grams *Radix Paeoniae Alba,* and 30 grams *Fructus Tritiei Levis.*

For cases with polyuria or incontinence of urine, add 9 grams *Oötheca Mantidis* and 9 grams *Fructus Corni.*

Other Common Methods of Treating Nephritis

PROVEN RECIPES

1. *Herba Ecliptae*	15 grams
Rhizoma Imperatae	30 "

Decoction given for acute nephritis marked by hematuria.

2. *Herba Leonuri*	30 grams
Exocarpium Benincasae	60 "

Decoction given for acute nephritis marked by hypertension.

3. *Herba Cephalanoploris*	9–15 grams
Cacumen Biotae	9–15 "
Herba Ecliplae	9–15 "
Radix Rubiae	9–15 "
Cortes Moutan Radicis	9–15 "

Decoction of one or two ingredients is given once daily for acute nephritis with hematuria.

4. *Fructus Rosae Laevigatae*	30 grams
Radix Astragali	15 "
Semen Glycine (black soybean)	15 "
Semen Euryales	15 "

CASE HISTORY
Male, age 15, admitted on November 13, 1972.

History

The patient had severe edema. Urinalysis showed protein + + +, granular casts, red blood cells +, and a few leukocytes. Blood pressure was 150/90 mm Hg. The condition was diagnosed as acute glomerulonephritis and renal hypertension. Treatment by modern medicine was ineffective, and the disease progressed to nephrotic syndrome, marked by puffiness of the face, pallor, edema of the lower limbs, distended abdomen, ascites, concentrated urine, shortness of breath, stuffiness in the chest, vomiting, and anorexia.

Diagnosis and Treatment

On examination, a pale tongue with white coating and a taut and slippery pulse were observed. The condition was thought to be due to deficiency of vital energy of the lung and spleen, causing retention of pathogenic dampness. It was considered advisable to activate the function of the lung and spleen and eliminate edema through diuresis. The ingredients given were as follows:

Herba Ephedrae (prepared with honey)	15	grams
Fructus Forsythiae	15	"
Ramulus Cinammomi	9	"
Cortex Mori	15	"
Exocarpium Benincasae (wax gourd peel)	15	"
Pericarpium Arecae	15	"
Cortex Poria	15	"
Rhizoma Dioscoreae Hypoglaucae	15	"
Polyporus Umbellatus	9	"
Rhizoma Alismatis	9	"
Herba Polygoni Avicularis	9	"
Herba Dianthi	15	"
Caulis Akebiae	9	"
Talcum (wrapped in gauze)	15	"
Semen Plantaginis (wrapped in gauze)	15	"
Herba Leonurus	15	"
Rhizoma Imperatae	30	"

Second visit.

After nine doses, the edema of the lower limbs and the ascites had decreased. But the patient complained of a cold sensation in the abdomen and legs, aching in the low back, dry mouth, and preference for hot drink. Therefore, the following ingredients were prescribed:

Herba Ephedrae Praeparata	21	grams
Polyporus Umbellatus	15	"
Poria	15	"
Rhizoma Alismatis	9	"
Rhizoma Atractylodis	6	"
Rhizoma Atractylodis Macrocephalae	6	"
Radix Astragali	15	"
Radix Codonopsis Pilosulae	15	"
Fructus Aconiti Praeparata	9	"
Cortex Cinnamomi	3	"

Radix Stephaniae Tetrandrae	9 grams	
Pericarpium Arecae	15	"
Rhizoma Dioscoreae Hypoglaucae	15	"
Semen Plantaginis	9	"
Semen Alpiniae Katsumadai	9	"
Endothelium Corneum Gigeriae Galli	9	"
Fructus Crataegi Praeparata	9	"
Herba Leonurus	15	"
Massa Fermentata Medicinalis	9	"

Third visit.

The ascites had been entirely eliminated after seven doses of the above prescription. The following ingredients were given to improve the patient's condition:

Radix Rehmannia	15 grams	
Radix Rehmannia Praeparata	15	"
Fructus Aconiti Praeparata	15	"
Cortex Cinnamomi	3	"
Fructus Rosae Laevigatae	15	"
Semen Euryales	15	"
Fructus Ligustri Lucidi	9	"
Poria	15	"
Rhizoma Alismatis	9	"
Radix Astragali	30	"
Rhizoma Dioscoreae Hypoglaucae	15	"
Radix Sanguisorbae	15	"
Caulus Akebiae	15	"
Rhizoma Imperatae	30	"
Herba Ephedrae	15	"

Folium Pyrrosiae, 30 grams daily, steeped in water and taken as a beverage; and Placenta Pills, 6 pills three times daily.

Fourth visit.

After 12 doses of the above prescription, the patient's condition had improved markedly. The doctor prescribed Restoring Kidney Pills Prescribed by the Golden Chamber, Bolus of Six Ingredients with Rehmannia, Nourishing Kidney Bolus, Decoction of Stephaniae and Astragali, Decoction of Four Noble Ingredients, and Placenta Pills. By the middle of November 1973, renal function had returned to normal. Blood pressure was 120/80 mm Hg. As of July 1979, there had been no relapse.

—Liu Yanchi, "The Treatment of Nephrotic Syndrome" *Journal of the Beijing College of Traditional Chinese Medicine* (1982), no. 4, pp. 33–34.

Radix Codonopsis Pilosulae	9	"
Rhizoma Atracylodis Macrocephalae	9	"
Rhizoma Dioscoreae	9	"

Decoction given for nephritis marked by progressive albuminuria.

  5. *Fructus Ligustri Lucidi*   15–30 grams
     Herba Ecliplae   15–30   "
     Fructus Rosae Laevigatae   15–30   "

Decoction of one or two ingredients given once daily for one month for chronic nephritis marked by progressive albuminuria.

  6. *Folium Pyrrosiae*   18 grams
     Semen Coicis   6   "

Decoction given for albuminuria.

ACUPUNCTURE TREATMENT

Main points: Shenshu (UB 23), Sanyinjiao (Sp 6), Guanyuan (Ren 4), Zusanli (St 36).
Points according to manifestations:

Fever—Quchi (LI 11)
Nausea, vomiting—Neiguan (P 6)
Headache—Taiyang (Extra 2)
Edema, scanty urine—Yinlingquan (Sp 9), Hegu (LI 4), Pishu (UB 20), Feishu (UB 13)

Reducing method is applied for acute nephritis and reinforcing method for chronic nephritis.

EAR-ACUPUNCTURE THERAPY. Lung, Kidney, Spleen, Ear-shenmen, Hypertension groove (for hypertension).
One or two points are selected for each treatment, and needles are embedded for three to five days.

LOW BACK PAIN

This term refers to unilateral or bilateral dorsolumbar pain accompanied by a heavy, cold sensation. Low back pain is closely related to the condition of kidney, which is located in this region. It is found in the conditions designated by modern medicine as urinary tract disorders, muscular rheumatism, spinal disorders, muscle strain, and bruises.

Etiology

Low back pain can be caused by the following:

- Retention of pathogenic damp-cold in the lumbar region and impairment of smooth flow of vital energy and blood after one has sat or lain on cold, damp ground or been caught in the rain.
- Impairment of the channels by pathogenic damp-heat (exogenous affection by pathogenic damp-heat or endogenous retention of damp-heat can cause obstruction of the channels).
- Consumption of kidney essence (due to hypofunction of the kidney in debilitated patients, senile deficiency of essence and blood, or intemperance in sexual life).
- Stagnation of vital energy and stasis of blood (due to strain, protracted illness, or trauma).

Essentials of Treatment

In patients affected by pathogenic factors, it is important to expel those factors and unblock the channels. In cases with deficiency of kidney essence, methods of tonifying the kidney and reinforcing vital energy are usually applied. Low back pain due to stagnation of vital energy and stasis of blood is relieved by promoting the smooth flow of vital energy and blood.

To relieve pain, herbs to promote the smooth flow of vital energy and to promote the smooth flow of blood are often administered simultaneously. Herbs to tonify the kidney are also used.

Treatment According to Differentiation of Symptom-Complexes

LOW BACK PAIN DUE TO COLD-DAMPNESS. Manifestations: Low back pain with cold and heavy sensation (intensified on cold, wet days and not relieved by bed rest), preference for warmth in the lumbar region, slimy white tongue coating, deep and slow pulse.

Principle of treatment: Dispelling pathogenic cold-dampness to unblock the channels.

Prescription: Decoction for Removing Dampness from the Kidney, with Modifications.

Poria	12 grams
Rhizoma Atractylodis Macrocephalae	9 "
Rhizoma Zingiberis	6 "
Radix Glycyrrhizae	6 "
Radix Angelicae Pubescentis	12 "
Rhizoma Atractylodis	9 "
Ramulus Cinnamomi	9 "
Radix Achyranthis Bidentatae	9 "
Cortex Eucommiae	9 "
Ramulus Loranthi	12 "
Radix Dipsaci (himalaya teasel root)	9 "
Rhizoma Cibotii (chain fern rhizome)	12 "
Fructus Chaenomelis	9 "

Modifications include: For cases with severe pain, intolerance of cold, and cold limbs, add 6 grams *Radix Aconiti* and 3 grams *Herba Asari.*

For cases with wandering pain and aching in the joints, substitute Decoction of Angelicae Pubescentis and Loranthi, with Modifications.

For cases with deficiency of vital energy and blood and weakness of the low back and knees, add 15 grams *Radix Codonopsis Pilosulae,* 15 grams *Radix Astragali,* and 15 grams *Radix Rehmannia Praeparata.*

LOW BACK PAIN DUE TO PATHOGENIC DAMP-HEAT. Manifestations: Pain and burning sensation in the lumbar region, bitter taste in the mouth, restlessness, concentrated urine, slimy yellow tongue coating, soft and rapid pulse.

Principle of treatment: Clearing away pathogenic damp-heat from the body to relieve pain.

Prescription: Decoction of Four Wonderful Herbs, with Modifications.

Rhizoma Atractylodis	12 grams
Cortex Phellodendri	9 "

Radix Achyranthis Bidentatae	9	grams
Semen Coicis	30	"
Radix Stephaniae Tetrandrae	9	"
Rhizoma Dioscoreae Hypoglaucae	9	"
Fructus Chaenomelis	9	"
Radix Dipsaci	9	"

Modifications include: For cases with a burning sensation of the urethra, add 9 grams *Polyporus Unbellatus,* 9 grams *Rhizoma Alismatis,* and 9 grams *Semen Plantaginis.*

For severe cases, add 6 grams *Resina Olibani* and 6 grams *Resina Myrrhae.*

LOW BACK PAIN DUE TO HYPOFUNCTION OF THE KIDNEY. Manifestations: Lumbar pain relieved by pressure, weakness of the legs and knees (intensified by strain and stress and alleviated by bed rest), dizziness, tinnitus, spermatorrhea, morbid leukorrhea, pallor, cold limbs, scanty urine, pale tongue with white coating, deep and thready pulse.

Principle of treatment: Strengthening vital function of the kidney to relieve pain.

Prescriptions: For low back pain due to lowered vital function of the kidney, Bolus for Reinforcing Deficiency of Vital Function *(yang)* of the Kidney, with Modifications.

Radix Rehmannia Praeparata	15	grams
Rhizoma Dioscoreae	12	"
Fructus Corni	9	"
Fructus Lycii	9	"
Cortex Eucommiae	9	"
Radix Aconiti Praeparata	6	"
Cortex Cinnamomi	6	"
Radix Angelicae Sinensis	9	"
Semen Cuscutae	9	"

For low back pain due to deficiency of vital essence of the kidney, Bolus for Reinforcing Deficiency of Vital Essence *(yin)* of the Kidney, with Modifications.

Radix Rehmannia Praeparata	15	grams
Radix Dioscorea	12	"

Fructus Corni	12 grams
Poria	9 "
Rhizoma Alismatis	6 "
Cortex Moutan Radicis	6 "
Fructus Lycii	12 "
Colla Plastrum Testudinis	15 "
Carapax Trionycis	15

Modifications include: For cases with fever accompanied by irritability and restlessness, add 9 grams *Rhizoma Anemarrhenae* and 6 grams *Cortex Phellodendri*.

For low back pain without marked symptoms of deficiencies of vital essence and/or vital energy, substitute 30 grams Green Moth Pills twice daily (made with equal amounts of *Cortex Eucommiae, Fructus Psoraleae,* and *Semen Juglandis*).

LOW BACK PAIN DUE TO STASIS OF BLOOD. Manifestations: Sharp fixed sting and rigidity in the lumbar region (aggravated by pressure and by turning of the body), dark red tongue or tongue with purpura on it, choppy pulse.

Principle of treatment: Promoting blood circulation to remove blood stasis and relieve pain.

Prescription: Decoction for Relieving Generalized Pain Due to Blood Stasis, with Modifications.

Radix Angelicae Sinensis	12 grams
Rhizoma Ligustici Chuanxiong	9 "
Semen Persicae	9 "
Flos Carthami	9 "
Rhizoma et Radix Notopterygii	9 "
Resina Myrrhae	6 "
Radix Achyranthis Bidentatae	12 "
Faeces Trogopterorum	6 "
Rhizoma Cyperi	9 "
Eupolyphaga sue Steleophaga	6 "

Modifications include: For cases with rheumatism, add 9 grams *Radix Angelicae Pubscentis,* 9 grams *Radix Clematidis,* and 9 grams *Radix Gentianae Macrophyllae.*

For cases with deficiency of the kidney, add 12 grams *Radix Dipsaci,* 9 grams *Cortex Eucommiae,* and 9 grams *Rhizoma Cibotii.*

For cases following trauma, add 6 grams *Radix et Rhizoma Rhei* and 3 grams *Pulvis Notoginseng.*

Other Common Methods of Treating Low Back Pain

PROVEN RECIPES

Decoction given for low back pain due to pathogenic wind-cold:

Radix Angelicae Pubscentis	15 grams
Herba Siegesbeckiae	30 "

Herbs soaked in spirits and used in treating low back pain due to deficiency of the kidney:

Cortex Eucommiae	15 grams
Fructus Lycii	15 "

Herb taken with hot rice wine and used in treating low back pain due to trauma and stasis of blood: *Pulvis Eupolyphaga seu Steleophage,* 1.5 grams, Taken thrice daily for two days.

ACUPUNCTURE TREATMENT

Main points: Shenshu (UB 23), Weizhong (UB 40) and Ashi point.

Points according to manifestations: Deficiency of the kidney—Taixi (K 3), moxibustion at Mingmen (Du 4).

Aching of the low back and legs—Huantiao (GB 30), Kunlun (UB 60). Uniform reducing and reinforcing method is applied.

EAR-ACUPUNCTURE THERAPY. Ear-Kidney and tender spots around Low Back. One or two points are selected for each treatment, and needles are embedded for three to five days.

SEMINAL EMISSION

This category includes nocturnal emission and spermatorrhea, both of which are caused by exhaustion of kidney essence. In modern medical terms, the causes include neurosis, prostatorrhea, and spermatocystitis.

Etiology

Causes of seminal emission include the following:

- Deficiency of the kidney (due to marrying too early, masturbation, excessive sexual activity resulting in exhaustion of the essence and diminished function of the kidney).
- Deficiency of vital essence and exuberance of fire (due to mental strain, consumption of vital essence of the heart, and breakdown of the normal coordination between the heart and kidney, so that heart or vital gate fire attacks the kidney and brings about seminal emission).
- Invasion of the kidney by pathogenic damp-heat (due to excessive intake of greasy food or of alcohol, which turns to damp-heat that drives downward into the kidney).

Essentials of Diagnosis and Treatment

Diagnosis should be based largely on the tongue picture and pulse condition. Because a number of factors cause seminal emission, it is inadvisable to treat it only with astringents. When there is deficiency of the kidney, blindly tonifying the kidney and strengthening its vital function is not enough. In addition, treating the root cause should be emphasized.

Treatment According to Differentiation of Symptom-Complexes

SEMINAL EMISSION DUE TO DEFICIENCY OF THE KIDNEY. Manifestations: Continual seminal emission, spermatorrhea, dizziness, tinnitus, aching of the low back, lassitude, reddened tongue, thready and rapid pulse.

Principle of treatment: Tonifying the kidney to check emission.

Prescription: Decoction of Six Ingredients with Rehmannia in Combination with Decoction for Seminal Consolidation, with Modifications.

Radix Rehmannia Praeparata	15	grams
Rhizoma Dioscoreae	12	"
Fructus Corni	12	"
Fructus Rosae Laevigatae	15	"
Semen Euryales	15	"
Fructus Tribuli	12	"
Fructus Schisandrae	9	"
Stigma Nelumbinis	9	"
Os Draconis Ustum	15	"
Concha Ostreae Usta	15	"

Modifications include: For cases with feverish sensation in the palms and soles, reddened tongue, and thready and rapid pulse (indicating deficiency of vital essence), add 15 grams *Radix Rehmanniae,* 15 grams *Radix Scrophulariae,* and 9 grams *Fructus Lycii.*

For cases with pallor, intolerance of cold, cold limbs, pale tongue with white coating, and deep and thready pulse (indicating lowered vital function), add 6 grams *Radix Aconiti Praeparata,* 6 grams *Cortex Cinnamomi,* and 9 grams *Colla Cornus Cervi.*

SEMINAL EMISSION DUE TO DEFICIENCY OF VITAL ESSENCE AND EXUBERANCE OF FIRE. Manifestations: Nocturnal emmission, excessive libido, dizziness, blurred vision, palpitation, insomnia, lassitude, reddened tongue, thready and rapid pulse.

Principle of treatment: Nourishing vital essence to quell exuberance of fire and calming the mind to arrest emission.

Prescription: Rehmanniae Decoction of Anemarrhenae and Phellodendri, with Modifications.

Radix Rehmannia Praeparata	15	grams
Rhizoma Dioscoreae	15	"
Fructus Corni	9	"
Poria	9	"

Rhizoma Anemarrhenae	6 grams	
Cortex Moutan Radicis	9	"
Rhizoma Alismatis	9	"
Cortex Phellodendri	6	"
Fructus Rosae Laevigatae	12	"
Semen Euryales	12	"
Os Drac..is Ustum	15	"
Concha Ostreae Usta	15	"
Semen Ziziphi Spinosae Praeparata	15	"

Modifications include: For cases with prominent deficiency of vital essence, add 15 grams *Plastrum Testudinis,* 15 grams *Radix Scrophulariae,* and 9 grams *Fructus Schisandrae.*

For cases with restlessness and insomnia, add 6 grams *Rhizoma Coptidis* and 12 grams *Radix Ophiopogonis.*

For seminal emission due to deficiency of both vital essence and energy, administer Pills for Consolidating Semen with Three Herbs (composed of *Radix Ginseng, Radix Rehmannia Praeparata, Radix Asparagi, Cortex Phelodendri, Fructus Amomi,* and *Radix Glycyrrhizae),* 30 pills daily.

SEMINAL EMISSION DUE TO DOWNWARD DRIVE OF PATHOGENIC DAMP-HEAT. Manifestations: Frequent seminal emission, sperm discharge on urination, restlessness, insomnia, bitter taste in the mouth, brown urine, slimy yellow tongue coating, soft rapid pulse or slippery pulse.

Principle of treatment: Clearing away pathogenic damp-heat to check seminal emission.

Prescription: Dioscoreae Decoction to Eliminate Damp-Turbidity, with Modifications.

Rhizoma Dioscoreae Hypoglaucae	15 grams	
Semen Plantaginis (wrapped in gauze)	9	"
Poria	9	"
Rhizoma Alismatis	9	"
Plumula Nelumbinis (lotus plumule)	9	"
Cortex Phellodendri	9	"
Rhizoma Atractylodis	15	"
Talcum	15	"
Rhizoma Acori Graminei	9	"

Modifications include: For cases with concentrated urine and pain on urination, add 9 grams *Fructus Gardeniae,* 6 grams *Caulis Akebiae,* and 9 grams *Fructus Forsythiae.*

For cases with distension of the lower abdomen and continuous dripping of urine, add 30 grams *Herba Patriniae* (patrinia) and 9 grams *Radix Paeoniae Rubra.*

Other Common Methods of Treating Seminal Emission

PROVEN RECIPES

Decoction given for seminal emission and spermatorrhea due to deficiency of the kidney:

Fructus Rosae Laevigatae	15 grams
Semen Euryales	15 "

Decoction given for seminal emission due to downward drive of pathogenic damp-heat:

Rhizoma Dioscoreae Hypoglaucae	12 grams
Cortex Phellodendri	6 "
Rhizoma Smilacis Glabrae (smilax glabra rhixome)	18 "

For any type of seminal emission, *Pulvis Corium Erinacei* (powder of dried hedgehog skin), 3 grams daily.

ACUPUNCTURE TREATMENT

Main points: Group 1, Guanyuan (Ren 4), Zusanli (St 36), Taixi (K 3).

Group 2, Shenshu (UB 23), Zhishi (UB 52), Sanyinjiano (Sp 6).

Two groups of points may be used on alternate days. Weak to moderate needle manipulation is applied.

IMPOTENCE

Impotence is characterized by inability of the penis to erect. It commonly occurs in sexual neurosis and in deficiency due to chronic illnesses.

Etiology

Impotence can result from:

- Lowered vital function of the kidney because of excessive sexual activity or frequent masturbation.
- Impeded generation of vital essence and blood because overexertion of the brain has injured the function of the heart and spleen.
- Impairment of the kidney by emotional strain leading to stagnation of vital energy.
- Dysfunction of the liver and kidney caused by downward drive of pathogenic damp-heat.

Essentials of Diagnosis and Treatment

It is inadvisable immediately to administer herbs that tonify the kidney and strengthen sexual ability. It is important first to know the nature of the impotence—deficiency or excess. In general, impotence occurring after excessive sexual activity, seminal emission, and ejaculatio praecox is considered to be due to lowered function of the kidney, whereas sudden onset of impotence is thought to result from damage to vital energy of the heart, spleen, and kidney.

Treatment According to Differentiation of Symptom-Complexes

IMPOTENCE DUE TO LOWERED VITAL FUNCTION OF THE KIDNEY. Manifestations: Impotence, pallor, dizziness, blurred vision, lassitude, aching of the low back and knees, white tongue coating, deep and thready pulse.

Principle of treatment: Tonifying the kidney to invigorate its vital function.

Prescription: Decoction for Supporting Impregnation, with Modifications.

Radix Rehmannia Praeparata	15	grams
Semen Cuscutae	12	"
Fructus Lycii	12	"
Rhizoma Curculiginis	12	"
Radix Morindae Officinalis	12	"
Herba Epimedii	9	"
Herba Cistanchis	12	"
Fructus Cnidii	9	"
Semen Allii Tuberose	9	"
Fructus Corni	12	"
Radix Aconiti Praeparata	6	"
Cortex Cinnamomi	6	"

IMPOTENCE DUE TO DEFICIENCY OF VITAL ESSENCE AND BLOOD. Manifestations: Impotence, ejaculatio praecox, depression, excessive dreaming during sleep, pallor, lassitude, palpitation, amnesia, pale tongue with thin coating, thready and weak pulse.

Principle of treatment: Tonifying the heart and spleen; replenishing vital energy of the kidney to invigorate its vital function.

Prescription: Decoction of Ginseng and Antler, with Modifications.

Radix Codonopsis Pilosulae	15	grams
or		
Radix Astragali	15	"
Radix Ginseng	6	"
Radix Rehmannia Praeparata	12	"
Herba Cistanchis	15	"
Rhizoma Dioscoreae	15	"
Radix Angelicae Sinensis	9	"
Semen Cuscutae	12	"
Herba Epimedii	12	"
Radix Morindae Officinalis	9	"
Pulvis Cornu Cervi Pantotrichum	1.5	"
(pilose antler taken separately)		

IMPOTENCE DUE TO EMOTIONAL DISTURBANCE. Manifestations: Impotence, depression, suspicion, palpitation, excessive dreaming during sleep, thin slimy tongue coating, taut and thready pulse.

Principle of treatment: Tonifying and invigorating vital function of the kidney; calming the mind.

Prescription: Decoction for Nourishing the Kidney, with Modifications.

Radix Codonopsis Pilosulae	15	grams
Rhizoma Dioscoreae Praeparata	12	"
Radix Rehmannia Praeparata	12	"
Cortex Eucommiae	9	"
Fructus Lycii	9	"
Radix Angelicae Sinensis	9	"
Fructus Corni	9	"
Semen Cuscutae	9	"
Herba Epimedii	12	"
Os Draconis Ustum	15	"
Concha Ostreae Usta	15	"
Semen Ziziphi Spinosae Praeparata	15	"

IMPOTENCE DUE TO DOWNWARD DRIVE OF PATHOGENIC DAMP-HEAT. Manifestations: Impotence, weakness and heaviness of the legs, concentrated urine, slimy yellow tongue coating, deep, slippery or taut, slippery, rapid pulse.

Principle of treatment: Clearing away damp-heat.

Prescription: Decoction of Two Wonderful Herbs in Combination with Decoction of Diuretic Ingredients, with Modifications.

Rhizoma Atractylodis	12	grams
Cortex Phellodendri	6	"
Talcum	15	"
Fructus Gardeniae	9	"
Caulis Akebiae	6	"
Semen Plantaginis (wrapped in gauze)	9	"
Poria	9	"
Rhizoma Dioscoreae Hypoglaucae	15	"
Radix Achyranthis Bidentatae	6	"
Radix Glycyrrhizae	6	"

CASE HISTORY
Male, age 28, first visit on June 20, 1980.

History

The patient had a history of masturbation. One month before his marriage, he developed impotence.

Diagnosis and Treatment

On examination, it was found that the patient was afflicted with loss of hair. A slightly reddened tongue with scanty coating and a deep and taut pulse were also observed. It was thus concluded that the patient's impotence was due to deficiency of vital essence and lowered functioning of the kidney. Therefore, it was considered advisable to replenish vital essence of the kidney to improve sexual ability. The patient was given the following prescription:

Radix Rehmannia Praeparata	15 grams
Fructus Corni	9 "
Fructus Lycii	15 "
Rhizoma Dioscoreae	15 "
Poria	12 "
Cortex Moutan Radicis	6 "
Radix Morindae Officinalis	9 "
Herba Epimedii	15 "
Herba Cistanchis	9 "
Semen Cuscutae	9 "
Radix Polygoni Multiflori Praeparata	15 "
Rhizoma Polygonati	15 "
Cornu Cervi Degelatinatum (deglued antler horn powder)	9 "

After 25 doses, impotence disappeared and sex life returned to normal. New hair growth was observed, and the patient's complexion became ruddy.

—From Chen Jiayang, *A Collection of Case Histories of Traditional Chinese Medicine* (Gansu People's Publishing House, 1981), pp. 532–33.

Other Common Methods of Treating Impotence

PROVEN RECIPES

1. *Herba Epimedii*   60 grams
   salt   3 "

Soaked in 300 grams alcohol; 30 grams given in the morning and evening.

2. Decoction of *Allium Chinenses*, 60 grams.

3. *Placenta Hominis*   1 portion
   Actinolitum (actinolite)   1   "

Six grams of powder given in the morning and evening.

ACUPUNCTURE TREATMENT

Main points: Group 1, Guanyuan (Ren 4), Zusanli (St 36), Taixi (K 3).
Group 2, Shenshu (UB 23), Zhishi (UB 52), Sanyinjiao (Sp 6).
Moxibustion may be applied to the above two groups of points on alternate days.

EAR-ACUPUNCTURE THERAPY. External Genitalia, Seminal Vesicle, Testis, Endocrine, Subcortex. One or two points are selected for each treatment, and needles are embedded for three days.

INSOMNIA

The term "insomnia" refers to difficulty in falling asleep and to disturbed sleep. Sometimes insomnia is accompanied by dizziness, headache, palpitation, and/or amnesia. It occurs commonly in conditions that modern medicine designates as neurosis and menopausal syndromes.

Etiology

Insomnia can result from:

• Insufficiency of vital energy and blood caused by mental strain and by dysfunction of the spleen and heart.
• Disharmony of the heart and kidney caused by protracted illness or asthenia that leads to consumption of vital essence of the kidney and exuberance of vital function of the heart.
• Deficiency of vital energy of the heart and gallbladder causing agitation of the mind.

- Upward flaring of liver fire because of mental depression.
- Retention of phlegm-heat because of improper diet and impairment of the stomach and intestines.

Essentials of Diagnosis and Treatment

It is important to determine whether the insomnia is of deficiency or excessiveness nature. Insomnia due to deficiency should be treated by reinforcing vital energy and blood; that due to excessiveness, by removing pathogenic factors. Sedatives and tranquilizing prescriptions may be administered to improve the effect.

Treatment According to Differentiation of Symptom-Complexes

INSOMNIA DUE TO LOWERED FUNCTIONING OF THE HEART AND SPLEEN. Manifestations: Insomnia, excessive dreaming during sleep, tendency to awake, palpitation, amnesia, dizziness, blurred vision, lassitude, poor appetite, pallor, pale tongue with thin coating, thready and weak pulse.

Principle of treatment: Tonifying the spleen and heart to ease the mind.

Prescription: Decoction for Acting on the Spleen, with Modifications.

Radix Codonopsis Pulosulae	12	grams
or		
Radix Ginseng	6	"
Rhizoma Atractylodis macrocephalae	9	"
Radix Astragali	9	"
Radix Angelicae Sinensis	9	"
Semen Ziziphi Spinosae	15	"
Arillus Longan (longan avil)	9	"
Lignum Pini Poriaferum	12	"
Radix Polygalae	9	"
Fructus Schisandrae	9	"
Semen Biotae	9	"
Cortex Albiziae	9	"

Modifications include: For cases with pallor due to deficiency of heart blood, add 15 grams *Radix Rehmanniae* and 6 grams *Colla Corii Asini.*

For cases with excessive dreaming during sleep, add 15 grams *Dens Draconis* (dragon's teeth), 15 grams *Concha Ostreae,* and 15 grams *Concha Margaritifera Usta.*

INSOMNIA DUE TO DEFICIENCY OF VITAL ESSENCE AND TO IN-TENSE HEAT. Manifestations: Restlessness, insomnia, palpitation, amnesia, dizziness, tinnitus, thirst, feverish sensation in the chest region, palms, and soles, low back pain, nocturnal emission, reddened tongue, thready and rapid pulse.

Principle of treatment: Replenishing vital essence to clear away heat and calm the mind.

Prescription: Mind-Easing Decoction, with Modifications.

Radix Rehmannia	15	grams
Radix Angelicae Sinensis	9	"
Radix Ophiopogonis	9	"
Semen Biotae	12	"
Semen Ziziphi Spinosae	12	"
Poria	9	"
Radix Polygalae	6	"
Fructus Schisandrae	6	"
Radix Salviae Miltiorrhizae	12	"
Rhizoma Coptidis	6	"
Concha Margaritifera Usta	30	"

Modifications include: For cases with seminal emission, add 9 grams *Fructus Rosae Laevigatae* and 9 grams *Semen Euryales.*

For cases with thirst, add 9 grams *Herba Dendrobii* and 9 grams *Rhizoma Polygonati Odorati.*

INSOMNIA DUE TO DEFICIENCY OF VITAL ENERGY OF THE HEART AND GALLBLADDER. Manifestations: Insomnia, excessive dreaming during sleep, propensity to awake with a start, palpitation, shortness of breath, lassitude, watery urine, pale tongue, taut and thready pulse.

Principle of treatment: Reinforcing vital energy to calm the mind.

Prescription: Bolus for Calming the Mind Combined with Decoction of Ziziphi Spinosae, with Modifications.

Radix Codonopsis Pilosulae	15 grams
or	
Radix Ginseng	6 "
Poria	12 "
Rhizoma Acori Graminei	9 "
Dens Draconis	15 "
Semen Ziziphi Spinosae	15 "
Rhizoma Anemarrhenae	6 "
Rhizoma Lugistici Chuanxiong	6 "
Magnetitum	15 "
Radix Glycyrrhizae Praeparata	6 "
Pulvis Cinnabaris (cinnabar powder, mixed with decoction)	9 "

Modifications include: For cases with thirst and feverish sensation, add 12 grams *Radix Paeoniae Alba,* 15 grams *Radix Rehmannia,* and 9 grams *Radix Ophiopogonis.*

For cases with spontaneous and night sweating, add 9 grams *Fructus Schisandrae* and 15 grams *Concha Ostreae.*

INSOMNIA DUE TO UPWARD FLARING OF LIVER FIRE. Manifestations: Insomnia, irritability, anorexia, thirst, pinkeye, bitter taste in the mouth, dark yellow urine, constipation, reddened tongue with yellow coating, taut and rapid pulse.

Principle of treatment: Soothing a depressed liver to eliminate intense heat and calm the mind.

Prescription: Decoction of Gentianae to Purge the Liver, with Modifications.

Radix Gentianae	12 grams
Radix Scutellariae	9 "
Fructus Gardeniae	9 "
Rhizoma Alismatis	9 "
Caulis Akebiae	6 "
Semen Plantaginis (wrapped in gauze)	9 "
Radix Angelicae Sinensis	9 "
Radix Rehmannia	12 "
Radix Bupleuri	6 "
Magnetitum	30 "
Dens Draconis	15 "
Semen Ziziphi Spinosae	15 "

Modifications include: For cases with distension of the chest and hypochondrium, add 9 grams *Rhizoma Cyperi,* 9 grams *Radix Curcumae,* and 9 grams *Fructus Aurantii.*

INSOMNIA DUE TO RETENTION OF PHLEGM-HEAT. Manifestations: Restlessness, insomnia, dizziness and heavy sensation in the head, bitter taste in the mouth, blurred vision, profuse sputum, suffocating feeling in the chest, slimy yellow tongue coating, slippery and rapid pulse.

Principle of treatment: Resolving phlegm and clearing away pathogenic heat to calm the mind.

Prescription: Gallbladder-Warming Decoction, with Modifications.

Pericarpium Citri Reticulatae	9	grams
Rhizoma Pinelliae Praeparata	9	"
Poria	12	"
Radix Glycyrrhizae	3	"
Caulis Bambusae in Taenis	9	"
Fructus Aurantii Immaturus	9	"
Rhizoma Coptidis	6	"
Fructus Gardeniae	9	"
Fructus Ziziphi Spinosae	15	"

Modifications include: For cases with palpitation, add 24 grams *Dens Draconis,* 15 grams *Magnetitum,* and 15 grams *Concha Margaritifera Usta.*

For cases with severe dizziness, add 9 grams *Bulbus Lilii,* 9 grams *Ramulus Uncariae cum Uncis,* and 9 grams *Flos Chrysanthemi.*

For cases with dyspepsia, add 9 grams *Massa Fermentata Medicinalis,* 9 grams *Fructus Crataegi,* and 15 grams *Semen Raphani.*

For cases with profuse sputum, substitute Phlegm Eliminating Pills of Chloriteschist.

Other Common Methods of Treating Insomnia

PROVEN RECIPES

1. *Fructus Ziziphi Spinosae,* 30 grams.
2. *Pulvis Fructus Ziziphi Spinosae,* 6 grams, administered before sleep.

3. Decoction of 30 grams *Bulbus Lilii* and 15 grams *Radix Rehmannia*.

4. Decoction of 18 grams *Caulis Polygoni Multiflori* (vine of multiflower knotweed) and 9 grams *Flos Albiziae* (flower of silktree).

ACUPUNCTURE TREATMENT

Main Points: Shenmen (H 7), Sanyinjiao (Sp 6).
Points according to manifestations:

Restlessness—Taichong (Liv 3)
Palpitation—Neiguan (P 6), Xinshu (UB 15)
Vertigo—Yintang (Extra 1)

Uniform reducing and reinforcing method is applied.

EAR-ACUPUNCTURE THERAPY. Ear-Shenmen, Heart, Kidney, Spleen, Subcortex.
One or two points are selected for each treatment, and needles are embedded for three to five days.

SYNCOPE

Syncope is the sudden loss of consciousness accompanied by cold limbs but without any sequelae such as hemiplegia, facial paresis, or loss of speech. It commonly occurs in shock, heatstroke, and hypertensive crises. Death may occur in severe cases.

Etiology

Syncope can result from:

• Deficiency of vital energy due to overwork or hunger.
• Adverse upward rush of vital energy and blood because of rage or because of deficiency of blood after childbirth.
• Adverse flow of vital energy in the channels because of emotional disturbance (such as rage or fright).

- Obstruction of the Heart Channel by phlegm because of deficiency of the spleen leading to generation of excessive phlegm.
- Obstruction of the channels due to retention of food and to dyspepsia.
- Obstruction of the channels because of summer heat.

Essentials of Diagnosis and Treatment

The nature and cause of syncope must be established first. In other words, one must determine whether an excess symptom-complex or a deficiency symptom-complex is present. Acupuncture treatment is the best method of treating syncope as soon as it occurs; then other methods to restore vital function by reinforcing vital energy are employed.

Treatment According to Differentiation of Symptom-Complexes

DEFICIENCY SYMPTOM-COMPLEXES

SYNCOPE DUE TO DEFICIENCY OF VITAL ENERGY. Manifestations: Sudden loss of consciousness, pallor, shallow breathing, cold limbs, perspiration, pale tongue, deep and feeble pulse.

Principle of treatment: Reinforcing vital energy to restore vital function from collapse.

Prescription: Decoction of Ginseng and Aconiti, with Modifications.

Radix Ginseng	9	grams
Radix Aconiti Praeparata	9	"
Radix Astragali	30	"
Rhizoma Atractylodis Macrocephalae	9	"
Cortex Cinnamomi	3	"

Modifications include: For cases with profuse perspiration, add 15 grams *Os Draconis,* 15 grams *Concha Ostreae,* and 9 grams *Fructus Schisandrae.*

For cases with palpitation and restlessness, add 9 grams *Radix Angelicae Sinensis,* 9 grams *Radix Polygalae,* and 15 grams *Semen Ziziphi Spinosae.*

SYNCOPE DUE TO DEFICIENCY OF BLOOD. Manifestations: Massive hemorrhage, syncope, pallor, pale lips, trembling limbs, sunken eyes, open mouth, spontaneous sweating, shallow breathing, pale tongue, hollow pulse or thready and rapid pulse.

Principle of treatment: Reinforcing vital energy and blood.

Prescription:

1. Decoction of Ginseng (30 grams *Radix Ginseng* simmered separately), administered at once to induce resuscitation.

2. Ginseng Nutrition Decoction, with Modifications.

Radix Ginseng	9	grams
Radix Angelicae Sinensis	9	"
Radix Paeoniae Alba	9	"
Radix Rehmannia Praeparata	12	"
Radix Aconiti Praeparata	6	"
Cortex Cinnamomi	3	"
Radix Astragali	30	"
Rhizoma Atractylodis Macrocephalae	9	"
Poria	9	"
Fructus Schisandrae	6	"
Pericarpium Citri Reticulatae	9	"
Radix Glycyrrhizae	6	"

Modifications include: For cases with massive hemorrhage, add 15 grams *Herba Agrimoniae,* 9 grams *Folium Biotae,* and 9 grams *Nodus Nelumbinis.*

For cases with palpitation and insomnia, add 15 grams *Arillus Longan,* 9 grams *Radix Polygalae,* and 15 grams *Semen Ziziphi Spinosae.*

For cases with spontaneous sweating and cold limbs, add 9 grams *Radix Aconiti Praeparata,* and 9 grams *Fructus Psoraleae.*

For cases with thirst and absence of saliva, add 9 grams *Radix Ophiopogonis,* 9 grams *Rhizoma Polygonati Odorati,* and 12 grams *Radix Glehniae.*

EXCESS SYMPTOM-COMPLEXES

SYNCOPE DUE TO ADVERSE FLOW OF VITAL ENERGY. Manifestations: Loss of consciousness as a result of rage or fright, clenched jaws, feeling of oppression in the chest, tachypnea, cold limbs, thin white tongue coating, deep and taut pulse.

Principle of treatment: Restoring normal flow of vital energy to dispel obstruction.

Prescription: Decoction for Removing Obstruction from the Five Internal Organs, with Modifications.

Lignum Aquilariae Resinatum (eaglewood)	6 grams
Radix Linderae	9 "
Semen Arecae	9 "
Fructus Aurantii Immaturus	9 "
Radix Aucklandiae	6 "
Radix Bupleuri	6 "
Radix Polygalae	6 "
Radix Curcumae	9 "

Modifications include: For cases with clenched jaws, administer a pill of Storax Bolus.

For cases with dizziness, distending headache, and malar flush due to exuberance of vital function of the liver, add 15 grams *Ramulus Uncariae cum Uncis,* 30 grams *Concha Haliotidis,* and 15 grams *Concha Margaritifera Usta.*

For cases with profuse sputum and impeded flow of vital energy, add 12 grams *Arisaema cum Bilis,* 9 grams *Bulbus Fritillariae,* and 9 grams *Exocarpium Citri Grandis.*

For cases with hysteria and insomnia, add 15 grams *Lignum Pini Poriaferum,* 9 grams *Radix Polygalae,* and 15 grams *Semen Ziziphi Spinosae.*

SYNCOPE DUE TO ADVERSE FLOW OF BLOOD. Manifestations: Constant headache, dizziness, loss of consciousness precipitated by rage, clenched jaws, malar flush, purple lips, dark red tongue, deep and taut pulse.

Principle of treatment: Promoting smooth flow of blood and vital energy.

Prescription: Decoction for Eliminating Blood Stasis, with Modifications.

Radix Angelicae Sinensis	12 grams
Fructus Crataegi	12 "
Flos Carthami	9 "
Semen Persicae	9 "
Rhizoma Cyperi	9 "
Radix Linderae	6 "
Radix Aucklandiae	6 "
Pericarpium Citri Reticulatae Viride (green orange peel)	9 "
Flos Chrysanthemi	9 "
Uncariae cum Uncis	15 "
Radix Achyranthis Bidentatae	9 "

Modifications include: For cases with irritability and excessive dreaming during sleep, add 30 grams *Concha Haliotidis* and 12 grams *Cortex Moutan Radicis.*

For cases with dizziness and headache, add 15 grams *Concha Margaritifera Usta* and 15 grams *Fructus Lycii.*

For cases with contracture or spasm of limbs, add 15 grams *Lumbricus* and 6 grams *Scorpio.*

SYNCOPE DUE TO OBSTRUCTION OF THE HEART CHANNEL BY PHLEGM. Manifestations: Sudden loss of consciousness, wheezing, coarse breathing with phlegm-like vomitus, slimy white tongue coating, deep and slippery pulse.

Principle of treatment: Promoting normal flow of vital energy to eliminate phlegm.

Prescription: Decoction for Expelling Phlegm, with Modifications.

Pericarpium Citri Reticulae	9 grams
Rhizoma Pinelliae Praeparata	9 "
Poria	12 "
Fructus Aurantii Immaturus	9 "
Arisaema cum Bilis	9 "
Rhizoma Acori Graminei	15 "
Frucus Perillae	6 "
Semen Sinapis Albae	6 "
Radix Curcumae	6 "
Radix Peucedani	9 "

Modifications include: For cases with thirst and constipation, add 9 grams *Radix Scutellariae,* 15 grams *Semen Trichosanthes,* and 3 grams *Natrii Sulfas Exsiccatus,* or substitute Phlegm Eliminating Pills of Chloriteschist, with Modifications.

SYNCOPE DUE TO OVEREATING. Manifestations: Loss of consciousness after overeating, fullness in the epigastric region and abdomen, thick slimy tongue coating, slippery and forceful pulse.

Principle of treatment: Promoting digestion and removing food retention.

Prescription: Decoction of Fermentata Medicinalis and Atractylodis in combination with Stomach Beneficial Bolus, with Modifications.

Pericarpium Citri Reticulatae	9	grams
Cortex Magnoliae Officinalis	9	"
Herba Agastachis	9	"
Poria	9	"
Rhizoma Pinelliae Praeparata	9	"
Fructus Crataegi	9	"
Massa Fermentata Medicinalis	9	"
Semen Raphani	15	"
Rhizoma Atractylodis	12	"
Fructus Amomi	6	"

Modifications include: For cases with sticky feeling in the mouth, add 9 grams *Herba Agastachis* and 9 grams *Herba Eupatorii.*

For cases with distended abdomen and constipation, add 9 grams *Radix et Rhizoma Rhei* and 6 grams *Natrii Sulfas Exsiccatus.*

SYNCOPE DUE TO SUMMER-HEAT. Manifestations: Loss of consciousness due to affliction by high temperature or summer heat, delirium, feverish sensation, perspiration, cold limbs, malar flush, reddened dry tongue, overflowing and rapid pulse or empty taut pulse.

Principle of treatment: Eliminating summer-heat, reinforcing vital energy, and removing intense heat from the heart by purgation.

Prescriptions:

1. Bezoar Bolus for Clearing Away Heart-Fire or Purple Snowy Powder (to restore consciousness).

2. Decoction for Invigorating Pulse-Beat, with Modifications.

CASE HISTORY

Female, age 32, first visit on November 4, 1972.

History

Because of rage, the patient had suddenly lost consciousness for a few minutes and developed cold limbs and pallor. After the incident, she complained of dizziness, feeling of oppression in the chest and hypochondria, frequent sighing, anorexia, restlessness, insomnia, and excessive dreaming during sleep.

Diagnosis and Treatment

On examination, a thin slimy tongue coating and deep and taut pulse were observed. The trouble was thought to be caused by adverse flow of vital energy due to a depressed liver. It was thus considered advisable to remove stagnancy of vital energy to ease the mind. The herbs administered were as follows:

Radix Bupleuri	6	grams
Rhizoma Cyperi	9	"
Radix Angelicae Sinensis	9	"
Radix Paeoniae Alba	9	"
Poria	12	"
Lignum Aquilariae Resinatum	3	"
Fructus Aurantii	9	"
Radix Polygalae	6	"
Semen Ziziphi Spinosae	9	"
Caulis Polygoni Multiflori	15	"
Herba Menthae (decocted later)	6	"

After four doses were taken, the feeling of oppression in the chest and hypochondria had almost disappeared, but excessive dreaming during sleep still remained. Then 24 grams *Concha Margaritifera Usta* were added to the prescription, which was taken for a few more days. Upon follow-up four months later, there had been no relapse and the patient's condition had improved markedly.

—From Luo Guojun, *Practical Traditional Chinese Internal Medicine* (Shanxi People's Publishing House, 1981), p. 328.

Radix Ginseng	6	grams
Radix Ophiopogonis	15	"
Fructus Schisandrae	9	"
Folium Nelumbilis	9	"
Flos Dolichoris	6	"

3. White-Tiger Decoction, with Ginseng (for cases with feverish sensation and malar flush after regaining consciousness).

Gypsum Fibrosum	30	grams
Rhizoma Anemarrhenae	9	"

Radix Ginseng Americana (decocted separately)	9 grams
Radix Ophiopogonis	15 "
Herba Dendrobii	12 "
Rhizoma Polygonati Odorati	9 "
Petiolus Nelumbilis (lotus petiole)	9 "
Herba Lophatheri	6 "
Radix Glycyrrhizae	6 "

Other Common Methods of Treating Syncope

ACUPUNCTURE TREATMENT

Main Points: Renzhong (Du 26), Yongquan (K 1), Neiguan (P 6), Zusanli (St 36).
Points according to manifestations:

Excess symptom-complex—Shixuan (Extra 30) prick to bloodlet (1–2 drops)
Deficiency symptom-complex—Baihui (Du 20), Qihai (Ren 6), Shenque (Ren 8).
Profuse sputum—Fenglong (St 40).
Adverse flow of vital energy—Shanzhong (Ren 17)

EAR-ACUPUNCTURE THERAPY. Subcortex, Adrenal, Sympathetic Nerve.
Two or three points are selected for each treatment. Needles are inserted swiftly and may be retained or attached to an electric stimulus until symptoms are relieved.

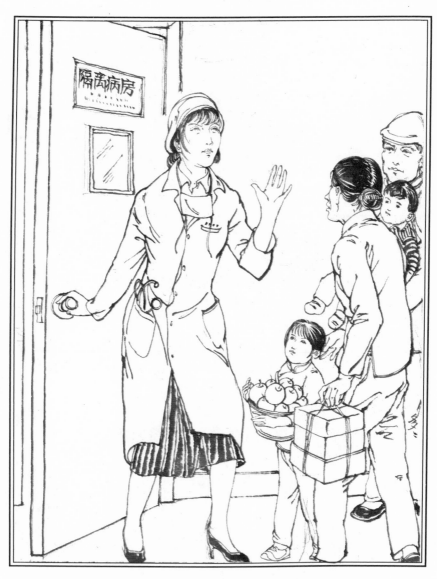

A doctor asking guests not to enter because of the infectious nature of the patient's disease.

CHAPTER FIVE

Treatment of
Common Communicable Diseases

THE EXISTENCE AND characteristic features of communicable diseases, including parasitoses, have long been recognized by traditional Chinese medicine. For example, the *Classic of Internal Medicine* states: "The five pestilences [a general term for all kinds of epidemic diseases] spread widely once they occur, and their symptoms are similar regardless of the patient's age."

Based on the method of analyzing and differentiating febrile diseases according to the theory of the Six Pairs of Channels, practitioners of the Ming and Qing Dynasties specializing in acute febrile disease established a new method to study communicable diseases: analyzing and differentiating febrile diseases according to the theories of the *wei* (superficial defensive), *qi* (secondard defensive), *ying* (nutient), and *xue* (blood) systems. With this method, it is easy to understand most of the common symptoms and signs of communicable disease—for example, fever, skin rash, and septicemia. Furthermore, the method has helped develop many effective prescriptions and other therapies and has contributed to the prevention of communicable disease.

Traditional Chinese medicine is experienced in treating and preventing communicable diseases. The rest of this chapter describes the current approaches to some of these diseases: viral hepatitis, epidemic

Japanese B encephalitis, epidemic parotitis (mumps), and ascariasis. In each disease, emphasis is placed on treatment according to the differentiation of symptom-complexes.

VIRAL HEPATITIS

Viral hepatitis is also known as infectious hepatitis. It is caused by hepatitis viruses and is marked by anorexia, nausea, sensation of fullness in the midabdominal region, dull pain in the liver area, and generalized weakness. In most cases, the liver is enlarged and tender; liver function can be impaired to various degrees. Some patients have jaundice or fever. According to the clinical manifestations and pathologic changes, the disease is divided into two classes: icteric (marked by jaundice) and anicteric (without jaundice).

In traditional Chinese medicine, acute icteric hepatitis is known as "jaundice of *yang* nature"; fulminant hepatitis, a severe version of this conditon, is known as "acute jaundice." Acute anicteric hepatitis is known as "costal pain due to stagnancy of vital energy of liver *qi*." Chronic persistent hepatitis or cirrhosis (traditionally known as abdominal mass caused by stasis of blood) is known as "jaundice of *yin* nature."

Etiology

Viral hepatitis is an exogenous affection due to epidemic toxins, pathogenic damp-heat, improper diet, emotional disturbances, and fatigue.

When drastic pathogens known as *epidemic toxins* infect the human body, they are readily converted into pathogenic fire, which impairs vital essence. They may be rapidly transmitted and attack the liver and gallbladder, injuring the *ying* and *xue* systems or the pericardium. As a result, fulminant hepatitis develops.

When *pathogenic damp-heat* invades the body, it may accumulate in the interior and affect the spleen and stomach, impeding the smooth flow of liver *qi* and the normal functioning of the spleen. As a result, anorexia, malaise, and pain in the hypochondriac region occur. Exuberant damp-heat in the interior may lead to escape of bile from the normal passages and thus cause jaundice.

Improper diet (including excessive intake of greasy, raw, or cold food or drink) often causes dysfunction of the spleen, liver, and gallbladder. Such dysfunction is marked by anorexia, diarrhea, a sensation of fullness in the midabdominal region, and nausea and vomiting due to adverse upward flow of stomach *qi*. *Emotional disturbances* and *fatigue* are internal causes conducive to invasion by toxins or pathogenic damp-heat.

Essentials of Diagnosis and Treatment

The first step is to determine the disease's characteristics and causative factors. Sudden onset, fever, and jaundice generally imply accumulation of pathogenic damp-heat. A slow onset and absence of fever and of jaundice usually indicate disharmony of the liver and spleen. The next step is to determine the location of the pathogenic factor (whether in the interior or exterior, or in the *qi* or *xue* systems) and the state of damp-heat.

When treating icteric hepatitis, it is advisable to clear away damp-heat or damp-cold; various methods and prescriptions are employed. In anicteric or chronic hepatitis, it is necessary to soothe the liver and invigorate the function of the stomach. If there is abundant dampness, the first choice is to strengthen the function of the spleen; if there is a deficiency of vital essence, it is advisable to replenish vital essence and soothe the liver.

Treatment Based on Differentiation of Symptom-Complexes

UPWARD ATTACK BY PATHOGENIC DAMP-HEAT (commonly found in acute icteric hepatitis). Manifestations: Jaundice, fever, restlessness, sensation of fullness in the midabdominal region, anorexia, nausea, vomiting, dryness and bitter taste in the mouth, pain in the right hypochondriac region, malaise, itching of the skin, brown urine, constipation or loose stools, slimy yellow tongue coating, taut, slippery, and rapid, or rapid and soft pulse.

Principle of treatment: Clearing away pathogenic damp-heat, soothing the liver, and invigorating the function of the gallbladder.

Prescription: Decoction of Artemisiae, with Modifications.

Herba Artemisiae Scopariae	30 grams
Fructus Gardeniae	9 "
Radix et Rhizoma Rhei	6 "
Radix Isatidis	12 "
Radix Gentianae	9 "
Flow Lonicerae	15 "
Fructus Forsythiae	15 "
Caulis Akebiae	6 "
Rhizoma Imperatae	30 "

Modifications include: For cases with headache, fever, and aversion to cold (suggesting an incipient case associated with exogenous affection), add 12 grams *Semen Sojae Practaratum,* 6 grams *Herba Eupatorii,* 6 grams *Herba Schizonepetae,* and 6 grams *Radix Ledebouriellae,* or administer Detoxicant Manna Pills 6 grams twice daily.

For cases with severe vomiting, add 9 grams *Caulis Bambusae in Taeniam,* 9 grams *Pericarpium Citri Reticulatae,* and 9 grams *Rhizoma Pinelliae.*

For cases with skin itching, add 6 grams *Periostracum Cicadae* and 12 grams *Fructus Kochiae* (broom cypress fruit).

For cases with pain in the hypochondriac region, add 9 grams *Radix Curcumae* and 12 grams *Fructus Meliae Toosendan.*

For cases with excessive dampness, add 12 grams *Rhizoma Atractylodis,* 9 grams *Rhizoma Pinelliae Praeparata,* 9 grams *Cortex Magnoliae Officinalis,* and 9 grams *Rhizoma Alismatis.*

For cases with excessive heat, add 15 grams *Folium Isatidis* and 15 grams *Herba Taraxaci.*

INTERNAL INVASION BY PATHOGENIC DAMP-HEAT (commonly seen in fulminant hepatitis or subacute hepatic necrosis). Manifestations: Swift and violent exacerbation of the disease, with progressive jaundice, high fever, thirst, delirium, convulsions, epistaxis, odontorrhagia, hematemesis, indistinct rash, distension and fullness in the chest and abdomen, ascites, scanty yellow urine, constipation, reddish dry tongue with yellow coating, rapid and slippery pulse.

Principle of treatment: Clearing away heat to cool the blood; removing heat toxins to resuscitate.

Prescription: Nutrient System Clearing Decoction, with Modifications.

Rhizoma Coptidis	6 grams
Cortex Moutan Radicus	6 "
Fructus Gardeniae Praeparata	9 "
Radix Ophiopogonis	9 "
Fructus Forsythiae	9 "
Radix Curcumae	9 "
Radix et Rhizoma Rhei	9 "
Radix Rehmannia	12 "
Radix Isatidis	15 "
Radix Salviae Miltiorrhiza	12 "
Flos Lonicerae	12 "
Herba Artemisiae Scopariae	12 "
Herba Taraxaci	12 "

Modifications include: For cases with hematemesis or epistaxis due to escape of blood from vessels, add 6 grams *Cornu Rhinocero,* 9 grams *Rhizoma Imperata,* 12 grams *Radix Rehmannia,* 9 grams *Cortex Moutan Radicis,* and 12 grams *Scrophulariae.*

For cases with indistinct rash, add 15 grams *Radix Arnebiae Seu Lithospermi* and 12 grams *Radix Scrophulariae.*

For cases with bloody stools, add 15 grams *Radix Sanguisorbae Carbonisatus* and 12 grams *Cacumen Biotae carbonisatus.*

For cases with ascites and scanty urine, omit *Radix Isatidis* and *Fructus Gardeniae,* and add 15 grams *Herba Verbenae* (European verbena), 12 grams *Pericarpium Arecae,* 12 grams *Spora Lygodii* (climbing fern), 15 grams *Poria Rubra,* 15 grams *Semen Plantaginis,* and 1.5 grams *Pulvis Lignum Aquilariae Resinatum.*

For cases with restlessness and delirium, omit *Rhizoma Imperata* and add 12 grams *Rhizoma Acori Graminei* or 1 Bezoar Resurrection Pill.

For cases with coma and delirium, add 30 grams *Radix Isatidis* and 1 Priceless Treasure Pill.

For cases with convulsions, add 9 grams *Lumbricus,* and 6 grams *Bombyx Batryticatus,* and dissolve 1.5 grams Purple Snowy Powder or 0.6 grams *Pulvis Cornu Antelopis* (antelope horn powder) in the decoction.

For cases with damage of fluids and reddened tongue with absence of coating, add 12 grams *Radix Glehniae,* 9 grams *Radix Ophiopogonis,* and 12 grams *Herba Dendrobii.*

DISTURBANCE OF THE SPLEEN BY PATHOGENIC DAMP-COLD (commonly seen in acute anicteric hepatitis and chronic hepatitis). Manifestations: Pain or dull pain in the right hypochondriac region, epigastric fullness and abdominal distension, nausea and vomiting, anorexia, lack of taste sensation, general malaise and feebleness, loose stools, slimy white tongue coating, deep and soft pulse.

Principle of treatment: Eliminating dampness and strengthening the function of the spleen; invigorating the spleen's vital function and regulating its vital energy.

Prescription: Stomachic Decoction of Poria, with Modifications.

Rhizoma Atractylodis	12	grams
Cortex Magnoliae Officinales	9	"
Pericarpium Citri Reticulatae	9	"
Rhizoma Cyperi	9	"
Herba Agastachis	9	"
Poria	12	"
Rhizoma Alismatis	9	"
Radix Curcumae	6	"
Semen Coicis	12	"
Rhizoma Atractylodis Macrocephalae	9	"
Semen Plantaginis (wrapped)	9	"

Modifications include: For cases with distension and oppressive feeling in the chest and stomach, add 1.5 grams *Fructus Amoni* and 6 grams *Radix Saussureae Laphae* (costus root).

For cases with pain in the hypochondriac region, add 9 grams *Fructus Meliae Toosendan* and 9 grams *Radix Paeoniae Alba*.

For cases with intolerance of cold, cold limbs, and pale complexion, add 6 grams *Radix Aconiti Alba praeparata* and 6 grams *Ramulus Cinnamomi*.

For cases with excessive heat transformed from accumulation of pathogenic dampness, add 30 grams *Herba Artemisiae Scopariae* and 9 grams *Cortex Phellodendri*.

STAGNANCY OF LIVER *qi* (commonly found in anicteric hepatitis or chronic hepatitis). Manifestations: Pain in the hypochondriac region, sensation of fullness in the chest and stomach, nausea, belching, abdominal distension, anorexia, moderate fever, bitter taste in the mouth, thin white tongue coating, taut pulse.

Principle of treatment: Soothing the depressed liver and rectifying the flow of its vital energy.

Prescription: Bupleuri Decoction for Soothing the Liver, with Modifications.

Radix Bupleuri	9	grams
Fructus Aurantii	9	"
Radix Paeoniae Abla	9	"
Rhizoma Cyperi	9	"
Radix Curcumae	9	"
Fructus Maliae Toosendan	6	"
Pericarpium Citri Reticulatae Viride	6	"
Radix Glycyrrhizae	6	"

Modifications include: For cases with severe pain in the hypochondriac region, add 9 grams *Rhizoma Corydalis,* 9 grams *Rhizoma Curcumae Longae* (turmeric rhizome) and 6 grams *Flos Carthami.*

For cases with anorexia and loose stools due to deficiency of the spleen, add 12 grams *Rhizoma Atractylodis Macrocephalae Praeparata* and 9 grams *Poria.*

For cases with fire transformed from stagnant *qi* (marked by irritability, bitter taste in the mouth, epistaxis, and rapid, taut pulse), add 9 grams *Fructus Gardeniae* and 9 grams *Cortex Moutan Radicis.*

DISHARMONY OF THE LIVER AND SPLEEN (commonly found at the convalescent stage of hepatitis). Manifestations: Distending pain or stinging located in the left hypochondriac region and often aggravated by emotional disturbance or fatigue, sensation of fullness in the stomach and abdomen, belching, anorexia, malaise, loose stools, concentrated urine, jaundice, thin white or slimy tongue coating, fine and taut pulse.

Principle of treatment: Soothing the depressed liver and invigoratinng gallbladder function; strengthening the function of the spleen and stomach.

Prescription: Combination of Bupleuri Decoction for Soothing the Liver, Decoction of Orange Peel and Pinellia, and Decoction of Four Noble Ingredients.

Radix Bupleuri	9	grams
Radix Paeoniae Alba	9	"

Radix Codonopsis Pilosulae	12 grams
Rhizoma Atractylodix Macrocephalae	9 "
Poria	12 "
Pericarpium Citri Reticulatae	9 "
Rhizoma Pinelliae Praeparata	6 "
Radix Angelicae Sinensis	9 "
Radix Curcumae	9 "
Fructus Meliae Toosendan	9 "
Rhizoma Corydalis	9 "
Rhizoma Ciperi Praeparata	9 "

Modifications include: For cases with irritability, bitter taste in the mouth, and occasional epistaxis, add 9 grams *Cortex Moutan Radicis* and 9 grams *Fructus Gardeniae.*

For cases with jaundice, add 15 grams *Herba Artemisiae Scopariae* and 6 grams *Radix Aconiti Praeparata.*

DEFICIENCY OF VITAL ESSENCE OF THE LIVER (frequently found in chronic hepatitis, or at the convalescent stage of acute icteric hepatitis). Manifestations: Dull pain in the hypochondriac region, occasional moderate fever, aching back, dry mouth, burning sensation of the palms and soles, irritability, disturbed sleep, deep-red tongue with little coating, fine, rapid, and taut pulse.

Principle of treatment: Replenishing vital essence of the liver and clearing away heat from the liver.

Prescription: Decoction for Adjusting the Flow of Vital Energy by Nourishing the Liver and Kidney, with Modifications.

Radix Glehniae	9 grams
Radix Ophiopogonis	9 "
Radix Angelica Sinensis	9 "
Radix Rehmannia	12 "
Fructus ligustri Lucidi	12 "
Herba Ecliptae	12 "
Radix Paeoniac Alba	12 "
Fructus Meliae Toosendan	6 "
Herba Dendrobii	12 "

Modifications include: For cases with severe pain in the hypochondriac region, add 9 grams *Rhizoma Corydalis,* 9 grams *Radix Curcumae,* and 9 grams *Fructus Citri Sarcodactylis* (citron).

For cases with constipation, add 15 grams *Fructus Cannabis* and 6 grams *Radix et Rhizoma Rhei*.

For cases with afternoon fever, add 9 grams *Cortex Moutan Radicis* and 9 grams *Fructus Gardeniae*.

STAGNANCY OF VITAL ENERGY AND BLOOD (commonly found in chronic hepatitis or early cirrhosis). Manifestations: Tender masses in the hypochondria, distension and oppressive feeling in the epigastric region, dry mouth, livid or pallid complexion, emaciation, malaise, reddened dry and shrunken tongue or tongue with purple spots at its border, deep, thready, and choppy pulse.

Principle of treatment: Activating blood circulation to eliminate blood stasis, nourishing blood to soothe the liver.

Prescription: Decoction of Trionycis, Ostreae, and Manitis for Removing Blood Stasis, with Modifications.

Carapax Trionycis	15	grams
Concha Ostreae	15	"
Squama Manitis	9	"
Radix Bupleuri	6	"
Radix Angelicae Sinensis	9	"
Radix Paeoniae Alba	12	"
Rhizoma Ligustici Chuanxiong	9	"
Radix Curcumae	9	"
Rhizoma Curcumae Longae	9	"
Semen Persicae	6	"
Flos Carthami	9	"
Radix Glycyrrhizae	6	"

Modifications include: For cases with pallor, dizziness, and weakness, add 15 grams *Radix Polygoni Multiflori* and 15 grams *Radix Rehmannia Praeparata*.

For cases with hard masses and with purple spots at the border of the tongue, add 6 grams *Eupolyphaga Seu Steleophaga* and 9 grams *Herba Lycopi* (bugleweed).

Other Common Methods of Treating Hepatitis

PROVEN RECIPES

Decoction given for treatment and prevention of jaundice.

Herba Artemisiae Scopariae	120 grams
Fructus Ziziphi Jujubae	30 "
Crystal sugar	30 "

Infusion given for hepatitis:

Radix Bupleuri	9 grams
Radix Angelicae Sinensis	9 "
Radix Paeoniae Rubra	9 "
Radix Paeoniae Alba	9 "
Pericarpium Citri Reticulatae	9 "
Fructus Aurantic	9 "
Radix Curcumae	9 "
Rhizoma Ciperi	12 "
Radix Salviae Miltiorrhizae	15 "
Radix Scrophulariae	15 "
Herba Artemisiae Scopariae	30 "
Radix Isatidis	30 "
Herba Patriniae	30 "

Powder given to normalize serum glutamic pyruvic transaminase (SGPT) level:

Fructus Schisandrae	120 grams
Radix Salviae Miltiorrhizae	60 "

Six grams powder thrice daily.
Powder given for acute hepatitis or chronic active hepatitis:

Alumen (alum)	3 grams
Indigo Naturalis	1.5 "

1.5 grams powder given thrice daily.

CASE HISTORY

Female, age 52, first visit on October 2, 1976.

History

The patient complained that she had been sluggish and anorexic for over half a month. Generalized itching, jaundice, severe abdominal distension, and yellow urine were present.

Diagnosis and Treatment

Laboratory findings included the following:

van den Bergh test: immediate direct reaction
Direct bilirubin: 12 mg per 100 ml
Icterus index: 120 units
Thymol turbidity test (TTT): 15 units
Thymol flocculation test: + + +
Serum glutamic pyruvic transaminase (SGPT): 36 units (normal value—0–21 units)

The patient's tongue was white-coated but had a yellow coating at its root; her pulse was slippery and taut. The diagnosis was invasion of the middle burner by damp-heat and acute icteric hepatitis. It was considered necessary to clear away damp-heat and promote blood circulation. The prescription used was as follows:

Herba Artemisiae Scopariae	90 grams
Radix Scutellariae	9 "
Rhizoma Coptidis	6 "
Rhizoma Cyperi	9 "
Herba Taraxaci	30 "
Herba Agastachis	9 "
Herba Eupatorii	9 "
Semen Armeniacae Amarum	9 "
Exocarpium Citri Grandis	9 "
Radix Paeoniae Rubra	15 "
Herba Lycopi	15 "
Herba Cephalanoploris	15 "
Semen Plantaginis (wrapped)	12 "
Six to One Powder (wrapped)	12 "
(composed of 6 portions talcum and 1 portion *Radix Glycyrrhizae*)	

One and one half months later, the laboratory findings were as follows:

Direct bilirubin: 0.3 mg per 100 ml
TTT: 2 units
Thymol flocculation: (−)
SGPT: 16.4 units

—From Guan Youbo, *Veteran Traditional Doctors' Experiences in Beijing,* (Beijing Publishing House, 1980), pp. 78–79.

ACUPUNCTURE TREATMENT

Main points: Zhigou (SJ 6), Yanglingquan (GB 34), Ganshu (UB 18), Yanggang (UB 48).
Points according manifestations:

Pain in the hypochondriac region—Zhangmen (Liv 13) and Qimen (Liv 14) with cupping applied after acupuncture.
Disharmony of the liver and stomach—Zhongwan (Ren 12) and Zusanli (St 36). Uniform reinforcing-reducing method is applied.

EAR-ACUPUNCTURE THERAPY. Points: Sympathetic nerve, Ear-Shenmen, Liver, Liver *Yang* 1 or Liver *Yang* 2.
Two or three points are selected for treatment.

JAPANESE B ENCEPHALITIS

Japanese B encephalitis is an acute infectious disease affecting the central nervous system. Traditionally known as "summer fever," "summer heat convulsion," or "heat exhaustion," it is marked by high fever, coma, and convulsions. The disease is most common in children under the age of 10 years, and the incidence is highest in summer and autumn.

Etiology

According to traditional Chinese medicine, this disease is caused mainly by the invasion of summer damp-heat. At the incipient stage of the disease, summer damp-heat affects the superficial part of the body and causes headache, aversion to cold, and fever. When invasion of the stomach and spleen causes dysfunction of these organs, somnolence, nausea and vomiting, and slimy white tongue coating appear.
The disease develops quickly, and the summer damp-heat transforms into fire and dryness and invades the interior, affecting the nutrient *(ying)* system. As a result of the extreme heat, high fever, restlessness, delirium, stiff neck, and tetany develop. When abundant heat invades the pericardium, coma occurs.

As the disease develops further, failure of body resistance to defeat pathogens may give rise to obstruction of the Heart Channel and collapse; manifestations include coma, wheezing, shortness of breath, faint respiration, profuse sweating, cold limbs, and hidden sunken pulse, indicating lowered vital function and depletion of vital energy. If pathogenic heat lingers in the Triple Burner, it may consume vital energy and vital essence, and hectic fever, dryness of the mouth and throat, and fatigue may occur, suggesting deficiencies of both vital energy and vital essence. Exhaustion of vital essence causes stirring up of endogenous wind, leading to tremor of the hands and feet. Malnourishment of vessels and blockage of the channels due to insufficiency of blood may produce paralysis of the limbs. Flaring up of fire due to deficiency of vital essence may turn body fluid into phlegm, obstructing channels and vessels and resulting in dementia and loss of speech and hearing.

Essentials of Diagnosis and Treatment

Because this disease is fulminant in nature, the progression of pathogenic heat through the *wei, qi, ying,* and *xue* systems occurs rapidly. The time spent by the pathogen in the primary defensive *(wei)* system is exceedingly short. Therefore, in treatment it is necessary to clear pathogenic heat from the secondary defensive *(qi)* system and dispel pathogenic factors from the exterior with drugs pungent in flavor and cool in property.

In treating pathogenic heat in the interior, it is advisable to remove toxic heat. To resuscitate patients unconscious because of invasion of the pericardium by pathogenic heat, treatment is aimed at removing toxic heat and resolving phlegm.

At the convalescent stage, after the pathogenic factors have been eliminated, lowered functioning and deficiency of vital essence usually occur. Thus, therapy is used to reinforce vital function and replenish vital essence.

In critical cases, combined traditional Chinese and western medicines are used. In patients in whom the sequelae include paralysis of the limbs, acupuncture treatment should be employed.

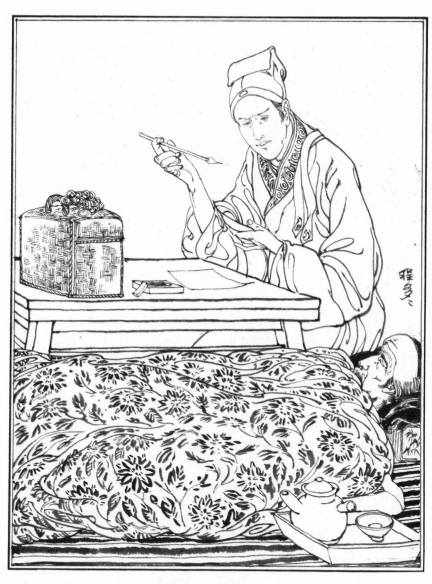

A doctor thinking about the prescription for his patient.

Treatment Based on Differentiation of Symptom-Complexes

AFFECTION OF BOTH *wei* AND *qi* SYSTEMS (usually seen in the early stage of mild Japanese B encephalitis). Manifestations: Fever, slight aversion to wind and cold, sweating or slight sweating, headache, somnolence or restlessness, slight rigidity of the neck, occasional moderate convulsions, thin white or yellow tongue coating, slippery and rapid pulse.

Principle of treatment: Removing toxic heat from the superficial portion of the body.

Prescription: Decoction of Lonicerae et Forsythiae, with Modifications.

Flos Lonicerae	15	grams
Folium Isatidis	15	"
Fructus Forsythiae	12	"
Radix Isatidis	30	"
Gypsum Fibrosum	30	"
Rhizoma Paridis	9	"
Herba Schizonepetae	6	"
Radix Scutellariae	6	"

Modifications include: For cases with concentrated urine, add 9 grams *Herba Lophatheri* and 9 grams *Talcum* (wrapped).

For cases with somnolence and slimy white tongue coating, add 9 grams *Herba Agastachis,* 6 grams *Herba Eupatorii,* and 6 grams *Cortex Magnoliae Officinalis.*

PATHOGENIC DAMP-HEAT IN THE *qi* SYSTEM (usually seen in the early stage of mild Japanese B encephalitis). Manifestations: Moderate fever, somnolence, lassitude, nausea, vomiting, absence of thirst, headache, slight rigidity of the neck, occasional mild convulsions, feeling of oppression in the chest, abdominal distension, anorexia, loose stools, sticky white or yellowish tongue coating, rapid soft pulse.

Principle of treatment: Expelling pathogenic damp-heat from the *wei* and *qi* systems.

Prescription: Detoxicant Manna Decoction, with Modifications.

Herba Agastachis	9	grams
Herba Eupatorii	9	"

Rhizoma Acori Graminei	9 grams
Herba Schizonepetae	6 "
Radix Scutellariae	9 "
Fructus Forsythiae	9 "
Herba Artemisiae Scopariae	15 "
Folium Isatidis	15 "
Pulvis Talcum	15 "
Radix Isatidis	30 "

Modifications include: For cases with nausea and vomiting, add 6 grams *Pericarpium Citri Reticulatae* and 6 grams *Rhizoma Pinelliae Praeparata*.

For cases with abdominal distension and loose stools, add 6 grams *Cortex Magnoliae Officinalis* and 12 grams *Semen Dolichoris Album*.

EXTREME HEAT IN BOTH THE *qi* AND THE *ying* SYSTEMS (commonly seen in moderate or severe Japanese B encephalitis). Manifestations: High fever, headache, stiff neck, tics of hands and feet, coarse breathing, somnolence, irritability, coma (in occasional cases), profuse sweating, thirst, scanty yellow urine, dry stools, deep-red tongue with dry yellowish coating, rapid overflowing pulse.

Principle of treatment: Expelling toxic heat from the nutrient system.

Prescription: Nutrient System Clearing Decoction, with Modifications.

Gypsum Fibrosum	60 grams
Folium Isatidis	15 "
Fructus Forsythiae	15 "
Rhizoma Anemarrhenae	9 "
Cortex Moutan Radicis	9 "
Cornu Rhinoceri Asiatici	3 "
Rhizoma Coptidis	6 "
Radix Rehmannia	12 "
Radix Scrophulariae	9 "
Herba Dendrobii	9 "

Modifications include: For cases with constipation, add 9 grams *Radix et Rhizoma Rhei* and 6 grams *Natrii Sulfas*.

For cases with severe convulsions, add 6 grams *Radix Gentianae,*

12 grams *Lumbricus*, 15 grams *Ramulus Uncariae cum Uncis*, 6 grams *Bombyx Batryticatus*, and 3 grams *Scorpio*.

For coma, administer 3 grams Purple Snowy Powder and 1 Bezoar Resurrection Bolus, or 1 Priceless Treasure Pill.

WIND STIRRED UP BY EXTREME HEAT (commonly seen in severe or critical Japanese B encephalitis). Manifestations: High fever, delirium, repeated spasms of the limbs, opisthotonus, coarse breathing, dry mouth and lips, oliguria, constipation, deep-red tongue, prickly tongue with dry black coating, deep, thready, and rapid pulse.

Principle of treatment: Calming the liver and subduing wind; clearing away extreme heat from the nutrient *(ying)* system to induce resuscitation.

Prescription: Decoction of Antelopis and Uncariae, with Modifications.

Pulvis Cornu Antelopis (mixed with the decoction)	3 grams
Radix Rehmannia	12 "
Radix Scrophulariae	12 "
Ramulus Uncariae cum Uncis	12 "
Flos Chrysanthemi	9 "
Radix Paeoniae Alba	9 "
Radix Isatidis	60 "
Gypsum Fibrosum (decocted first)	60 "
Rhizoma Acori Graminei	15 "
Cortex Moutan Radicis	9 "
Rhizoma Coptidis	3 "

Modifications include: For cases with tics of the limbs and with opisthotonus, add 30 grams *Concha Margaritifera Usta*, 12 grams *Ramulus Uncariae cum Uncis*, 12 grams *Plastrum Testudinis*, and 12 grams *Carapax Trionicis*.

For cases with constipation, add 9 grams *Radix et Rhizoma Rhei*, 6 grams *Natrii Sulfas*, and 3 grams *Radix Glycyrrhizae*.

THE COLLAPSE SYNDROME (usually seen in critical Japanese B encephalitis). Manifestations: High fever, coma, repeated intense spasms of the limbs, generalized rigidity, opisthotonus, trismus, wheezing, shortness of breath, sudden pallor, profuse sweating, cold limbs, deep, hidden, and rapid pulse.

Principle of treatment: Restoring vital energy from collapse; re-solving phlegm for resuscitation.

Prescription: Decoction of Ginseng and Aconiti in Combination with Decoction for Invigorating Pulse Beat, with Modifications.

Radix Ginseng (decocted separately)	6 grams
Radix Aconiti Praeparata	9 "
Radix Ophiopogonis	9 "
Fructus Schisandrae	9 "
Concha Ostreae	15 "
Plastrum Testudinis	15 "
Carapax Trionicis	15 "
Radix Isatidis	60 "
and *Purple Snowy Powder* (take separately)	1.5 "
Pills of Six Magic Ingredients (take separately)	10 pills

Modifications include: For cases with wheezing and shortness of breath, add 6 grams *Concretio Silicea Bambusae* and 30 grams *Succum Bambusae* (take with the decoction).

For cases with deep coma, add 3 grams *Arisaeme cum Bile* and 9 grams *Rhizoma Acori Graminei.*

DEFICIENCY OF BOTH VITAL ENERGY AND VITAL ESSENSE (com-monly seen in the convalescent stage of Japanese B encephalitis). Manifestations: Slight afternoon fever, flushed face, irritability, sweating of the head, anorexia, thirst, deep-red tongue with yellow coating or no coating, thready, rapid pulse (and sometimes mental aberration, mania, dementia, tremor of hands and feet, and/or flaccid paralysis of the lower limbs).

Principle of treatment: Replenishing vital essence to relieve fever; calming the liver to subdue endogenous wind.

Prescription: Pulse Activating Decoction of Trionycis, Ostreae, and Manitis, with Modifications.

Radix Glehniae	15 grams
Radix Rehmannia	15 "
Radix Scrophulariae	15 "
Radix Cynanchi Atrati	15 "
Carapax Trionycis	15 "
Colla Corii Asini	9 "

Radix Ophiopogonis	9 grams
Rhizoma Coptidis	3 "
Cortex Moutan Radicis	9 "
Cortex Lycii Radicis	9 "

Modifications include: For cases with mania, add 9 grams *Rhizoma Anemarrhenae,* 9 grams *Bulbus Lilii,* 30 grams *Magnetitum,* and 30 grams *Concha Margaritifera Usta.*

For cases with hand tremor, add 15 grams *Plastrum Testudinis,* 15 grams *Concha Ostreae,* and one egg yolk.

For cases with persistent moderate fever, add 9 grams *Herba Artemisiae Chinghao* and 9 grams *Radix Stellariae.*

For cases with anorexia, dry mouth, and reddened tongue, add 9 grams *Herba Dendrobii,* 6 grams *Fructus Mume,* and 6 grams *Herba Agastachis.*

Other Common Methods of Treating Japanese B Encephalitis

PROVEN RECIPES

Decoction given for mild Japanese B encephalitis:

Folium Isatidis	30 grams
Radix Isatidis	30 "
Rhizoma Paridis	30 "
Fructus Forsythiae	15 "

Decoction given for sequalae of Japanese B enchephalitis (e.g., contraction of the limbs):

Scorpio	4.5 grams
Herba Schizonepetae	4.5 "
Ramulus Uncariae cum Uncis	12 "
Herba Menthae (decocted later)	3 "

Powder given for mild cases due to extreme heat in the secondary defensive *(qi)* and nutrient *(ying)* systems:

Gypsum Fibrosum (decocted first)	30 grams
Radix Scutellariae	9 "

Fructus Gardeniae Praeparata	9 grams
Radix Curcumae	4.5 "
Radix et Rhizoma Rhei	4.5 "

Prepared powder rubbed on the teeth for sequelae of Japanese B encephalitis:

Radix Aconiti Alba Praeparata	18 grams
Radix Aconiti Nigri Praeparata	12 "
Realgar (elutriated)	12 "
Moschus	6 "
Radix Angelica Dahuricae	9 "

Powder is applied thrice daily for 2–7 days.

ACUPUNCTURE TREATMENT

Acupuncture is commonly used for sequelae of Japanese B encephalitis. During the acute stage it is used as a supplementary therapy for cases with high fever, coma, or convulsions.
Points according to symptoms:

High fever, loss of consciousness—Quchi (LI 11), Renzhong (Du 26), Shixuan (Extra 30; prick to bloodlet) and Hegu (LI 4)
Convulsions caused by stirring of endogenous wind—Neiguan (P 6), Yanglingquan (GB 34), Taichong (Liv 3) and Yongquan (K 1)
Hypopnea—Huiyin (Ren 1) (strong stimulus with needle retained for 10–12 minutes and twirling once), and Respiration point (located at lower third on the midline of the posterior margin of the musculus sternocleidomas-toideus)
Facial paralysis (deviation of the eyes and mouth)—Dicang (St 4) and Hegu (LI 4)
Difficulty in swallowing—Tianrong (SI 17), Neiting (St 44), Renying (St 9), Lianquan (Ren 23), Hegu (LI 4) and Sanyinjiao (Sp 6)
Insomnia—Zanzhu (UB 2) needle through to Yuyao (Extra 3), Jingming (UB 1), Qiuhou (Extra 4), Hegu (LI 4), Guangming (GB 37) and Taixi (K 3), needles are retained for 30 minutes.
Loss of consciousness—Baihui (Du 20), Sishencong (Extra 6), Fengchi (GB 20), Fengfu (Du 16), Dazhui (Du 14) and Shenmen (H 7).
Paralysis of the upper limbs—Jianzhen (SI 9), Jianyi (LI 15), Dazhui

CASE HISTORY

Female, age 4, first visit on August 15, 1964.

History

Three days before admission, the patient developed a fever, which decreased during sweating and then rose again. The patient had a severe headache, was dysphoric and lethargic, and had scanty urine and dry stools.

Diagnosis and Treatment

The patient had a pale tongue with a slimy yellowish coating; her pulse was floating, slippery, and rapid. The diagnosis was affection by a combination of pathogenic wind, heat, and dampness, or Japanese B encephalitis. It was considered imperative to eliminate wind-dampness and regulate the functioning of the middle burner. The prescription was as follows:

Herba Agastachis	6 grams
Semen Armeniacae Amarum	6 "
Semen Coicis	12 "
Semen Cardamomi Rotundi	3 "
Cortex Magnoliae Officinalis	6 "
Rhizoma Pinelliae Praeparata	6 "
Fructus Tribuli	9 "
Flos Chrysanthemi	6 "
Bombyx Batryticatus	6 "
Semen Sojae Praeparata	9 "
Caulis Allii Fistulosi (added to decoction later)	3.5 inches
Six to One Powder	15 grams
(six portions of talcum and one portion of glycyrrhizae)	
Herba Lophatheri	4.5 "

On the second visit (on August 17), the only manifestations of illness were dry stools and slight sweating. The patient's temperature was returning to normal, and her headache had subsided. It was considered advisable to continue using the above prescription with some modifications. Therefore, 4.5 grams medicated leaven and 4.5 grams *Semen Arecae* were added, and *Semen Sojae Praeparata* and *Caulis Allii Fistulosi* were omitted. The patient soon recovered.

—From *Medical Experiences of Dr. Pu Fuzhou*, compiled by Academy of Traditional Chinese Medicine (People's Medical Publishing House, 1976), pp. 227–28.

(Du 14), Shousanli (LI 10) and Outer Laogong (point on dorsum of hand opposite to Laogong, P 8)

Paralysis of the lower limbs—Huantiao (GB 30), Yangling-quan (GB 34), Xuanzhong (GB 39), Sanyinjiao (Sp 6), Jiexi (St 41), Dachangshu (UB 25), and Shenshu (UB 23)

EAR-ACUPUNCTURE THERAPY. Hypopnea—Lung, Sympathetic nerve, Occiput, Adrenal, and Ear-Asthma. Strong stimulus is applied for three to five minutes, twirling once.

Insomnia—Kidney, Liver, Eye, Eye 1, and Eye 2. Needles are embedded for three to five days.

Paralysis of the lower limbs—Subcortex, Brain point, Occiput, Forehead, Ear-Shenmen, and Heart. Two or three points are selected for each treatment in conjunction with body points.

EPIDEMIC PAROTITIS (MUMPS)

Epidemic parotitis, or mumps, is an acute viral infection. It is marked by swelling and pain in one or both parotid glands. The disease may occur throughout the year but is most common in the spring and winter, and it occurs mainly in children. Traditionally, it is known as "swollen cheek," "suppurative infection of the cheek," and "infection with a toadlike head."

Etiology

The disease is due to pathogenic wind-heat and is closely related to accumulation of heat in the stomach and intestines. The pathological changes usually affect the region along the course of the Gallbladder and Liver Channels.

In epidemic parotitis, pathogenic wind-heat that has invaded through the mouth and nose and combined with the accumulated heat in the stomach and intestines goes upward through the Gallbladder Channel to the ear; therefore, painful local swelling occurs. Flooding of pathogenic wind-heat in the Triple Burner may produce headache, fever, and slight aversion to wind-cold. Accumulation of heat in the stomach causes vomiting due to disturbance of the stomach. Because the liver is exteriorly-interiorly related to the gallbladder and the Liver Channel is connected downward with the external genitalia, toxic heat can go down through the Liver Channel into the external genitalia and produce pain and swelling of the testes. Furthermore, if body resistance fails to defeat the pathogenic factors, endogenous wind may be stirred up in the liver or there may be inward attack of the pericardium by the epidemic toxins.

Essentials of Diagnosis and Treatment

The disease is usually of excess symptom-complex. In mild cases, the only manifestations are slight swelling and pain in the parotid. In more severe cases, there is usually a complication of the exogenous affection, such as invasion of heat into the pericardium or stirring up of endogenous wind. In milder cases, external application of drugs for eliminating heat and relieving swelling suffices; in more severe cases, a combination of internal and external treatment based on differentiation of symptom-complexes is required.

Treatment Based on Differentiation of Symptom-Complexes

UPWARD ATTACK BY PATHOGENIC WIND AND HEAT (usually seen in mild cases). Manifestations: Swelling and slight pain in the parotid area (usually occurring first on one side and then spreading to the other side within two or three days), absence of redness over the skin of the area, sometimes a moderate fever, slight aversion to wind and cold, no particular change in the tongue coating or pulse.

Principle of treatment: Eliminating toxicity and relieving swelling.

Prescription: Decoction of Five Detoxicants, with Modifications.

Flos Lonicerae	15	grams
Flos Chrysanthemi	12	"
Herba Taraxaci	12	"
Herba Violae	12	"
Radix Scrophulariae	12	"
Radix Semiaquilegiae	6	"
Herba Menthae	6	"
Fructus Arctii	6	"

Herbs for external application:

1. *Folium seu Flos Hibisci* (cottonrose leaf or flower) pounded with *Yellow Golden Pulvis* (a patent drug). Paste prepared and applied to the swollen area once or twice daily.

2. *Indigo Naturalis*, mixed with vinegar and applied to the swollen area.

ACCUMULATION OF WARM TOXINS (usually seen in more serious cases or cases complicated by orchitis). Manifestations: Swelling and pain in the parotid area, scattered hard lumps on the neck, cheeks, and jaw, fever, headache, vomiting, anorexia, sore throat, concentrated urine, constipation, reddened tongue with yellow coating, floating, overflowing, slippery, and rapid pulse, swelling and bearing-down pain of one testis in some patients.

Principle of treatment: Clearing away toxic heat and swelling.

Prescription: Detoxicant Decoction for Universal Relief, with Modifications.

Radix Scrophulariae	15	grams
Radix Isatidis	30	"
Lasiosphaera seu Calvatia	6	"
Herba Menthae (decocted later)	6	"
Radix Platycodi	6	"
Radix Scutellariae	9	"
Fructus Actii	9	"
Fructus Forsythiae	9	"
Rhizoma Cimicifugae	3	"
Radix Bupleuri	6	"
Rhizoma Coptidis	6	"
Pericarpium Citri Reticulatae	6	"
Radix Glycyrrhizae	3	"

Modifications include: For cases with constipation, add 3 grams *Radix et Rhizoma Rhei* and 6 grams *Natrii sulfas Exsiccatus.*

For cases with swelling and bearing-down pain of one testis, add 15 grams *Semen Litchi* (lychee-pit) and 9 grams *Fructus Meliae Toosendan.*

Apply externally to the parotid area any of the following: Yellow Golden Pulvis, crushed *Folium seu Flos Hibisci,* or *Indigo Naturalis.*

INVASION OF THE INTERIOR BY PATHOGENIC HEAT (usually seen in cases complicated by purulent parotitis or meningoencephalitis). Manifestations: Redness, swelling, heat, and pain in both parotids, headache, vomiting, persistent high fever, dry mouth, thirst, restlessness, sore throat, choking on drinking, somnolence, wheezing, tics of the hands and feet, semi-consciousness or unconsciousness, dark, reddened, prickly tongue with dry black coating, deep, thready, taut, and rapid pulse.

Principle of treatment: Clearing away toxic heat from the nutrient system and cooling the blood; resolving phlegm to restore consciousness.

Prescription: Nutrient System Clearing Decoction, with Modifications.

Flos Lonicerae	15 grams	
Herba Taraxaci	15	"
Radix Isatidis	30	"
Radix Rehmannia	15	"
Radix Scrophulariae	15	"
Radix Ophiopogonis	9	"
Fructus Forsythiae	9	"
Rhizoma Coptidis	6	"
Radix Paeoniae Rubra	6	"
Cortex Moutan Radicis	9	"

Modifications include: For cases with high fever, add 30 grams *Gypsum Fibrosum* and 9 grams *Rhizoma Anemarrhenae*.

For tics of the hands and feet, add 9 grams *Bombyx Batryticatus* and 6 grams *Paeoniae Alba*.

For cases with semiconsciousness or unconsciousness, administer 1 Bezoar Resurrection Bolus through nasal feeding.

Other Common Methods of Treating Epidemic Parotitis

PROVEN RECIPES

For mild epidemic parotitis, any of the following herbs is crushed and applied to the swollen area once for four hours: *Herba Taraxaci, Herba Portulacae, Rhizoma Paridis, Herba Houttuyniae, Herba Commelinae* (dayflower), *Flos Chrysanthemi Indici, Herba Plantaginis, Herba Violae, Herba Opuntia Dillenii* (cactus), or *Folium Isatidis*.

Decoction given for epidemic parotitis:

Spica Prunellae	9 grams	
Radix Isatidis	15	"
Radix Glycyrrhizae	3	"

CASE HISTORY
Male, age 7, first visit on May 18, 1964.

History

The patient had a high fever for three days. There was swelling, soreness, and distending pain of both parotid glands. Prior to lapsing into unconsciousness, the patient had headache, anorexia, vomiting, constipation, and yellow urine and was restless.

Diagnosis and Treatment

The patient had a flushed face, reddened and swollen throat, yellow tongue coating, and rapid floating pulse. His temperature was 40.2°C, Babinski's sign and Kernig's sign were negative, and the cremasteric reflex was absent. White blood cell count was 10,400 (55% neutrophils, 1% eosinophils, 40% lymphocytes, 4% monocytes). The diagnosis was blockage of the Shaoyang Channels by pathogenic wind and seasonal epidemic factors and invasion of the pericardium by exuberant noxious heat, (i.e., parotitis complicated by encephalitis). It was considered necessary to clear away toxic heat, remove the blockage of the channels, and revive the patient. The prescription was as follows:

Herba Menthae (added to decoction toward end of heating process)	4.5 grams	
Rhizoma Phragmitis Recens	24	"
Flos Lonicerae	12	"
Fructus Forsythiae	9	"
Folium Isatidis	9	"
Radix Isatidis	9	"
Bombyx Batryticatus	9	"
Herba Lophatheri	6	"
Fructus Gardeniae Praeparata	6	"
Ramulus Uncariae cum Uncis	9	"
Gypsum Fibrosum	18	"
Flos Chrysanthemi Alba	12	"
Purple Snowy Powder (added to the decoction in two equal doses)	2.4	"

Second visit: May 19.

After one dose of the above prescription, heat was eliminated through perspiration, the patient regained consciousness, his temperature fell to 37°C, and the headache was relieved. However, restlessness, anorexia, vomiting, constipation, yellow urine, yellow tongue coating, and rapid pulse remained. The findings suggested unrelieved exuberant toxic heat. The original treatment method was continued with the following prescription:

Herba Menthae	3 grams	
Flos Lonicerae	9	"
Fructus Forsythiae	9	"
Gypsum Fibrosum (decocted first)	18	"
Folium Isatidis	9	"
Radix Scutellariae	6	"
Fructus Gardeniae Praeparata	6	"
Flos Chrysanthemi	12	"
Caulis Bambusae in Taeniam	6	"
Herba Lophatheri	6	"

Radix Isatidis		9 grams
Bulbus Cremastrae		6 "
Purple Snowy Powder (added to the decoction in two equal doses)	2.1 "

Third visit: May 20.
The patient's temperature had returned to normal (36.8°C). The remaining manifestations of disease were anorexia, slight swelling and pain in the cheeks, white tongue coating, and rapid pulse. Seasonal toxic heat was believed to remain in the body. It was considered advisable to allow the patient to recuperate while removing toxic heat. The prescription was as follows:

Folium Isatidis	9 grams
Spica Prunellae	4.5 "
Radix Scrophulariae	9 "
Charred Fructus Crataegi	9 "
Radix Isatidis	9 "
Radix Scutellariae	4.5 "
Gypsum Fibrosum (decocted first)	15 "
Herba Taraxaci	6 "
Fructus Forsythiae	9 "
Rhizoma Anemarrhenae	4.5 "
Fructus Gardeniae praeparata	6 "

Fourth visit: May 22.
After two doses of the above decoction, the swelling and pain of the cheeks disappeared, and the tongue picture and pulse condition returned to normal. White blood cell count was 8,200 (69% neutrophils, 1% eosinophils, 27% lymphocytes, 3% monocytes).

—From *Selected Successful Case Records of Traditional Doctors,* compiled by Beijing Traditional Chinese Medical Hospital (Beijing Institute of Traditional Chinese Medicine, 1965), pp. 241–42.

ACUPUNCTURE TREATMENT

Main points: Hegu (LI 14), Jiache (St 6), and Yifeng (SJ 17)
Points according to manifestations:

Fever—Quchi (LI 11)
Severe swelling and pain—Shaoshang (Lu 11) and Shangyang (LI 1)
Orchitis—Xuehai (Sp 10), Ququan (Liv 8), Sanyinjiao (Sp 6) and Xingjian (Liv 2)
Reducing method is usually used.

EAR-ACUPUNCTURE THERAPY. Parotid, Cheek, Subcortex, and Tender spots. Strong stimulus is applied daily, and needles are retained for 70 minutes per treatment. All points are used for each treatment.

ASCARIASIS

Ascariasis is a parasitic disease caused by ascarids (a kind of roundworm) in the human intestines. Clinically, it is marked by repeated bouts of periumbilical pain that may remit spontaneously, livid complexion, emaciation, hunger, and a tendency to eat peculiar substances. Descriptions of ascariasis are contained in early Chinese medical works such as the *Classic of Internal Medicine,* the *Discussion of Cold-Induced Diseases,* and the *Synopsis of the Golden Chamber.* Medical works of later dynasties include monographs on various parasites, especially ascarids, cestodes, and oxyurids. In *General Collection of Wise Healing,* it was noted that "ascarids are more harmful to people than are other parasites."

Etiology

This disease results from ingestion of the parasites' eggs. When in the small intestine, the ascarids may cause dysfunction of the spleen and stomach, marked by epigastric upset and/or desire to eat peculiar substances (e.g., earth or uncooked rice). Protracted parasitosis impedes the function of the spleen and stomach in digestion and absorption, so that malnutrition and deficiency of vital energy and blood result. The diminished function of the spleen leads to a livid complexion, emaciation, and pot belly. Insufficiency of the spleen function may affect the kidney, resulting in deficiency of vital function of the kidney in children and finally to maldevelopment. In cases with vomiting of ascarids, presence of ascarids in the biliary tract should be considered. Colicky abdominal pain and constipation suggest intestinal obstruction by ascarids; this conditon is known as "ascarid mass" in traditional Chinese medicine.

Essentials of Diagnosis and Treatment

Ascariasis is not difficult to diagnose, for it has the following manifestations: intermittent pain around the umbilicus, white "wormspots" on the face, bluish dots on the whites of the eyes, white granules on the inner side of the lower lip, reddish spots on the tongue surface, desire to eat peculiar substances, history of ascarid excretion, and finding of worm eggs in the stools.

Treatment is aimed mainly at expelling the worms. Ascarids prefer warmth and dislike cold and acid. They became inactive when they encounter pungent flavor, and bitter drugs drive them from the body. Therefore, drugs that are sour, pungent, or bitter are effective in expelling worms.

In cases with acute abdominal pain, it is advisable to tranquilize the worms first and then to expel them. Otherwise, they may rush into the bile duct and cause perforation.

Treatment Based on Differentiation of Symptom-Complexes

Manifestations: Intermittent pain around the umbilicus, addiction to eating peculiar substances, livid complexion, emaciation, grinding of teeth in sleep, itching of the nostrils, thin white tongue coating, and taut or deep and tight pulse.

Principle of treatment: Tranquilizing and expelling ascarids.

Prescriptions: 1. Black Plum Bolus, with Modifications.

Fructus Mume	18 grams	
Herba Asari	3	"
Fructus Capsici (hot pepper)	6	"
Rhizoma Zingiberis	6	"
Cortex Phellodendri	6	"
Cortex Meliae (Chinaberry bark)	15	"
Fructus Quisqualis	18	"

2. Decoction for Destroying Worms, with Modifications.

Cortex Meliae	12 grams	
Semen Arecae	15	"

CASE HISTORY
Female, age 8, first visit on October 5, 1978.

History

The patient complained of intermittent abdominal pain that had been present for more than a year and had become worse recently. Two weeks previously, ascaris eggs had been found on fecal examination. Piperazine was then administered; only one ascarid was excreted, and the distending pain in the lower abdomen became sharper. There had been no bowel movement for five days.

Diagnosis and Treatment

X-ray examination showed distension of the intestine with gas. There was a lump alongside the umbilicus, aggravated by pressure; other manifestations included hiccuping and acid regurgitation, slimy yellow tongue coating, and slippery and rapid pulse. The diagnosis was blockage of the middle burner by worms and undigested food, or ascariasis. It was considered advisable first to relieve the acute symptoms. The prescription used was Magnoliae Decoction with Seven Ingredients, with Modifications:

Cortex Magnoliae Officinalis	6	grams
Fructus Aurantii Immaturus	6	"
Radix Glycyrrhizae	6	"
Radix et Rhizoma Rhei Praeparata	3	"
Semen Raphani Praeparata	12	"
Pericarpium Citri Reticulatae Viride	6	"
Rhizoma Coptidis	3	"
Fructus Mume	6	"
Semen Arecae Praeparata	9	"
Pericarpium Zanthoxyli (peppertree pricklyash)	6	"
Charred Fructus Crataegi	6	"
Charred Massa Fermentata Medicinalis	6	"
Charred Fructus Hordei Germinatus	6	"
Fructus Cannabis	21	"
Juice of Allium Fistuloxum (mixed with decoction)	18	"

Second visit: October 18.

After the decoction was taken, a mass of decayed ascarids was excreted in the stools, and the abdominal distension was immediately relieved. The patient had a dry yellow tongue coating and a floating and rapid pulse. The prescription then used was Coptidis and Mume Decoction for Tranquilizing Ascarids, with Modifications:

Rhizoma Coptidis	3	grams
Fructus Mume	6	"
Semen Torreyae (Chinese torreya seed)	6	"
Omphalia Lapidescens	6	"
Fructus Ulmus Macrocarpa	6	"
Semen Arecae	9	"
Fructus Quisqualis	9	"
Cortex Meliae	9	"
Radix et Rhizoma Rhei Praeparata	3	"
Pericarpium Zanthoxyli	6	"

Charred Fructus Crataegi	6 grams
Charred Massa Fermentata Medicinalis	6 "
Charred Fructus Hordei Germinatus	6 "
Pericarpium Citri Reticulatae Viride	6 "
Pericarpium Citri Reticulatae	6 "

Third visit: October 12.
After the patient took this decoction, more than thirty ascarids were excreted, the patient's appetite improved, and the abdominal pain subsided. A prophylactic anthelmintic was given. Six months later, fecal examination was negative, and the patient had completely recovered.

—From Pei Shenyi, *A Collection of Case Histories of Traditional Chinese Medicine* (Gansu People's Publishing House, 1981), pp. 363–64.

Fructus Quisqualis	18 grams
Fructus Ulmus Macrocarpa	9 "
Omphalia Lapidescens	9 "

Modifications include: For cases with deep pulse and cold limbs due to cold of the viscera, add 6 grams *Radix Axoniti Praeparata* and 6 grams *Ramulus Cinnamomi.*

For cases with prominent heat symptoms, add 6 grams *Rhizoma Coptidis* and 9 grams *Gentianae.*

For cases with debility, add 12 grams *Radix Codonopsis Pilosulae* and 9 grams *Radix Angelicae Sinensis.*

For cases with constipation, add 6 grams *Radix et Rhizoma Rhei.*

OTHER PROVEN RECIPES

Decoction given to expel ascarids: *Cortex Meliae,* 45–60 grams. The amount is reduced for children (5 grams for under age 3, 15 grams for ages 5–7, adult dose for for over 7).

Fructus Quisqualis, stir-baked, 15–20 grains for adults, one grain per year of age for children, given once daily for 3–5 successive days.

Decoction taken 2–3 days in succession to expel ascarids:

Fructus Quisqualis	9 grams
Semen Arecae	9 "
Fructus Mume	9 "
Cortex Meliae	15 "

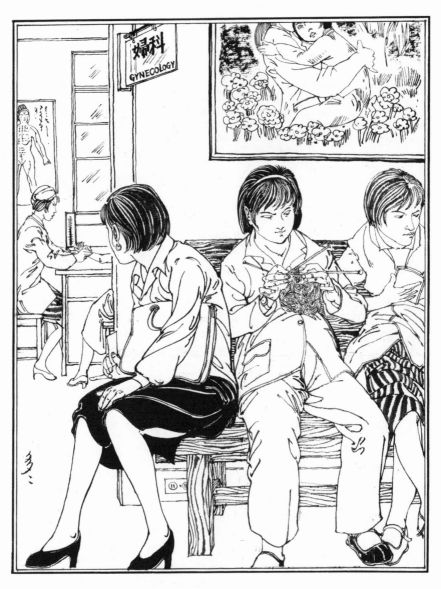

Women patients waiting for clinical care.

---◆·●———

CHAPTER SIX

Treatment of
Common Gynecologic Disorders

TRADITIONAL CHINESE MEDICINE holds that the physiologic and pathologic condition of the female is closely related to the state of the Ren (Conception) and Chong (Vital) Channels and the vital energy of the kidney. The Ren and Chong Channels originate in the pelvis (uterus) and directly influence menstruation and pregnancy; it is said that "the Chong Channel is the reservoir of blood" and "the Ren Channel governs development of the fetus." Abundant vital energy of the kidney is the basis of growth and development of the human body. Therefore, normal menstruation and fetal development depend on harmonious functioning of the *zang-fu* organs and smooth flow of vital energy and blood, as well as a substantial reservoir of blood.

Gynecologic disorders are caused by such factors as the six exogenous pathogenic factors, emotional disturbance, fatigue, sexual intemperance, improper diet, and abrupt environmental changes. The pathogenic mechanism is believed to be derangement of vital energy and blood, disharmony of the five *zang* organs, and injury of the Chong and Ren Channels.

In diagnosing and treating gynecologic disorders, information on menstruation, vaginal discharge, pregnancy, and childbirth must be considered. Generally, in diagnosing and treating menstrual disorders, one must note the menstrual cycle and the amount, color, smell,

and quality of menstrual blood, as well as the character of any abdominal pain, in order to determine the nature of the trouble (i.e.,
whether it is of cold, heat, deficiency, excess, or disorder of vital
energy and blood).

Morbid vaginal discharge or leukorrhea usually is related to pathogenic dampness and dysfunction of the spleen and stomach. In differentiating the symptom-complexes, it is important to note the
amount, color, smell, and quality of the discharge. In addition, it is
necessary to ascertain if there is itching of the vulva. Thus, one may
determine the nature of the disease (whether it is of damp-heat, deficiency in the spleen or in the kidney).

During pregnancy, the woman's physical condition must be noted.
If the woman is short of vital energy and blood, abortion may occur.
If the fetal vital energy is so abundant that it impedes the normal
function of the liver, kidney, spleen, and stomach of the woman,
there may be morning sickness, edema during pregnancy, and
eclampsia of pregnancy.

Illness after delivery is often related to debility and stasis. It is
essential to take note of any pain in the lower abdomen and to determine whether lochia is present, to notice bowel movements in
order to tell the condition of body fluid, and to observe lactation and
food intake in order to tell the state of digestion.

In treating gynecologic disorders, regulating the function of the
spleen and stomach and nourishing the liver and kidney are common
methods. For young girls, treatment of the kidney is the basic method
because they have enough vital energy in the kidney and the Chong
and Ren Channels are not yet connected. But for middle-aged women,
treatment of the liver should be stressed because loss of blood has
occurred as a result of menstruation, pregnancy, delivery, and lactation.

After menopause, treatment of the stomach becomes of primary
importance because when kidney function is declining, food intake
is the only source of nourishment for the body.

The rest of this chapter describes how the above concepts are applied to the diagnosis and treatment of the following gynecologic
disorders: amenorrhea, uterine hemorrhage, dysmenorrhea, threatened abortion, agalactia, salpingitis, and menopause.

AMENORRHEA

Amenorrhea is defined as the absence of menses or the abnormal stoppage of menses for more than three cycles.

Etiology

Amenorrhea can be caused by either deficiencies or excesses. The former include deficiencies of both vital energy and blood, lowered functioning of the liver and kidney, and impairment of the Chong and Ren Channels, resulting in stoppage of menstrual flow. These deficiencies usually are due to such factors as abortion, too many pregnancies, massive loss of blood after delivery, protracted illness, improper diet, and fatigue, all causing impeded growth of blood because the spleen and stomach are injured. A prolonged deficiency of blood may produce impairment of the liver and kidney. Excesses include retarded flow of vital energy and blood and collection of phlegm-dampness in the Chong and Ren Channels, leading to stoppage of menstrual flow. These excesses are due to exogenous affection by pathogenic wind-cold, which invades the uterus and solidifies the blood; to emotional disturbance causing stagnancy of vital energy and blood; or to obesity and collection of phlegm-dampness in the uterus, impeding menstrual flow.

Essentials of Diagnosis and Treatment

It is important to know the nature of the symptom-complex. Deficiency symptom-complexes often produce pallor, lassitude, afternoon fever, night sweats, and an irregular menstrual cycle. In contrast, excess symptom-complexes often produce distending abdominal pain that is aggravated by pressure.

Tonifying is good for deficiency symptom-complexes, and attacking blood stasis is used for excess symptom-complexes. If amenorrhea is caused by tuberculosis or diabetes mellitus, it is necessary first to remove the causative factors.

Treatment Based on Differentiation of Symptom-Complexes

DEFICIENCIES OF BOTH VITAL ENERGY AND BLOOD (usually found in amenorrhea due to such factors as massive loss of blood after delivery, prolonged lactation, too many pregnancies, and malnutrition). Manifestations: Livid complexion, dizziness, blurred vision, palpitation, shortness of breath, lassitude, pale tongue with thin coating, deep and thready pulse.

Principle of treatment: Reinforcing vital energy and blood to regulate menstruation.

Prescription: Decoction of Eight Precious Ingredients, with Modifications.

Radix Codonopsis Pilosulae	15	grams
Radix Astragali	15	"
Rhizoma Rehmannia Praeparata	15	"
Colla Corii Asini	6	"
Herba Leonuri	15	"
Poria	9	"
Rhizoma Atractylodis Macrocephalae	9	"
Radix Angelicae Sinensis	9	"
Radix Paeoniae Alba	9	"
Rhizoma Ligustici Chuanxiong	6	"
Radix Glycyrrhizae Praeparata	3	"

Modifications include: For cases with distending pain, anorexia, and loose stools, omit *Radix Paeoniae Alba* and *Radix Rehmannia* and add 3 grams *Radix Aucklandiae,* 6 grams *Pericarpium Citri Reticulatae,* 9 grams *Massa Fermentata Medicinalis,* and 9 grams *Fructus Oryzae Germinatus.*

DEFICIENCY OF VITAL ESSENCE OF THE SPLEEN AND KIDNEY (usually seen in amenorrhea due to tuberculosis or diabetes mellitus). Manifestations: Primary amenorrhea (or retarded menstrual flow at puberty and then amenorrhea), dizziness, tinnitus, weakness of the loins and legs, dry mouth, feverish sensation in the palms, soles, and chest, afternoon fever, night sweats, livid complexion, malar flush, reddened or pale tongue with scanty coating, thready taut or thready choppy pulse.

Principle of treatment: Tonifying the liver and kidney; nourishing the blood to regulate menstruation.

Prescription: Angelicae Decoction for Acting on the Kidney, with Modifications.

Radix Rehmannia Praeparata	15	grams
Cortex Eucommiae	9	"
Semen Cuscutae	9	"
Fructus Lycii	9	"
Radix Angelicae Sinensis	9	"
Fructus Corni	9	"
Rhizoma Dioscoreae	12	"
Poria	9	"
Plastrum Testudinis	12	"
Colla Corii Asini	6	"
Caulis Spatholobi	15	

Modifications include: For cases with chills, anorexia, lassitude, polyuria, and deep and weak pulse, add 9 grams *Radix Morindae Officinalis,* 9 grams *Cornu Cervi Degelatinatum,* and 6 grams *Pulvis Placenta Hominis.*

For cases with heat sensation, restlessness, and afternoon fever, add 9 grams *Cortex Lycii Radicis* and 3 grams *Cortex Phellodendri.*

For cases with expectoration of bloody sputum, add 30 grams *Rhizoma Imperatae* and 9 grams *Nodus Nelumbinis Rhizomatis.*

RETARDED FLOW OF VITAL ENERGY AND BLOOD (usually seen in amenorrhea due to emotional disturbances). Manifestations: Livid complexion, depression, irritability, stuffy sensation in the chest and hypochondria, distending lower abdominal pain aggravated by pressure, dark red tongue border or tongue with petechiae on it, deep-taut or deep-choppy pulse.

Principle of treatment: Promoting smooth flow of vital energy and blood; removing blood stasis to regulate menstruation.

Prescription: Decoction of Four Herbs with Persicae and Carthami, with Modifications.

Semen Pericae	6	grams
Radix Paeoniae Rubra	9	"
Rhizoma Ligustici Chuanxiong	6	"

Flos Carthami	9 grams
Radix Bupleuri	9 "
Radix Linderae	9 "
Radix Angelicae Sinensis	9 "
Rhizoma Cyperi Praeparata	9 "
Rhizoma Corydalis	9 "
Radix Rhemannia	12 "
Faeces Trogopterorum	9 "

Modifications include: For cases with distending pain in the hypochondria, add 6 grams *Fructus Meliae Toosendan* and 9 grams *Radix Curcumae.*

For cases with distending pain and cold sensation in the lower abdomen and cold limbs, add 3 grams *Cortex Cinnamomi,* 3 grams *Fructus Evodiae,* and 9 grams *Folium Artemisiae Argyi.*

COLLECTION OF PHLEGM-DAMPNESS (usually found in amenorrhea due to affliction with cold during menstruation or due to obesity). Manifestations: Abdominal distension, nausea, profuse sputum, lassitude, profuse leukorrhea, lack of taste sensation, slimy white tongue coating, thready and slippery pulse.

Principle of treatment: Eliminating dampness and phlegm; activating blood flow to regulate menstruation.

Prescription: Decoction of Atractylodis and Cyperi for Removing Phlegm, with Modifications.

Rhizoma Atractylodis	9 grams
Rhizoma Cyperi Praeparata	9 "
Pericarpium Citri Reticulatae	6 "
Rhizoma Pinelliae Praeparata	6 "
Poria	9 "
Arisaema cum Bile	6 "
Rhizoma Zingiberis Recens	3 "
Fructus Aurantii Immuturus	9 "

Modifications include: For cases with profuse, thick, foul-smelling leukorrhea, add 6 grams *Cortex Phellodendri* and 12 grams *Cortex Ailanthi* (heaven tree bark).

For cases with dizziness, nausea, and profuse sputum, add 9 grams *Caulis Bambusae in Taenis* and 6 grams *Semen Raphani.*

CASE HISTORY

Female, age 18, first visit on July 2, 1973.

History

The patient had been amenorrheic since April 1972. Since then, she had had profuse clear vaginal discharge, lower abdominal pain, and a sensation of weakness in the lower back.

Diagnosis and Treatment

The patient had a pale tongue and a taut and deep pulse. Western medicine diagnosed the case as hypoplasia (underdevelopment) of the uterus and secondary amenorrhea. Traditional Chinese medicine considered the condition deficiency of the kidney and amenorrhea due to deficiency of the blood. The principle of treatment was to tonify the kidney by replenishing its essence and to nourish the blood to stimulate menstrual flow. The prescription used was as follows:

Radix Angelicae Sinensis	9	grams
Rhizoma Ligustici Chuanxiong	4.5	"
Radix Paeoniae Alba	9	"
Radix Rehmannia Praeparata	12	"
Rhizoma Curculiginis	4.5	"
Herba Epimedii	9	"
Semen Cuscutae	9	"
Fructus Rubi	9	"
Semen Plantaginis (wrapped)	9	"
Fructus Lycii	12	"
Fructus Schisandrae	9	"
Radix Achyranthis Bidentatae	9	"

Fourteen doses were given over a period of fourteen days.

At the second visit (on July 30), the patient complained of dizziness, restlessness, abdominal distension, an oppressive sensation in the epigastric region, and flushed cheeks. She had a white tongue coating and a deep, taut, and slippery pulse. This time the patient was diagnosed as having amenorrhea due to flaring up of pathogenic heat in the liver, resulting in adverse flow of blood.

The principle of treatment was changed to nourishing essence by dissipating pathogenic heat from the liver, and activating blood to stimulate menstrual flow. The following prescription was administered:

Radix Angelicae Sinensis	15	grams
Radix Paeoniae Alba	15	"
Rhizoma Ligustici Chuanxiong	4.5	"
Radix Rehmannia	15	"
Radix Ophiopogonis	12	"
Herba Lycopi	9	"
Herba Leonuri	12	"
Radix Acyranthis Bidentatae	12	"
Flos Carthami	9	"
Aloë (aloe)	4.5	"
Radix Scrophalaria	9	"
Semen Plantaginis (wrapped)	9	"

At the next visit (on August 5), the patient reported that after one dose of the second prescription, she menstruated. The menstrual period had lasted from July 31 to August 4, and the flow had been normal in amount and color.

—From *Liu Fengwu's Experience in Gynecology*, compiled by Beijing College of Traditional Chinese Medicine (People's Medical Publishing House, 1977), pp. 116–17.

Other Common Methods of Treating Amenorrhea

PROVEN RECIPES

The following patent drugs are useful for amenorrhea due to deficiency of vital energy and blood:

Pills for Acting on the Spleen
Universal Tonic Bolus with Ten Ingredients
Ginseng Nutrition Pills

The following patent drugs are effective for amenorrhea due to deficiency of vital essence of the liver and kidney:

Major Bolus for Tonifying Vital Essence
Placenta Compound Restorative Pills

The following herbs are good for amenorrhea due to retention of vital energy and blood:

Herba Leonuri	60	grams
Herba Artemisia Anomalas	30	"
Radix Rubiae	30	"
Herba Verbenae	30	"
Excrementum Bombycis	120	"
Caulis Spatholobi	120	"

Choose one or two ingredients, and cook with brown sugar and 120 grams rice wine.

ACUPUNCTURE TREATMENT

Main points: Guanyuan (Ren 4), Sanyinjiao (Sp 6), Hegu (LI 4)
Points according to manifestations:

Deficiency symptom-complexes—Zusanli (St 36), Xuehai (Sp 10), Shenshu (UB 23). Uniform reinforcing-reducing or reinforcing alone is applied.

Excess symptom-complexes—Taichong (Liv 3), Zhongji (Ren 3). Reducing method is applied.

EAR-ACUPUNCTURE THERAPY. Uterus, Endocrine, Ovary, Subcortex, Ear-Shenmen, Sympathetic Nerve.

One or two points are selected for each treatment, and needles are embedded for three to five days.

UTERINE HEMORRHAGE

Uterine hemorrhage is defined as abnormal uterine bleeding due to functional disturbance of the ovary. It includes sudden profuse uterine bleeding and chronic bloody vaginal discharge.

Etiology

Uterine hemorrhage is due to derangement of vital energy and blood and hypofunction of the Chong and Ren Channels. Pathogenic heat in the blood system, blood stasis, and deficiency of vital energy are considered the three causative factors.

Essentials of Diagnosis and Treatment

During hemorrhage, it is necessary to determine the character of the bleeding, including such features as the amount of blood loss and the color of the blood. To distinguish deficiency from excess symptom-complexes, one must notice whether distending pain in the abdomen and other symptoms are present.

In treatment of sudden profuse uterine bleeding, it is essential to stop escape of blood. For chronic bloody vaginal discharge, treatment should be aimed at nourishing blood and regulating the smooth flow of vital energy. In both conditions, when the hemorrhage stops, it is necessary to strengthen the function of the kidney and Chong Channel to consolidate the effect.

Treatment Based on Differentiation of Symptom-Complexes

ESCAPE OF BLOOD DUE TO PATHOGENIC HEAT IN THE BLOOD SYS-
TEM. Manifestations: Massive uterine bleeding with dark red blood
that is thick or clotted or mild persistent bloody vaginal discharge,
fever, irritability, thirst, dizziness, flushed face, reddened tongue with
yellow coating, slippery and rapid pulse.
   Principle of treatment: Removing heat from the blood.
   Prescription: Decoction for Checking Menstruation, with Modifications.

Plastrum Testudinis (decocted first)	15–30 grams
Radix Scutellariae	9 "
Cortex Phellodendri	9 "
Fructus Gardeniae Praeparata	9 "
Radix Rehmannia	15 "
Herba seu Radix Cirsii Japonici	9 "
Herba Cephalanoploris	9 "
Radix Sanguisorbae Carbonisatus	9 "
Concha Ostreae Usta	15 "

Modifications include: For cases with dizziness, headache, and distending pain in the abdomen and hypochondria due to intense heat
brought about by a depressed liver, add 9 grams *Cortex Moutan Radicis,* 9 grams *Radix Curcumae,* and 9 grams *Herba Schizonepetae Carbonisatus.*
   For cases with massive hemorrhage, administer 9 grams *Petiolus
Trachycarpi Carbonisatus,* 15 grams *Radix Sanguisorbae Carbonisatus,*
and 12 grams *Cortex Phellodendri Carbonisatus.*

UTERINE BLEEDING DUE TO BLOOD STASIS. Manifestations: Mild
persistent bloody vaginal discharge or sudden profuse uterine bleeding with dark red clotted blood, lower abdominal pain aggravated
by pressure and alleviated by discharge of clots, livid complexion,
dark red tongue with petechiae on its tip, deep choppy or taut tight
pulse.
   Principle of treatment: Soothing the liver to normalize the flow of
vital energy; activating blood circulation to eliminate blood stasis.

Prescription: Decoction for Removing Blood Stasis, with Modifications.

Pollen Typhae	9 grams
Pollen Typhae Praeparata	9 "
Faeces Trogopterorum	6 "
Faeces Trogopterorum Praeparata	6 "
Radix Angelicae Sinensis	9 "
Radix Paeoniae Rubra	9 "
Rhizoma Cyperi Praeparata	6 "
Herba Leonuri	30 "
Radix Rubiae Carbonisatus	9 "
Colli Corii Asini Praeparata	9 "
Pulvis Notoginseng (infused)	3 "

Modifications include: For cases with stuffy sensation in the lower abdomen, add 9 grams *Fructus Meliae Toosendan* and 12 grams *Radix Salviae Miltiorrhizae*.

For cases with distending pain in the lower abdomen, add 9 grams *Radix Linderae* and 9 grams *Rhizoma Corydalis*.

FAILURE OF VITAL ENERGY TO CONTROL BLOOD. Manifestations: Sudden profuse uterine bleeding or mild persistent bloody vaginal discharge with thin light-colored blood, pallor, lassitude, palpitation, shortness of breath, dizziness, anorexia, loose stools, pale tongue with thin coating, thready and empty pulse.

Principle of treatment: Reinforcing vital energy to arrest blood; nourishing blood to stop hemorrhage.

Prescription: Decoction for Acting on the Spleen, with Modifications.

Radix Codonopsis Pilosulae	15 grams
Radix Astragali	15 "
Rhizoma Atractylodis Macrocephalae	9 "
Radix Glycyrrhizae Praeparata	6 "
Lignum Pini Poriaferum	9 "
Radix Rehmannia Praeparata	9 "
Petiolus Trachycarpi Carbonisatus	9 "
Os Sepiae	15 "

Concha Ostreae Usta	30 grams
Rhizoma Cimicifugae	3 "
Radix Bupleuri	3 "

Modifications include: For cases with dizziness, backache, and frequent urination, add 9 grams *Colla Cornu Cervi,* 9 grams *Fructus Rubi* (red raspberry), 12 grams *Semen Cuscutae,* and 9 grams *Radix Dipsaci.*

For cases with loose stools, add 9 grams *Radix Puerariae,* 6 grams *Fructus Schisandrae,* and 9 grams *Rhizoma Dioscoreae.*

For cases with cold limbs, hidden pulse, and profuse sweating (indicating collapse), add 9 grams *Radix Ginseng* and 9 grams *Radix Aconiti Praeparata.*

DEFICIENCY OF VITAL ENERGY OF THE KIDNEY. Manifestations: Cessation of uterine bleeding, dizziness, tinnitus, weakness in the back and legs, thin tongue coating, deep and thready pulse.

Principle of treatment: Strengthening the function of the kidney to reinforce vital energy.

Prescription: Restoring Kidney Pills Prescribed by the Golden Chamber, with Modifications.

Radix Rehmannia Praeparata	15 grams
Rhizoma Dioscoreae	12 "
Fructus Corni	9 "
Poria	9 "
Cortex Moutan Radicis	6 "
Radix Aconiti Praeparata	6 "
Ramulus Cinnamomi	6 "
Semen Cuscutae	9 "
Radix Dipsaci	9 "
Ramulus Loranthi	9 "

Modifications include: For cases with deficiency of vital essence of the kidney (marked by afternoon fever, feverish sensation in the palms, soles, and chest, dry mouth, reddened tongue without coating, thready and rapid pulse), add 15 grams *Radix Rehmannia,* 9 grams *Fructus Ligustri Lucidi,* 9 grams *Herba Ecliptae,* 9 grams *Fructus Lycii,* and 9 grams *Radix Polygoni Multiflori.*

For cases with lowered vital function of the kidney (marked by thin white leukorrhea, frequent urination, pale tongue with thin

---

CASE HISTORY

Female, age 48, first visit on October 20, 1974.

History

The patient was suffering from severe vaginal bleeding due to overwork. She had a weak physique, pale complexion, and soft voice and suffered lassitude, dyspnea, spontaneous perspiration, and abnormal appetite. She also experienced a sinking sensation in the lower abdomen.

Diagnosis and Treatment

Upon examination, the patient was found to have a pale tongue with white coating and a deep and feeble pulse. The diagnosis was failure of the spleen to maintain blood circulating in the vessels. The principle of treatment adopted was replenishing the vital energy of the spleen. The prescription was as follows:

Radix Astragati sue Hedysari	30 grams
Radix Codonopsis Pilosulae	24 "
Radix Paeoniae Alba	24 "
Radix Rehmannia	30 "
Colla Corii Asini (melted)	24 "
Radix Glycyrrhizae Praeparata	6 "
Herba Agrimoniae	18 "
Nodus Nelumbinis Rhizomatis Carbonisatus	30 "

After three doses, the bleeding was reduced. Another four doses of the above prescription were administered. Upon further consultation, the vaginal bleeding had stopped, the patient's appetite had improved, and her pulse was normal. Pills for Acting on the Spleen were prescribed to consolidate the curative effect.

—From Pan Yangzhi, *A Collection of Case Histories of Traditional Chinese Medicine* (Gansu People's Publishing House, 1981), p. 209.

---

coating, empty and thready pulse), add 9 grams *Rhizoma Curculiginis*, 9 grams *Herba Epimedii*, 9 grams *Herba Cistanchis*, and 9 grams *Fructus Psoraleae*.

Other Common Methods of Treating Uterine Bleeding

Proven Recipes

Decoction given for various kinds of uterine bleeding: *Petiolus Trachycarpi Carbonisatus*, 15 grams.

Powder; 6 grams taken twice daily for uterine bleeding due to intense heat:

Flos Celosiae Cristatae (common cockscomb flower)   1 portion
Cacumen Biotae Carbonisatus   1   "

Decoction given for uterine bleeding due to intense heat: *Radix Sanguisorbae Carbonisatus,* 60 grams.
Decoction for uterine bleeding due to blood stasis:

Herba Leonuri   60 grams
or
Herba Verbenae   30   "

or *Pulvis Receptaculum Nelumbinis Carbonisatus,* 6–9 grams twice daily.

ACUPUNCTURE TREATMENT

Main points: Yinbai (Sp 1), Sanyinjiao (Sp 6), Zusanlu (St 36), Xuehai (Sp 10), Guanyuan (Ren 4), Qihai (Ren 6).
Moxibustion is also applied to Yinbai (Sp 1) and Guanyuan (Ren 4). Uniform reinforcing-reducing method is generally applied.

EAR-ACUPUNCTURE THERAPY. Endocrine, Uterus, Ovary, Kidney. One or two points are selected for each treatment, and needles are embedded for three to five days.

DYSMENORRHEA

Dysmenorrhea is defined as painful menstruation. It sometimes is accompanied by such signs and symptoms as pallor, cold sweat and cold limbs, and nausea.

Etiology

Dysmenorrhea occurs when impeded flow of vital energy and blood causes retardation of menstrual flow. Such impeded flow can be caused by exogenous affliction by pathogenic wind-cold, intake of excessive cold raw matter, or emotional disturbance. It also can follow serious illness or result from lowered vital function.

Essentials of Diagnosis and Treatment

It is necessary to know the character of the pain (including location and time of attack) and the causative factors. In excess symptom-complexes, the trouble is due to collection of cold, stagnancy of vital energy, or blood stasis, and the pain occurs before and during menstruation. There is usually sharp lower abdominal pain aggravated by pressure. The pain is relieved when the clots are discharged. Deficiency symptom-complexes are associated with lack of vital energy and blood, and pain occurs during and after menstruation. There is usually mild lower abdominal pain that is alleviated by pressure.

In treating excess symptom-complexes, it is advisable to restore the normal flow of vital energy and blood and dispel pathogenic cold. Before menstruation, treatment is aimed at restoring smooth flow of vital energy; during menstruation, it is necessary to activate blood circulation. In deficiency symptom-complexes, it is advisable to tonify the body and regulate menstruation.

Treatment Based on Differentiation of Symptom-complexes

STAGNANCY OF VITAL ENERGY AND BLOOD. Manifestations: Delayed menstruation, distending pain or cramping that is present in the lower abdomen for one to two days before menstruation or during menstruation and is aggravated by pressure, dark red menstrual discharge with clots, alleviation of pain after discharge of clots, dark red tongue with petechiae on its border, deep taut or taut choppy pulse.

Principle of treatment: Regulating the flow of vital energy and blood to remove stasis and pain.

Prescription: Decoction for Removing Stagnant Blood and Promoting Hemogenesis, with Modifications.

Radix Angelicae Sinensis	15 grams
Faeces Trogopterorum	12 "

Radix Salviae Miltiorrhizae	12 grams
Herba Leonuri	15 "
Rhizoma Ligustici Chuanxiong	6 "
Semen Persicae	6 "
Radix Paeoniae Rubra	6 "
Rhizoma Cyperi Praeparata	9 "
Radix Bupleuri	6 "
Pollen Typae	9 "

Modifications include: For cases with prominent distension in the lower abdomen, add 9 grams *Fructus Meliae Toosendan,* 9 grams *Radix Linderae,* and 9 grams *Rhizoma Corydalis.*

For cases with cyanosis and prominent cramping in the lower abdomen due to blood stasis, add 4.5 grams *Resina Olibani* and 4.5 grams *Resina Myrrhae.*

For cases with cold sensation and pain in the lower abdomen due to collection of cold, add 3 grams *Fructus Evodiae,* 3 grams *Cortex Cinnamomi,* and 9 grams *Folium Artemisiae Argyi.*

For cases with bitter taste and dry mouth, restlessness, yellow tongue coating, and taut and rapid pulse due to excessive heat in the liver, add 6 grams *Fructus Gardeniae Praeparata* and 6 grams *Radix Scutellariae.*

DEFICIENCY OF BOTH VITAL ENERGY AND BLOOD . Manifestations: Delayed menstruation, dull pain that is present during or after menstruation and is alleviated on pressure, scanty light-colored menstrual blood without clots, livid complexion, dizziness, palpitation, pale tongue, thready and weak pulse.

Principle of treatment: Reinforcing vital energy and blood to regulate menstruation.

Prescription: Decoction of Eight Precious Ingredients, with Modifications.

Radix Codonopsis Pilosulae	12 grams
Rhizoma Astractylodis Macrocephalae	9 "
Radix Astragali	12 "
Radix Angelicae Sinensis	9 "
Radix Paeoniae Alba	9 "
Rhizoma Ligustici Chuanxiong	4.5 "
Radix Glycyrrhizae Praeparata	3 "

Radix Rehmannia Praeparata	9 grams
Folium Artemisiae Argyi	4.5 ″

Modifications include: For cases with persistent profuse menstrual blood, add 9 grams *Colli Corii Asini* and 12 grams *Petiolus Trachycarpi Carbosatus.*

For cases with weakness of the back and legs, add 9 grams *Cortex Eucommiae* and 9 grams *Semen Cuscutae.*

Other Methods of Treating Dysmenorrhea

PROVEN RECIPES

Dysmenorrhea powder:

Radix Angelicae Sinensis	12 grams
Rhizoma Ligustici Chuanxiong	6 ″
Radix Salviae Miltiorrhizae	15 ″
Faeces Trogopterorum	9 ″
Rhizoma Cyperi Praeparata	9 ″
Pollen Typhae	9 ″
Radix Paeoniae Alba	9 ″
Semen Persicae	9 ″
Aspongopus (stink-bug)	4.5 ″

Take 6–9 grams of the powder twice daily for either three days before or three days during menstruation.

Decoction prepared with brown sugar and given for dysmenorrhea: *Herba Leonuri,* 30 grams.

Preparation for dysmenorrhea:

Pollen Typhae	9 grams
Faeces Trogopterorum	9 ″
Rice Wine	30 ml

Cook together and give two doses daily.

Decoction given for dysmenorrhea:

Radix Angelicae Sinensis	12 grams
Radix Salviae Miltiorrhizae	12 ″

Fructus Foeniculi (common fennel fruit)	6 grams
Rhizoma Cyperi	6 "
Herba Lycopi	6 "

ACUPUNCTURE TREATMENT

Main points: Sanyinjiao (Sp 6), Hegu (LI 4), Guanyuan (Ren 4), Qihai (Ren 6) (apply needling first and then moxibustion).

All points are used for each treatment. Needles are retained for 15 to 20 minutes.

EAR-ACUPUNCTURE THERAPY. Uterus, Sympathetic Nerve, Ear-Shenmen.

One or two points are selected for each treatment. Needles are retained for 15 to 30 minutes.

THREATENED ABORTION

Threatened abortion is defined as signs and symptoms of impending expulsion of the embryo or fetus during the first 28 weeks of pregnancy. It can be characterized by bloody discharge from the uterus and lower abdominal pain or by continuous movement of the fetus, abdominal pain, and scanty bloody discharge. In traditional Chinese medicine, it is known as "fetal leakage" and "abdominal pain during pregnancy."

Etiology

Threatened abortion is due to weakness of the Chong and Ren Channels, which leads to failure to control blood and nourish the fetus. Such weakness is caused by deficiency of vital energy and blood, weakened kidney function, intense heat in the blood system, or trauma.

Essentials of Diagnosis and Treatment

If bloody discharge is present, it is necessary to tonify the kidney to stop bleeding and reinforce vital energy and blood to prevent miscarriage. In treatment of continuous fetal movement and abdominal pain, it is essential to remove intense heat and nourish blood to support the fetus.

Treatment Based on Differentiation of Symptom-Complexes

DEFICIENCY OF VITAL ENERGY AND BLOOD. Manifestations: Downward movement of the fetus in early pregnancy, scanty light red bloody discharge from the uterus, lassitude, pallor, palpitation, shortness of breath, backache, distended abdomen, pale tongue with thin white coating, thready slippery pulse.

Principle of treatment: Reinforcing vital energy and blood, strengthening the function of the kidney to prevent miscarriage.

Prescription: Decoction for Prevention of Miscarriage, with Modifications.

Radix Ginseng (simmered separately)	9	grams
Cortex Eucommiae	9	"
Radix Paeoniae Alba	6	"
Radix Rehmannia Praeparata	15	"
Rhizoma Atractylodis Macrocephalae	9	"
Radix Glycyrrhizae Praeparata	3	"
Pericarpium Citri Reticulatae	6	"
Radix Astragali	12	"
Colli Corii Asini (melted)	6	"

LOWERED FUNCTIONING OF THE KIDNEY. Manifestations: Aching loins during pregnancy, lower abdominal pain with tenesmus, a sensation of the fetus prolapsing, bloody discharge from the uterus, dizziness, tinnitus, weak legs, aching heels, frequent urination, pale tongue with thin coating, deep weak pulse, history of habitual abortion.

Principle of treatment: Tonifying the kidney and reinforcing vital energy to prevent miscarriage.

Prescription: Fetus-Saving Decoction, with Modifications.

Ramulus Loranthi	15	grams
Semen Cuscutae	9	"
Cortex Eucommiae	9	"
Radix Dipsaci	9	"

Radix Rehmannia Praeparata	9 grams
Colli Corii Asini	6 "
Folium Artemisiae Carbonisatus	6 "
Radix Glycyrrhizae Praeparata	3 "
Radix Boehmeriae	9 "

CONTINUOUS FETAL MOVEMENT DUE TO INTENSE HEAT IN THE BLOOD SYSTEM. Manifestations: Bright red bloody discharge from the uterus, sensation of the fetus prolapsing, restlessness, flushed face and lips, dry mouth, afternoon fever, heat sensation of the palms, concentrated urine, constipation, reddened tongue with dry yellow coating, slippery, rapid, or taut slippery pulse.

Principle of treatment: Replenishing vital essence to remove intense heat, nourishing blood to prevent miscarriage.

Prescription: Decoction for preserving Vital Essence, with Modifications.

Radix Rehmannia	15 grams
Radix Paeoniae Alba	9 "
Radix Scutellariae	6 "
Cortex Phellodendri	6 "
Radix Dipsaci	9 "
Radix Glycyrrhizae	3 "
Colli Corii Asini (melted)	9 "
Radix Sanguisorbae	9 "
Herba Ecliptae	9 "
Radix Boehmeriae	9 "

CONTINUOUS FETAL MOVEMENT DUE TO TRAUMA. Manifestations: Sensation of the fetus prolapsing, aching and distending pain in the lower back, bloody discharge from the uterus, slippery, weak pulse, all occurring after trauma.

Principle of treatment: Reinforcing vital energy and blood; strengthening the functioning of the kidney to prevent miscarriage.

Prescription: Fetus-Easing Decoction, with Modifications.

Radix Ginseng (simmered separately)	9 grams
Radix Astragali	15 "
Radix Angelicae Sinensis	9 "

CASE HISTORY

Female, age 27, first visit on April 16, 1970.

History

The patient had a history of eight miscarriages in five years. Each time that abortion threatened, she was admitted to the hospital but failed to continue the pregnancy. During the first trimester of the ninth pregnancy, she suffered from vaginal bleeding for thirteen consecutive days. The discharge was scanty and purple. The patient complained of a sinking sensation and pain in the lower back and confined herself to bed because of the previous miscarriages.

Diagnosis and Treatment

The patient appeared weak and spoke in a soft voice. She had a pink tongue with a thin coating and a deep, thready, and slippery pulse. The diagnosis was threatened abortion and habitual abortion due to deficiencies of both the spleen and kidney. The principle of treatment was invigorating the spleen and tonifying the kidney to consolidate the fetus and arrest bleeding. The prescription administered was:

Radix Pseudostellariae (pseudostellaria root)	9 grams
Rhizoma Dioscoreae	9 "
Semen Nelumbinis	9 "
Cortex Eucommiae	9 "
Radix Dipsaci	9 "
Semen Cuscutae	9 "
Ramulus Loranthi	9 "
Petiolus Trachycarpi Carbonisatus	9 "
Colla Corii Asini (melted)	12 "

After three doses, the vaginal bleeding gradually stopped, and the pain and sinking sensation in the lower back were relieved. The previous prescription was continued with the omission of

Peliolus Trachycarpi Carbonisatus
Colla Corii Asini

and addition of 9 grams *Fructus Psoraleae.*

The patient was informed that although the pain was relieved and the fetus appeared well, the second prescription should be taken four or five times per month for the rest of the pregnancy.

Delivery was in October 1970; both mother and child did well.

—From Chen Jiayang, *A Collection of Case Histories of Traditional Chinese Medicine)* (Gansu People's Publishing House, 1981), pp. 526–27.

Radix Rehmannia Praeparata	12 grams
Radix Paeoniae Alba	9 "
Semen Cuscutae	9 "
Ramulus Loranthi	12 "

Radix Dipsaci	9 grams
Folium Artemisiae Argyi Carbonisatus	9 "
Colli Corii Asini (melted)	6 "

Additional Decoction for Treating Threatened Abortion: *Radix Boehmeriae,* 30–90 grams.

MOXIBUSTION TREATMENT

Moxibustion of Tianshu (St 25) and Sanyinjiao (Sp 6) is sometimes used to treat threatened abortion.

AGALACTIA

Agalactia is the absence of milk in the breasts following delivery. Traditional Chinese medicine calls this disorder "absence of lactation" or "nonflowing of milk."

Etiology

In postpartum women, milk is formed from *qi* and blood. The production of these latter two substances depends on the digestion and transport functions of the spleen and stomach. Therefore, the absence of lactation is due to deficiency of *qi* and/or blood after delivery, or due to deficiency of the spleen and stomach resulting in their inability to distribute enough nutrients and water to form milk in the breasts. Agalactia may be caused by emotional stress and depression of liver *qi* inducing blockage of lactation. It is said: "Absence of the secretion of milk may be due to emotional stress, such as crying, weeping, sorrow, anger, grief, and depression" (*Confucians' Duties to Their Parents* by Zhang Congzheng, A.D. 1228).

Essentials of Diagnosis and Treatment

The symptom-complexes of agalactia include those of insufficiency and excessiveness. Patients presenting with a strong constitution and fullness and pain of the breasts have an excessiveness symptom-complex; those with a weak constitution and without fullness and pain of the breasts have a deficiency symptom-complex. Excessiveness symptom-complexes are treated by regulating *qi* and clearing the channels to improve the flow of milk. Insufficiency symptom-complexes are treated by reinforcing *qi* and nourishing blood to induce lactation.

Treatment Based on Differentiation of Symptom-Complexes

DEFICIENCY OF *qi* AND BLOOD. Manifestations: Agalactia, absence of fullness and pain of the breasts, pale complexion, dizziness, palpitation, pale tongue, feeble pulse.

Principle of treatment: Reinforcing vital energy and nourishing the blood.

Prescription: Powder for Inducing Lactation, with Modifications.

Radix Codonopsis Pilosulae	15	grams
Radix Astragali	15	"
Radix Angelicae Sinensis	15	"
Radix Paeoniae Alba	9	"
Radix Ophiopogonis	9	"
Caulis Akebiae	6	"
Radix Platycodi	6	"
Medulla Tetrapanacis	3	"

The decoction is prepared in 200 ml of stew made from one pig trotter.

Modifications include: for cases with poor appetite, dyspepsia, and other manifestations of deficiency of the spleen and stomach, such as belching, nausea, and diarrhea, add 9 grams *Rhizoma Atractylodis Macrocephalae* and 9 grams medicated leaven.

STAGNANCY OF LIVER *qi*. Manifestations: Absence of milk secretion, fullness sensation of the breasts, emotional distress, oppressive feeling in the chest, epigastrium, or hypochondriac region, poor appetite, thin tongue coating, wiry tight pulse.

Principle of treatment: Soothing the liver, regulating the flow of *qi*.

Prescription: Powder for the Welling Up of Lactation, with Modifications.

Radix Bupleuri	9	grams
Pericarpium Citri Reticulatae Viride	6	"
Radix Angelicae Sinensis	12	"
Radix Paeoniae Alba	9	"
Radix Platycodi	6	"
Medulla Tetrapanacis	3	"
Radix Trichosanthis	9	"
Squama Manitis	9	"
Semen Vaccariae (seed of cowherb)	9	"
Radix Rhapontici seu Echinopsis (globethistle root)	9	"

Other Common Methods of Treating Agalactia

PROVEN RECIPES

Beverage given for agalactia: Two pig trotters and two carps stewed with 9 grams of *Medulla Tetrapanacis* to make a salt-free soup.

Decoction given for agalactia:

Radix Angelicae Sinensis	15	grams
Semen Vaccariae	9	"

ACUPUNCTURE TREATMENT

Main points: Tanzhong (Ren 17), Hegu (LI 4), Shaoze (SJ 1), Zusanli (St 36), Sanyinjiao (Sp 6). All points are used for each treatment. Uniform reinforcing-reducing method is applied.

SALPINGITIS

Salpingitis, or pelvic inflammatory disease, is an infection of the fallopian tubes. In traditional Chinese medicine, acute salpingitis is known as "hot hernia" or "cord-like swellings on both sides of the umbilicus." Chronic salpingitis is known as "menstrual irregularity," "abnormal vaginal discharge," or "swelling of the abdomen."

Etiology

Salpingitis generally results from neglecting personal hygiene around time of menstruation, delivery, sexual intercourse, or abortion. When such hygiene is neglected, heat- and damp-producing pathogenic factors can invade and be retained in the lower burner. The resulting heat and dampness stagnate in the womb and its connected channels and collaterals. This impedes the normal flow of *qi* and blood, resulting in injury to the Chong and Ren Channels.

During the initial stages of the disease, when the invading pathogenic factors are actively resisted by the antipathogenic *qi,* a symptom-complex of excess is manifested. If treatment is not thoroughly effective or is delayed, antipathogenic *qi* decreases in strength and the pathogenic factors, as well as stagnated *qi* and blood, are retained in the Chong and Ren Channels, resulting in a chronic condition manifested by a deficiency symptom-complex or by a more complicated symptom-complex of the coexistence of insufficiency and excess.

Diagnosis and Treatment

At the onset of the disease, treatment should emphasize dispelling heat and dampness as well as dispersing blood stasis. In the later stages, when manifestations of *qi* and blood stasis are prominent, treatment should be aimed at promoting the flow of *qi* and blood; before therapy, the substance that is more stagnated should be carefully determined. Treatment should be flexible, taking into consideration the strength and nature of the pathogenic factors as well as the strength of the antipathogenic *qi*.

Treatment Based on Differentiation of Symptom-Complexes

DAMP-HEAT COMPLICATED BY BLOOD STASIS (usually seen in acute salpingitis or excerbation during chronic salpingitis). Manifestations:

Fever and mild chills, lower abdominal pain exacerbated by pressure, lower abdominal distension, mass and swelling in the lower abdomen, yellowish foul-smelling blood-stained vaginal discharge, yellowish greasy tongue coating, rapid and taut pulse.

Principle of treatment: Removing heat and dampness, dispersing blood stasis.

Prescription: Decoction of Rhei and Cortex Moutan and Decoction of Sargentodoxae, with Modifications.

Radix et Rhizoma Rhei	9	grams
Cortex Moutan Radicis	9	"
Caulis Sargentodoxae (sargentgloryvine stem)	30	"
Herba Patriniae	30	"
Semen Coicis	9	"
Semen Corydalis	9	"
Fructus Meliae Toosendan	9	"
Semen Plantaginis (wrapped)	9	"

Modifications include: For cases with severe abdominal distension, add 9 grams *Rhizoma Cyperi* and 9 grams *Pericarpium Citri Reticulatae Viride.*

For cases with severe abdominal pain and masses, add 9 grams *Faeces Trogopterorum,* 9 grams *Radix Salviae Miltiorrhizae,* 9 grams *Rhizoma Sparganii,* 9 grams *Rhizoma Zedoariae,* 6 grams *Resina Olibani Praeparata,* 6 grams *Resina Myrrhae Praeparata,* and 6 grams *Flos Carthami.*

For cases with high fever and yellowish vaginal discharge, add 24 grams *Herba Violae,* 15 grams *Flos Lonicerae,* and 9 grams *Cortex Phellodendri.*

For cases with downward drive of dampness manifested by profuse vaginal discharge and greasy thick tongue coating, add 9 grams *Poria* and 9 grams *Rhizoma Alismatis.*

STAGNANCY IN THE LIVER LEADING TO STASIS OF *qi* (usually seen in chronic salpingitis). Manifestations: Severe abdominal pain before and during menstruation, sensation of oppression in the chest, pain in the costal region, distension of breasts, thin tongue coating, taut and thready pulse.

Principle of treatment: Soothing the liver, regulating the flow of *qi*, and relieving pain.

Prescription: Pills of Tangerine Seed.

Semen Citri Reticulatae	15	grams
Radix Linderae	9	"
Rhizoma Cyperi	9	"
Fructus Meliae Toosendan	9	"
Radix Bupleuri	9	"
Pericarpium Citri Reticulatae Viride	6	"
Pericarpium Citri Reticulatae	9	"
Rhizoma Corydalis	9	"
Radix Curcumae	9	"

Modifications include: For cases with downward drive of damp-heat manifested by yellowish vaginal discharge, add 9 grams *Rhizoma Alismati* and 9 grams *Semen Coicis*.

RETENTION OF BLOOD STASIS (usually seen in chronic salpingitis). Manifestations: Lower abdominal mass, dull pain that is more severe during menstruation, increase or decrease in the amount of menstrual flow, dark or clotted menstrual blood, lumbar pain, purple tongue, taut or choppy pulse.

Principle of treatment: Activating the blood circulation to eliminate blood stasis and relieve pain.

Prescription: Decoction for Removing Blood Stasis Under the Thoracic Diaphragm, with Modifications.

Semen Persicae	9	grams
Flos Carthami	9	"
Radix Angelicae Sinensis	9	"
Radix Paeoniae Rubra	9	"
Rhizoma Ligustici Chuanxiong	6	"
Eupolyphaga seu Steleophaga	9	"
Rhizoma Corydalis	9	"
Rhizoma Cyperi Praeparata	9	"
Radix Linderae	9	"

Modifications include: For cases with low fever and yellowish vaginal discharge, replace *Flos Carthami* and *Radix Angelicae Sinensis* with

9 grams *Caulis Sargentodoxae.* 15 grams *Herba Patriniae.* 9 grams *Cortex Phellodendri.* and 9 grams *Rhizoma Alismatis.*

For cases with debility, dizziness, and lassitude, add 15 grams *Radix Astragali seu Hedysari* and 15 grams *Radix Codonopsis Pilosulae.*

ACUPUNCTURE TREATMENT OF SALPINGITIS

Main points: Dazhui (Du 14), Guanyuan (Ren 4), Qihai (Ren 6), Zhongwan (Ren 12), Shenshu (UB 23), Hegu (LI 4), Zusanli (St 36)

Reinforcing only is applied. Needles are retained for 20–30 minutes.

MENOPAUSE

Menopause is the transitional phase in a woman's life when menstrual function ceases. Menopause may be asymptomatic or associated with symptoms (primarily due to estrogen deficiency resulting from age-related decline in ovarian function), which may be severe. Traditional Chinese medicine calls menopause "menstrual irregularity," "dizziness," or "palpitations" in the older woman.

Etiology

The kidney is in charge of reproduction. At the end of the reproductive period, kidney *qi* declines, as do the functions of the Chong and Ren Channels. Therefore, menstruation is irregular, and menopause begins.

The kidney is also the foundation of congenital essence and congenital vital function. When the *qi* of the kidney declines, its *yin* and *yang* become imbalanced, influencing other organs. If the menopausal woman is of weak or nervous constitution and cannot adapt to the physiological changes during this period, she may thus show manifestations of disturbances of other organs.

Diagnosis and Treatment

For the different symptom-complexes of menopause, diagnosis and treatment should be made with the decline of the kidney in mind. Treatment therefore should emphasize reinforcing the kidney. For deficiencies of kidney and liver *yin*. therapy should be aimed at reinforcing the vital essence of both organs. For exuberance of liver *yang*. treatment should be designed to reinforce the kidney along with subduing hyperactivity of the liver. Deficiencies of spleen and kidney *yang* should be treated by using tonics and drugs warm in property.

Treatment Based on Differentiation of Symptom-Complexes

DEFICIENCY OF *yin* OF THE LIVER AND KIDNEY. Manifestations: Abnormal scanty menstruation that is red or dark-red, flushed cheeks, feverishness in the palms and soles, hectic fever, night sweats, palpitation, restlessness, dizziness, tinnitus, thirst, irritability, melancholy, weakness of the lower back and knees, reddened tongue with thin coating, fine taut and rapid pulse.

Principle of treatment: Nourishing *yin* of the liver and kidney.

Prescription: Bolus of Six Ingredients with Rehmannia, with Modifications.

Radix Rehmannia	15	grams
Rhizoma Dioscoreae	9	"
Fructus Corni	9	"
Poria	9	"
Rhizoma Alismatis	9	"
Cortex Moutan Radicis	9	"
Radix Paeoniae Rubra	9	"
Radix Paeoniae Alba	9	"
Fructus Ligustri Lucidi	9	"
Concha Haliotidis (decocted first)	24	"
Radix Scrophulariae	9	"

Modifications include: For cases with deficiency of *yin* accompanied by flaring up of inner-fire (due to exuberance of liver *yang*), with symptoms such as flushed cheeks, restlessness, and scanty concentrated urine, add 9 grams *Cortex Phellodendri* and 9 grams *Rhizoma Anemarrhenae.*

For cases with profuse sweating, add 15 grams *Fructus Tritici Levis.*

For cases with insomnia, add 30 grams *Caulis Polygoni Multiflori* and 24 grams *Magnetitum* (decocted first).

For cases with pain in the lower back, add 12 grams *Radix Dipsaci,* 12 grams *Ramulus Loranthi,* and 9 grams *Fructus Psoraleae.*

DEFICIENCY OF *yang* OF THE SPLEEN AND KIDNEY. Manifestations: Profuse menstruation of light color, pale complexion, lassitude, intolerance of cold, weak sensation of lower back, anorexia, loose stools, frequent urination, pale tongue with thin coating, feeble deep and fine pulse.

Principle of treatment: Warming and tonifying the spleen and kidney.

Prescription: Bolus for Reinforcing Deficiency of Vital Function of the Kidney, with Modifications.

Radix Rehmannia Praeparata	15	grams
Rhizoma Dioscoreae	9	"
Fructus Corni	9	"
Fructus Lycii	9	"
Radix Dipsaci	9	"
Radix Codonopsis Pilosulae	12	"
Rhizoma Atractylodis Macrocephalae	9	"
Rhizoma Curculiginis	9	"
Herba Epimedii	9	"
Cortex Cinnamomi	3	"

Modifications include: For cases with profuse menstruation, add 9 grams *Cacumen Biotae,* 9 grams *Petiolus Trachycarpi Carbonisatus* and 3 grams *Pulvis Radix Notoginseng* (dissolved in the decoction).

For cases with edema of the face and feet, replace *Radix Rehmannia Praeparata* with 12 grams *Cortex Poria* (tuckahoe bark), 9 grams *Radix Astragali seu Heydysari,* and 6 grams *Radix Stephaniae Tetrandrae.*

ACUPUNCTURE TREATMENT OF MENOPAUSE

Main points: Guanyuan (Ren 4), Zhongji (Ren 3), Guilai (St 29), Shuidao (St 28), Sanyinjiao (Sp 6), Ligou (Liv 5), Zhongdu (Liv 6)

Points according to manifestations:

Lower abdominal masses—Fushe (Sp 13)
Lower abdominal pain—Qichong (St 30)
Lower backache—Shenshu (UB 23), Ciliao (UB 32)
Leukorrhea—Diji (Sp 8), Yinlingquan (Sp 9), Daimai (GB 26)

Uniform reinforcing-reducing method is applied. Needles are retained for 20 minutes. Treat once daily; one course of therapy is 20 days.

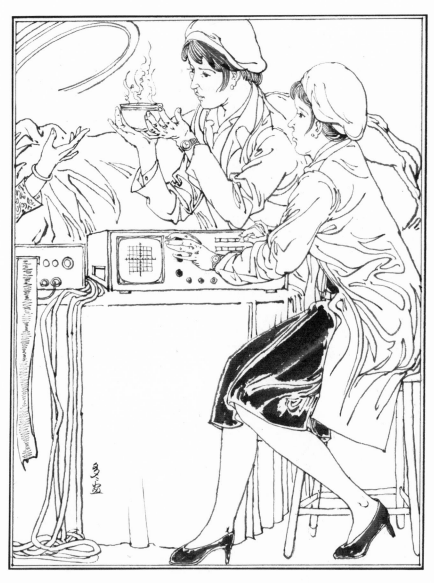

Two physicians combining Chinese and Western medicine in treating their patient.

CHAPTER SEVEN

Treatment of
Other Selected Conditions

ORAL ADMINISTRATION OF medicinal herbs has been shown to be quite effective in treating various disorders such as inflammations, dermatological conditions, and diseases of the sense organs. This chapter presents various common disorders in these categories. As in the previous chapters, the names of the diseases are in western medicine terminology, whereas etiology, diagnosis, and treatment are according to traditional Chinese medicine.

ACUTE CHOLECYSTITIS AND CHOLELITHIASIS

Acute cholecystitis (inflammation of the gallbladder) and cholelithiasis (gallstones) are common abdominal conditions. Manifestations include sharp pain in the upper abdomen, nausea, vomiting, alternate spells of fever and chills, and jaundice. Cholecystitis often leads to formation of biliary calculi (stones), and cholelithiasis often brings on cholecystitis. In traditional Chinese medicine, these conditions are known as "pain due to stagnation of the liver and stomach," "vomiting," and "jaundice."

Etiology

These conditions can result from emotional strain, such as depression, worry, or anger, that leads to dysfunction of the liver and gallbladder and stagnancy of vital energy. They also can occur when improper diet impedes function of the spleen and stomach and causes collection of pathogenic damp-heat and dysfunction of the liver and gallbladder. Accumulation of pathogenic damp-heat over a long period can then lead to formation of gallstones.

Essentials of Diagnosis and Treatment

Diagnosis can easily be made on the basis of the location of tenderness and the x-ray examination. The symptom-complexes can be divided into three kinds: stagnancy of vital energy due to a depressed liver, accumulation and brewing of pathogenic damp-heat, and pathogenic fire produced by intense heat.

The aims of the treatment are to soothe the liver, to invigorate the functioning of the gallbladder, and to eliminate heat and stones by purgation. In acute cholecystitis complicated by toxic shock, pyogenic obstructive cholecystitis, gallbladder perforation, or empyema of the gallbladder, timely surgery is necessary when medicinal herbs are ineffective.

Treatment Based on Differentiation of Symptom-Complexes

STAGNANCY OF VITAL ENERGY DUE TO A DEPRESSED LIVER (usually found in simple cholecystitis, cholelithiasis, and chronic cholecystitis. Manifestations: Repeated dull or distending pain in the right upper abdomen, bitter taste and dryness in the mouth, anorexia, abdominal distension after meals, nausea at times, moderate fever, thin white or light yellow tongue coating, taut, rapid or thready pulse.

Principle of treatment: Eliminating heat to invigorate the functioning of the gallbladder; soothing the liver to normalize the flow of vital energy.

Prescription: Bupleurum Decoction for Soothing the Liver, with Modifications.

Radix Bupleuri	9 grams
Rhizoma Ligustici Chuanxiong	6 "
Fructus Aurantii Immaturus	9 "
Radix Paeoniae Alba	9 "
Rhizoma Cyperi Praeparata	9 "
Radix Curcumae	9 "
Fructus Gardeniae Praeparata	9 "
Radix Scutellariae	9 "
Herba Lysimachiae	30 "

Modifications include: For cases with jaundice, add 30 grams *Herba Artemisiae Scopariae* and 12 grams *Spora Lygodii*.

For cases with constipation, add 9 grams *Radix et Rhizoma Rhei* and 6 grams *Natrii Sulfas Exsiccatus* (dissolved in the decoction).

For cases with bitter taste and dryness in the mouth and reddened tongue with yellow coating, add 6 grams *Rhizoma Coptidis* and 9 grams *Radix Gentianae*.

GATHERING AND BREWING OF PATHOGENIC DAMP-HEAT (usually found in acute cholangitis, acute cholecystitis, and calculi in the common bile duct). Manifestations: Sharp distending upper right abdominal pain radiating into the right shoulder and hypochondrium, restlessness, profuse sweating, alternate spells of fever and chills, moderate fever, stuffy sensation in the chest and abdomen, bitter taste in the mouth, nausea and vomiting, thirst without desire for beverages, jaundice, concentrated urine, constipation, reddened tip and border of the tongue, slimy or rough yellow tongue coating, taut, slippery, and rapid pulse.

Principle of treatment: Clearing away pathogenic heat from the liver through purgation to invigorate the functioning of the gallbladder.

Prescription: Major Decoction of Bupleurum, with Modifications.

Radix Bupleuri	9 grams
Radix Scutellariae	9 "
Rhizoma Pinelliae Praeparata	9 "
Fructus Aurantii Immaturus	9 "

Radix Paeoniae Rubra	9 grams
Radix Curcumae	9 "
Herba Artemisiae Scopariae	30 "
Herba Lysimachiae	30 "
Spora Lygodii	12 "
Radix et Rhizoma Rhei	9 "
Natrii Sulfas Exsiccatus (dissolved in the decoction)	9 "

Modifications include: For cases with high fever and dry yellow tongue coating (suggesting intense heat), add 3 grams *Rhizoma Coptidis*, 9 grams *Fructus Gardeniae Praeparata*, 9 grams *Fructus Forsythiae*, and 15 grams *Flos Lonicerae*.

For cases with moderate fever, stuffy sensation in the chest, heavy feeling in the head, thirst without desire for beverages, and slimy white tongue coating, add 9 grams *Rhizoma Atractylodis*, 6 grams *Fructus Amomi Tsaoko* (amomum tsao-ko fruit), 9 grams *Herba Agastachis*, and 9 grams *Herba Eupatorii*.

PATHOGENIC FIRE RESULTING IN INTENSE HEAT (usually seen in acute obstructive pyogenic cholecystitis and in cholelithiasis complicated by gangrenous cholecystitis). Manifestations: Persistent upper right abdominal distending pain aggravated by pressure, sometimes with a palpable lump at the site of pain, alternate spells of fever and chills or high fever without chills, bitter taste and dryness in the mouth, restlessness, delirium, jaundice, vomiting, constipation, red urine, reddened prickly tongue with dry yellow coating, taut and rapid pulse.

Principle of treatment: Soothing the liver to invigorate the functioning of the gallbladder; removing intense heat by purgation.

Prescription: Decoction of Gentianae to Purge the Liver, with Modifications.

Radix Gentianae	9 grams
Radix Scutellariae	9 "
Fructus Gardeniae	9 "
Radix Bupleuri	9 "
Fructus Meliae Toosendan	9 "
Cortex Phellodendri	9 "
Fructus Aurantii	9 "
Flos Lonicerae	15 "

Herba Houtuyniae	15 grams
Herba Patriniae	15 "
Herba Lysimachiae	30 "
Radix Rehmannia	30 "
Radix et Rhizoma Rhei	9 "

Modifications include: For cases with prominent jaundice, add 30 grams *Herba Artemisiae Scopariae* and 9 grams *Spora Lygodii*.

Other Common Methods of Treating Cholecystitis and Cholelithiasis

PROVEN RECIPES

Decoction for treating cholelithiasis: Decoction for Expelling Stones from the Bile Ducts.

Herba Lysimachiae	30 grams
Herba Artemisiae Scopariae	15 "
Radix Curcumae	15 "
Fructus Aurantii	9 "
Radix Aucklandiae	9 "
Radix et Rhizoma Rhei	9 "

Bolus for cholelithiasis: Bolus for Invigorating the Function of the Gallbladder.

Herba Artemisiae Scopariae	120 grams
Radix Gentianae	90 "
Radix Curcumae	90 "
Radix Aucklandiae	90 "
Fructus Aurantii	90 "

The above ingredients are ground into a powder and cooked with 500 ml pig, sheep, or cow bile into a 250 ml concentrate. The concentrate is then mixed with honey to make boluses. Nine grams of the boluses are taken three times daily for chronic cholelithiasis.

Decoction given for cholelithiasis: Calculus-Expelling Decoction.

CASE HISTORY
Female, age 40, first visit on January 24, 1973.

History

The patient had epigastric pain of about six months' duration. The pain radiated to the shoulders and sometimes was not relieved by injections of demerol hydrochloride. Cholecystography revealed cholelithiasis. The patient declined surgery and asked for traditional Chinese medicine treatment.

Diagnosis and Treatment

The patient's tongue was pink with a thin coating; her pulse was taut. The pain was thus believed to be caused by obstruction in the liver and biliary tract due to overeating of greasy· food. The resulting stagnation of damp-heat had induced stagnation of vital energy and stasis of blood in the liver region and blocked the flow from liver to gallbladder; thus stones were formed. It was considered necessary to relieve stagnancy of vital energy of the liver and dissolve and/or expel stones to relieve internal stasis. Decoction for Expelling Stones from the Bile Ducts was prescribed:

Herba Lysimachiae	30 grams
Calculus Psuedosciaena Encephalon (yellow croaker ear stone)	9 "
Radix Curcumae	9 "
Endothelium Corneum Gigeriae Galli	9 "
Fructus Crataegi (charred)	9 "
Pericarpium Citri Reticulatae Viride	4.5 "
Pericarpium Citri Reticulatae	4.5 "
Fructus Aurantii (stir-fried)	6 "
Caulis Bambusae (boiled with ginger)	6 "
Rhizoma Corydalis	9 "
Fructus Meliae Toosendan	9 "
Radix Bupleuri	4.5 "
Radix et Rhizoma Rhei	9 "
Radix et Rhizoma Rhei Praeparata	9 "
Natrii Sulfas Exsiccatus (dissolved in the decoction)	9 "

After three doses, the patient had three bowel movements in one day and the pain was relieved. She found three soybean-size stones in the stools.

Another three doses, without the *Natrii Sulfas*, were ordered. Later consultation found complete alleviation of the pain in the right costal region. Another 12 doses were prescribed to consolidate the curative effect. Follow-up over five years revealed no recurrence.

—From Li Zunwu, *Shanghai Veteran
Traditional Doctors' Experiences*, compiled by
Shanghai Bureau of Health (Scientific and
Technical Publishing House of Shanghai,
1980), p. 514.

Herba Artemisiae Scopariae	15 grams	
Radix Aucklandiae	9	"
Fructus Aurantii	9	"
Rhizoma Ciptidis	6	"
Radix Scutellariae	6	"

Decoction given for cholelithiasis: *Herba Lysimachiae,* 60–120 grams.

ACUPUNCTURE TREATMENT

GENERAL TREATMENT. Main points: Yanglingquan (GB 34), Zhigou (SJ 6), Zusanli (St 36).

Alternate points: Neiguan (P 6), Zhangmen (Liv 13), Qimen (Liv 14), Danshu (UB 19), Qiuxu (GB 40).

Points according to manifestations:

Vomiting—Shangwan (Ren 13)
Severe pain—Zhongwan (Ren 12)
Backache—Ganshu (UB 18), Danshu (UB 19)
High fever—Quchi (LI 11), Hegu (LI 4)
Jaundice—Zhiyang (Du 9), Yanggang (UB 48)
Abdominal distension and constipation—Dachangshu (UB 25), Tianshu (St 25)

Strong stimulus with needle retention is generally applied. Needle the alternative points if use of the main points does not yield relief.

EXPELLING STONES BY ACUPUNCTURE. Main points: Danshu (UB 19), Zhongwan (Ren 12), Zusanli (St 36).

Strong stimulus is applied once a day. A prominent tender spot in the right hypochondrium may appear after needling Zhongwan (Ren 12). The day after it appears, needle the Ashi point 1.5 *cun* lateral to the middle of the abdomen and parallel to the tender spot; Danshu (UB 19) and Zusanli (St 36) are also needled. One course lasts 10 days; the stone usually is discharged in two courses.

EAR-ACUPUNCTURE THERAPY. Sympathetic Nerve, Ear-Shenmen, Gallbladder, Liver, Subcortex.

One or two points are selected for each treatment, and needles are retained for 15 minutes or embedded for 3 to 5 days.

ACUTE APPENDICITIS

Acute appendicitis is one of the most common acute abdominal conditions. In traditional Chinese medicine it is termed "carbuncle of the intestine."

Etiology

This condition can be caused by improper diet, irregular weather, or walking too swiftly after meals, resulting in disturbance of the transport function of the intestine and blockage of the functional activities of vital energy. *Qi* and blood stagnate in the appendix region, causing inflammation.

At onset, pain appears around the umbilicus. Later the pain is localized in the right lower quadrant and accompanied by nausea and vomiting. If *qi* and blood stagnate over a long period, then fever appears; if the stagnation is not dispersed, masses may develop. If exuberant heat accumulates, an abscess is formed. If the condition progresses, extreme heat may bring on noxious fire, which spreads the inflammation to the peritoneum. This type of pathogenic fire consumes vital energy and blood; therefore deficiencies of both occur in the advanced stage of acute appendicitis.

Essentials of Diagnosis and Treatment

Since the main cause of acute appendicitis is stasis of *qi* and blood that results in stagnancy of noxious heat in the intestine, the symptom-complexes are of heat and excessiveness. Therefore, diagnosis differentiating these two symptom-complexes is of priority. Treatment is aimed at eliminating internal heat by clearing the intestine and activating blood flow to disperse stasis. Modifications of the prescription are according to the degree of stagnation of *qi* or blood and of the toxicity of heat. In the advanced stage, treatment should be supported with tonics for reinforcing vital energy and strengthening body resistance.

Treatment Based on Differentiation of Symptom-Complexes

ONSET OF ACUTE APPENDICITIS. Manifestations: Abdominal distension, nausea and vomiting, loss of appetite, abdominal pain and guarding, constipation or loose stools, thirst, fever, scanty and concentrated urine, tenderness and rebound pain over the right lower abdomen; red or dark red tongue with yellowish and greasy tongue coating, rapid slippery or rapid taut pulse.

Principle of treatment: Removing pathogenic heat by clearing the intestine, activating the circulation of blood to disperse stasis.

Prescription: Decoction of Rhei and Cortex Moutan, with Modifications.

Radix et Rhizoma Rhei	9 grams
Cortex Moutan Radicis	9 "
Semen Persicae	9 "
Caulis Sargentodoxae (sargentgloryvine stem)	30 "
Herba Patriniae	30 "

Modifications include: For cases with migratory pain around the umbilicus or appendicular colic, borborygmus, and abdominal distension, add 9 grams *Fructus Meliae Toosendan,* 9 grams *Rhizoma Corydalis,* and 9 grams *Radix Aucklandiae.*

For cases with severe blood stasis, fixed continuous pain in the right lower abdomen, or a fixed mass, add 9 grams *Radix Paeoniae Rubra* and 9 grams *Radix Angelicae Sinensis.*

For cases with suppurative appendicitis, high fever, severe abdominal pain, guarding upon pressure or even touch, and distinct rebound pain, add 30 grams *Flos Lonicerae,* 30 grams *Fructus Forsythiae,* 30 grams *Herba Violae,* and 30 grams *Herba Taraxaci.*

For cases with noxious heat, high fever, and intolerance of cold, thirst, flushed cheeks and red eyes, severe abdominal pain with muscular tension, distinct rebound pain, and yellowish dry tongue coating, add 3 grams *Rhizoma Coptidis,* 9 grams *Radix Scutellariae,* 9 grams *Cortex Phellodendri,* and 9 grams *Fructus Gardeniae.*

For cases with severe pathogenic dampness, nausea and vomiting, thirst without desire to drink, abdominal distension, loose stools, and yellowish greasy and thick tongue coating, add 30 grams *Semen Coicis* and 30 grams *Semen Benincasae.*

For cases in the advanced stage with deficiency of both *qi* and blood, marked by lassitude, dizziness, pale tongue, and rapid and thready pulse, add 15 grams *Radix Codonopsis Pilosulae,* 15 grams *Radix Astragali seu Hedysari,* 9 grams *Radix Angelicae Sinensis,* and 15 grams *Radix Rehmannia.*

CHRONIC APPENDICITIS. Manifestations: Recurrent dull pain over the right lower abdomen, poor appetite, nausea, constipation, thin yellowish tongue coating, taut or rapid pulse.

Principle of treatment: Regulating vital energy and activating blood to disperse stasis.

Prescription: Powder for Cold Limbs, with Modifications.

Radix Bupleuri	6 grams
Fructus Aurantii Immaturus	9 "
Pericarpium Citri Reticulutae Viride	9 "
Radix Paeoniae Rubra	9 "
Radix Angelicae Sinensis	9 "
Semen Persicae	9 "
Caulis Sargentodoxae	30 "

Modifications include: For cases with constipation, add 9 grams *Radix et Rhizoma Rhei Praeparata.*

For cases with deficiency symptom-complex, add 15 grams *Radix Codonopsis Pilosulae.*

For cases with cold symptom-complex, add 9 grams *Radix Aconiti Praeparata.*

Other Common Methods of Treating Appendicitis

PROVEN RECIPES

Decoction for acute appendicitis:

Caulis Sargentodoxae	30 grams
Herba Taraxae	30 "
Radix et Rhizoma Rhei Praeparata	12 "
Cortex Magnoliae Officinalis	9 "

CASE HISTORY

Female, age 17, admitted on August 7, 1977.

History

The patient had had pain in the right lower abdomen for one day. Two days previously, she had had over ten purulent stools after overeating raw fruits. The diarrhea had been relieved by syntomycin.

Diagnosis and Treatment

Physical examination on the day of admission revealed muscular tension over the right lower abdomen, and tenderness at McBurney's point but no rebound pain. The psoas sign was positive. The patient's temperature was 38.6°C. White blood cell count was 12,100/mm^3, with 81% neutrophils. The patient had a red tongue with yellowish greasy coating and a rapid slippery pulse. The diagnosis was acute appendicitis, and according to traditional Chinese medicine damp-heat had stagnated in the intestine. The principle of treatment was to clear toxic heat with febrifugals and detoxicants and activate blood circulation and remove dampness through diuresis. The prescription was as follows:

Flos Lonicerae	30	grams
Fructus Forsythiae	15	"
Herba Taraxaci	30	"
Herba Violae	30	"
Herba Patriniae	30	"
Cortex Moutan Radicis	9	"
Radix et Rhizoma Rhei	9	"
Semen Benincasae	30	"
Radix Paeoniae Rubra	9	"
Radix Salviae Miltiorrhizae	9	"
Fructus Meliae Toosendan	12	"
Radix Aucklandiae	9	"
Radix Scutellariae	9	"
Semen Coicis	30	"
Radix Glycyrrhizae	6	"

The day following admission, after the first dose had been taken, the patient's fever subsided, and the pain was reduced; white blood cell count was 6,300/mm^3, with 74% neutrophils.

By the third day, there was only mild pain over the abdomen and at McBurney's point, and there was no rebound pain; the tongue was yellowish with a greasy coating, and the pulse was taut. The prescription was modified by omitting *Semen Benincasae* and adding:

Massa Fermentata Medicinalis	9	grams
Fructus Crataegi	9	"
Herba Agastachis	9	"
Pericarpium Citri Reticulatae	9	"

Three doses were given, after which all the symptoms and signs disappeared. The patient was discharged on August 13, 1977.

—From Zhao Shanghua, *Insights Into Traditional Chinese Surgery* (Shanxi People's Publishing House, 1982), pp. 116–17.

Decoction for appendicular abscess:

Caulis Sargentodoxae	60 grams
Herba Violae	30 "

Pills of Rhei and Eupolyphuga may be taken with this decoction.

ACUPUNCTURE TREATMENT.

General treatments for relieving pain. Main points: Appendicular point, between Zusanli (St 36) and Shangjuxu (St 37); Tianshu (St 25).
Alternative point: Neiguan (P 6).
Points according to manifestations:

Vomiting—Shangwan (Ren 13)
High fever—Quchi (Li 11), Xingjain (Liv 12), Hege (LI 14)

Reducing method is applied, followed by moxibustion on the point of rebound pain for about 5–15 minutes; one or two moxibustion treatments are administered daily. If symptoms and signs are not relieved, timely surgery should be undertaken.

THROMBOANGIITIS OBLITERANS

Thromboangiitis obliterans is a disease of the blood vessels of the extremities. It probably is of inflammatory nature, and it most commonly affects the lower extremities. Ischemia of the tissue and gangrene occur. In traditional Chinese medicine, the condition is known as "gangrene of the extremities."

Etiology

Thromboangiitis obliterans can result from emotional strain that lowers vital function of the spleen and kidney and thus impedes the flow of blood and vital energy. It also can result from prolonged affliction with pathogenic damp-cold, which hinders the normal circulation of blood in the lower extremities.

Essentials of Diagnosis and Treatment

Treatment is aimed at reinforcing vital energy and activating blood flow to remove obstruction. If there is a deficiency symptom-complex marked by abundant pathogenic cold, it is advisable initially to warm the channels and dispel cold from them. If there are symptoms of intense toxic heat, suggesting a deficiency symptom-complex complicated by an excess symptom-complex, it is advisable to remove toxic heat.

Treatment Based on Differentiation of Symptom-Complexes

DEFICIENCY OF VITAL ENERGY AND GATHERING OF PATHOGENIC COLD. Manifestations: Pain and cold sensation in the affected limb, pallid or dark red color of the limb, preference for warmth, muscle atrophy, limping after a period of walking, thin tongue coating, deep, slow, thready, and weak pulse.

Principle of treatment: Reinforcing vital energy and nourishing blood; warming the channels to remove obstruction from the vessels.

Prescription: Decoction for Restoring the Ability to Walk, with Modifications.

Radix Astragali	15	grams
Radix Codonopsis Pilosulae	15	"
Radix Angelicae Sinensis	30	"
Radix Salviae Miltiorrhizae	15	"
Ramulus Cinnamomi	6	"
Radix Aconiti Praeparata	6	"
Radix Achyranthis Bidentatae	9	"
Herba Dendrobii	9	"

Modifications include: For cases with prominent blood stasis and sharp pain, add 9 grams *Semen Persicae,* 6 grams *Resina Myrrhae,* and 6 grams *Resina Olibani* (olibanum).

CASE HISTORY

Male, age 27, first visit on June 20, 1979.

History

The patient had a four-year history of intermittent claudication (limping) of the right leg, following exposure to cold on an automobile drive on January 1, 1975. Initially his right foot had been swollen, painful, and purple; apparently it was frost-bitten. The patient had been admitted to several hospitals and was diagnosed as having Buerger's disease, or thromboangiitis obliterans. Treatment with western medicine proved ineffective.

Diagnosis and Treatment

Upon examination, the right leg was purple and cold to the touch; there was little hair on the leg, the toenails were pale or broken, and the skin at the toe tips was cracked. The right calf was slightly atrophied, and the pulse of the anterior tibial artery was absent. Rheography showed high tensity and low elasticity of the arteries in the right leg; there was 72% difference in the arterial flow amplitudes between the two legs. The patient's tongue was red with white coating, and his pulse was slow and choppy. Diagnosis according to traditional Chinese medicine was stagnation of *qi* and blood stasis accompanied by deficiency of vital energy and symptoms of cold. The principle of treatment was to activate blood circulation and clear the vessels by reinforcing the flow of vital energy with tonics. The prescription used was as follows:

Radix Salviae Miltiorrhizae	30 grams
Caulis Spatholobi	30 "
Flos Carthami	9 "
Radix Codonopsis Pilosulae	9 "
Radix Astragali	30 "
Rhizoma Atractylodis Macrocephalae	9 "
Radix Angelicae Sinensis	30 "
Radix Paeoniae Rubra	15 "
Radix Paeoniae Alba	15 "
Ramulus Cinnamomi	9 "
Squama Manitis (stir-baked)	9 "
Radix Glycyrrhizae	30 "

Also prescribed was local steaming with a decoction of red pepper and Chinese mugwort leaf:

Fructus Capsici (hot pepper)
Folium Artemisiae Argyi
Ramulus Cinnamomi
Radix Ledebouriellae
Herba Speranskia
Ramulus Sophorae (Chinese scholartree twig)
Bulbus Allii (garlic)
Radix Angelicae Sinensis
Lignum Sappan (sappan caesalpinia)
Flos Carthami
Ramulus Mori
Radix Aconiti

The dose and processing method of this prescription are an official trade secret. The prescription's actions are warming the channels and dispelling cold, activating blood circulation, and expelling pathogenic wind. The indication for use is gangrene of the fingers or toes due to stagnation of pathogenic cold in the channels.

After 9 doses of the above prescriptions, the patient was able to walk with ease. After 21 doses there was marked improvement, with the skin of the right leg assuming a healthy appearance. The pain and cold sensation had disappeared, there was new nail growth, and the patient was walking freely.

—From Zhao Shanghua, *Insights Into Traditional Chinese Surgery* (Shanxi People's Publishing House, 1982), pp. 203–5.

DEFICIENCY OF VITAL ENERGY AND BLOOD. Manifestations: Mild pain, scaling, necrosis, and pallid granulation tissue with slow healing, all of the affected leg; livid complexion, pale and swollen tongue with thin coating, thready pulse.

Principle of treatment: Reinforcing vital energy and nourishing blood.

Prescription: Ginseng Nutrition Decoction, with Modifications.

Radix Ginseng (simmered separately)	6 grams	
Poria	9	"
Rhizoma Atractylodis Macrocephalae Praeparata	9	"
Radix Glycyrrhizae Praeparata	6	"
Radix Angelicae Sinensis	9	"
Radix Rehmannia Praeparata	15	"
Radix Paeoniae Alba	9	"
Pericarpium Citri Reticulatae	9	"
Radix Astragali	15	"
Cortex Cinnamomi	3	"
Radix Polygalae	9	"
Fructus Schisandrae	6	"
Rhizoma Zingiberis Recens	3 pieces	
Fructus Ziziphi Jujubae	4	"

GATHERING AND BREWING OF TOXIC HEAT. Manifestations: Burning sensation and swelling of the limb, deep ulcer, necrosis, and sharp pain of the affected leg; fever, thirst, concentrated urine, reddened tongue with thin yellow coating, taut and rapid pulse.

Principle of treatment: Removing toxic heat; reinforcing vital energy to activate blood circulation.

Prescription: Decoction of Four Miraculous Herbs for Relief of Disorders, with Modifications.

Flos Lonicerae	30	grams
Herba Violae	15	"
Herba Taraxaci	15	"
Cortex Phellodendri	9	"
Radix Scrophulariae	15	"
Radix Glycyrrhizae	6	"
Radix Astragali	15	"
Radix Angelicae Sinensis	30	"
Radix Salviae Miltiorrhizae	15	"
Radix Achyranthis Bidentatae	9	"
Herba Dendrobii	9	"

ACUPUNCTURE TREATMENT

Main points: Yanglingquan (GB 34), Yinlingquan (Sp 9), Sanyinjiao (Sp 6), Chengshan (UB 57), Juegu (GB 39).

One treatment is given every day or every other day; needles are retained for 15 to 20 minutes. The points may be selected in turn.

BURNS

This category includes scalds and injuries resulting from exposure to fire or extreme heat.

Etiology

Burns by such agents as fire and heat may lead to decay of the skin and flesh. Extensive burns can injure vital energy, blood and body fluid, and internal organs. Serious complications include inward attack of toxic heat, which may invade the cardiac and nervous systems, depletion of body fluid, derangement of vital essence, and collapse due to depletion of vital energy and essence.

Essentials of Diagnosis and Treatment

In treating burns, drugs are given orally to help replenish vital essence and enrich body fluid, remove toxic heat, restore vital function from collapse, and/or strengthen body resistance and speed up healing. Drugs cool in nature are applied externally to help eliminate toxic heat. In emergency cases, burns must be treated by both traditional and modern medicine.

Treatment Based on Differentiation of Symptom-Complexes

BURNS CAUSED BY EXPOSURE TO FIRE AND RESULTING IN INJURY OF VITAL ESSENCE (usually moderate burns). Manifestations: Fever, restlessness, thirst, dry mouth, concentrated urine, constipation, yellow and reddened tongue with or without coating, taut, rapid or thready, rapid pulse.

Principle of treatment: Removing toxic heat and replenishing vital essence to enrich body fluid.

Prescription: Decoction of Five Detoxicants in Combination with Decoction for Enriching the Body Fluid, with Modifications.

Flos Lonicerae	30	grams
Herba Violae	30	"
Radix Rehmannia	30	"
Radix Scrophulariae	12	"
Fructus Forsythiae	15	"
Herba Dendrobii	9	"
Radix Ophiopogonis	9	"
Radix Glycyrrhizae	6	"
Rhizoma Anemarrhenae	9	"
Radix Trichosanthis (snakegourd root)	9	"

COLLAPSE DUE TO DEPLETION OF VITAL ESSENCE AND VITAL ENERGY (usually seen in the shock stage of burns). Manifestations: Thirst, restlessness, oliguria or anuria, lassitude, pallor, shortness of breath, cold limbs, cold sweats, fall in blood pressure and body temperature, pale dry tongue, empty, weak or fine, thready, rapid pulse.

Principle of treatment: Replenishing vital essence and reinforcing vital energy to restore vital function from collapse.

Prescription: Decoction for Invigorating Pulse-Beat in Combination with Decoction of Ginseng and Aconiti.

Radix Rehmannia	30	grams
Radix Ophiopogonis	9	"
Radix Aconiti Praeparata	6	"
Radix Ginseng American (simmered separately)	6	"
Radix Codonopsis Pilosulae	12	"
Fructus Schisandrae	9	"

INWARD ATTACK OF TOXIC HEAT (usually found in septicemia due to burns). Manifestations: High fever, restlessness, shortness of breath, abdominal distension, oliguria, delirium, convulsions, bleeding of the dermis, increased fluid exudation into the wound, local edema, reddened tongue with yellow coating, overflowing, rapid or thready pulse.

Principle of treatment: Removing toxic heat.

Prescription: Decoction of Five Detoxicants in Combination with Detoxicant Decoction of Coptidis, with Modifications.

Flos Lonicerae	30	grams
Fructus Forsythiae	15	"
Herba Violae	30	"
Flos Chrysanthemi Indici	12	"
Herba Taraxaci	30	"
Cortex Moutan Radicis	6	"
Gypsum Fibrosum (decocted first)	30	"
Radix Scutellariae	9	"
Fructus Gardeniae	9	"
Rhizoma Coptidis	3	"

DEFICIENCIES OF BOTH VITAL ENERGY AND BLOOD (usually found in the convalescent stage). Manifestations: Subsidence of fever, healing by granulation, emaciation, lassitude, livid complexion, pale tongue, weak, thready pulse.

Principle of treatment: Reinforcing vital energy and nourishing blood.

Prescription: Universal Tonic Decoction with Ten Ingredients, with Modifications.

Radix Codonopsis Pilosulae	9 grams
Radix Astragali	9 "
Rhizoma Atractylodis Macrocephalae	9 "
Radix Angelicae Sinensis	9 "
Radix Paeoniae Alba	9 "
Radix Rehmanni Praeparata	18 "
Fructus Oryzae Germinatus (rice sprout)	12 "
Pericarpium Citri Reticulatae	4.5 "
Radix Glycyrrhizae Praeparata	6 "

Other Common Methods of Treating Burns

PROVEN RECIPES FOR EXTERNAL APPLICATION

Ointment prepared and applied to second degree burns:

Burn Oleol:	
Radix Sanguisorbae	5 grams
Rhizoma Polygoni Cuspidati (giant knotweed)	5 "
Pericarpium Granati	5 "
Radix Arnebiae seu Lithospermi	5 "
Borneolum	2–4 "
Arachis oleum (vegetable oil)	100 ml

Extract used for early treatment of burns:

Burn Extract:	
Radix Rehmannia	60 grams
Radix Sanguisorbae	60 "
Cortex Phellodondri	60 "
Rhizoma Coptidis	45 "
Radix Arnebiae sue Lithospermi	15 "
Radix et Rhizoma Rhei	30 "
Rhizoma Corydalis	30 "
Sesame oil	900 ml

Powder prepared and applied with concentrated tea or sesame oil to first- or second-degree burns: *Rhizoma Polygoni Cuspidati* (giant knotweed).

URTICARIA

This condition is a vascular reaction of the skin. It is marked by the sudden transient appearance of smooth, slightly elevated patches that are redder or paler than the surrounding skin and often are accompanied by severe itching. The eruption may subside rapidly, leaving no signs.

Etiology

Urticaria is due to exogenous affliction by pathogenic wind-cold or wind-heat, causing impeded flow of vital energy of the *ying* and *wei* systems. Certain foods (such as fish, shrimp, and crab) and intestinal parasitosis sometimes produce urticaria.

Essentials of Diagnosis and Treatment

It is important to distinguish urticaria from other eruptions; this can easily be done by inspection. Treatment is aimed at dispersing wind and removing toxic heat and cold.

Treatment Based on Differentiation of Symptom-Complexes.

COLLECTION OF PATHOGENIC WIND-HEAT. Manifestations: Red eruption, burning sensation, itching, restlessness, fever, thin yellow tongue coating, floating, rapid pulse.

Principle of treatment: Dispersing wind and removing pathogenic heat.

Prescription: Decoction for Dispersing Pathogenic Wind, with Modifications.

Herba Schizonepetae	6	grams
Radix Ledebouriellae	6	"
Fructus Arctii	6	"
Periostracum Cicadae	6	"
Radix Rehmannia	15	"

Gypsum Fibrosum (decocted first)	30 grams
Cortex Moutan Radicis	9 "
Radix Paeoniae Rubra	9 "
Radix Angelicae Sinensis	9 "

INVASION OF THE SKIN BY PATHOGENIC WIND-COLD (usually seen following an attack of wind-cold). Manifestations: Light red or pallid eruption, thin white tongue coating, floating, tight pulse.

Principle of treatment: Dispersing wind-cold; regulating the *ying* and *wei* systems.

Prescription: Decoction of Ramulus Cinnamomi, with Modifications.

Ramulus Cinnamomi	4.5 grams
Herba Ephedrae	3 "
Folium Perillae	9 "
Herba Schizonepetae	6 "
Radix Ledebouriellae	6 "
Radix Paeoniae Alba	9 "
Rhizoma Zingeberis Recens	6 "

PATHOGENIC DAMP-HEAT IN THE INTESTINES AND STOMACH. Manifestations: Patches of eruption, epigastric pain upon attack of urticaria, lassitude, anorexia, constipation or diarrhea, slimy yellow tongue coating, slippery and rapid pulse.

Principle of treatment: Clearing away pathogenic damp-heat; dispersing pathogenic wind.

Prescription: Decoction of Ledebouriellae for Dispersing Superficial Wind.

Herba Schizonepetae	6 grams
Radix Ledebouriellae	6 "
Rhizoma Atractylodis	12 "
Radix et Rhizoma Rhei Praeparata	9 "
Fructus Gardeniae Praeparata	9 "
Radix Sophorae Flavescentis	12 "
Cortex Poria	12 "
Pulvis Talcum	15 "
Radix Glycyrrhizae	3 "

Modifications include: For cases with abdominal pain, suggesting intestinal parasites, add 12 grams *Fructus Mume,* 9 grams *Fructus Quisqualis,* and 9 grams *Semen Arecae.*

DEFICIENCY OF VITAL ENERGY AND LOWERED FUNCTIONING OF THE *wei* SYSTEM. Manifestations: Repeated patches of pallid eruption occurring upon exertion or affection by wind-cold; pallor, pale tongue coating, thready, fine pulse.

Principle of treatment: Reinforcing vital energy and strengthening superficial resistance to disperse wind.

Prescription: Jade Screen Decoction, with Modifications.

Radix Astragali	12 grams
Semen Coicis	12 "
Rhizoma Atractylodis Macrocephalae	9 "
Radix Ledebouriellae	9 "
Radix Codonopsis Pilosulae	9 "
Ramulus Cinnamomi	6 "
Poria	9 "
Pericarpium Citri Reticulatae	6 "
Fructus Ziziphi Jujubae	4 pieces

PRESENCE OF PATHOGENIC WIND DUE TO DEFICIENCY OF BLOOD. Manifestations: Repeated light red patches of eruption during menstrual periods and pregnancy, irregularities of menstruation, reddened tongue tip with thin white coating, thready and rapid pulse.

Principle of treatment: Nourishing blood to disperse wind.

Prescription: Angelicae Decoction, with Modifications.

Radix Angelicae Sinensis	9 grams
Herba Schizonepetae	6 "
Rhizoma Ligustici Chuanxiong	6 "
Radix Paeoniae Alba	9 "
Radix Rehmannia Praeparata	15 "
Radix Polygoni Multiflori	15 "
Radix Ledebouriellae	6 "
Radix Astragali	9 "
Fructus Tribuli	12 "
Radix Glycyrrhizae	3 "

Modifications include: For obstinate chronic urticaria, add 9 grams *Bombyx Batryticatus,* 9 grams *Lumbricus,* 6 grams *Scorpio,* and 9 grams Zaocys (black snake).

Other Common Methods of Treating Urticaria

PROVEN RECIPES

Decoction given for urticaria due to deficiency of blood:

Lumbricus	9 grams
Radix Glycyrrhizae	9 "

Decoction given for urticaria due to deficiency of blood: *Folium Kaki* (persimmon leaf), 60 grams.

Decoction given for collection of pathogenic wind-heat:

Herba Spirodelae (duckweed)	30 grams
Fructus Kochiae	30 "
Periostracum Cicadae	9 "

ACUPUNCTURE TREATMENT

Main points: Dazhui (Du 14), Xuehai (Sp 10), Quchi (LI 11), Sanyinjiao (Sp 6); Dachangshu (UB 15) for chronic urticaria.

Points according to manifestations:

Urticaria precipitated by food and accompanied by diarrhea—Zusanli (St 36)
Sensation of oppression in the chest and shortness of breath—Hegu (LI 4), Neiguan (P 6)

EAR-ACUPUNCTURE THERAPY. Lung, Adrenal, Ear-Shenmen, Endocrine.

One or two points are selected for each treatment. Needles are retained for 15 minutes or embedded for three to five days.

MENIERE'S DISEASE

Meniere's disease is a disorder characterized by recurrent prostrating vertigo, tinnitus, and hearing loss. The attacks of vertigo appear suddenly and are associated with nausea and vomiting. This disorder is known as "vertigo" in traditional Chinese medicine.

Etiology

"The liver is an organ involved in all wind syndromes," the symptoms of which are vertigo, tremor, and sometimes convulsions. Deficiency symptom-complexes may be due to deficiency of vital essence of the liver and kidney or deficiency of liver blood. Excess symptom-complexes may be caused by exuberance of vital function of the liver or flaring up of liver fire. Also, traditional Chinese medicine views vertigo as usually due to phlegm; thus patients with Meniere's disease often have an overabundance of phlegm.

Essentials of Diagnosis and Treatment

Symptom-complexes solely of deficiency or excess are not commonly seen. Usually deficiency symptom-complexes complicated by symptoms of excessiveness predominate. This should be kept in mind when diagnosing Meniere's disease.

Treatment should resolve excessiveness through dispelling pathogenic factors, while also replenishing deficiency. This may be accomplished by using blood tonics or tonics for deficiency of vital essence of both the liver and kidney. The same prescription should also have the action of subduing hyperfunction of the liver and eliminating wind, while also dispelling phlegm. For exuberance of liver fire, treatment should remove intense fire from the liver by purgation.

Treatment Based on Differentiation of Symptom-Complexes

EXUBERANCE OF VITAL FUNCTION OF THE LIVER RESULTING IN STIRRING UP OF WIND. Manifestations: Vertigo and tinnitus that are aggravated by overwork or anger, vomiting, bitter taste in the mouth, thirst, excessive dreaming during sleep, irritability, fullness or pressure in the ear, red tongue, taut thready or rapid pulse.

Principle of treatment: Subduing hyperfunction of the liver and dispelling wind; after the vertigo is alleviated the curative effect is consolidated by reinforcing vital essence through nourishing the liver and kidney.

Prescription: Decoction of Gastrodia and Uncariae Cum Uncis, with Modifications.

Rhizoma Gastrodiae	9	grams
Ramulus Uncariae cum Uncis	12	"
Poria (stirred with cinnabaris)	12	"
Ramulus Loranthi	12	"
Cortex Eucommiae	12	"
Radix Achyranthis Bidentatae	9	"
Herba Leonuri	12	"
Caulis Polygoni Multiflori	12	"
Radix Scutellariae	9	"
Fructus Gardeniae	6	"
Concha Haliotidis (decocted first)	15	"

PROFUSE ENDOGENOUS PHLEGM-DAMPNESS. Manifestations: Vertigo and tinnitus, nausea and vomiting, sensation of oppression in the chest, palpitation, somnolence, poor appetite, profuse spitting of phlegm in the morning, greasy tongue coating, slippery pulse.

Principle of treatment: Resolving dampness and dispelling phlegm.

Prescription: Decoction of Orange Peel and Pinellia, with Modifications.

Pericarpium Citri Reticulatae	9	grams
Rhizoma Pinelliae	9	"
Poria	12	"
Rhizoma Alismatis	9	"
Pulvis Talci (wrapped)	15	"
Herba Agastachis	9	"
Herba Eupatorii	9	"
Rhizoma Atractylodis	9	"
Radix Glycyrrhizae	6	"

Modifications include: For cases with yellowish greasy tongue coating, dry and bitter taste in the mouth, concentrated urine, restlessness, and constipation, add 9 grams *Caulis Bumbusae in Taeniam,* 9 grams *Fructus Aurantii Immaturus,* 6 grams *Lumbricus,* 2 grams *Concha Margaritifera Usta,* and 6 grams *Rhizoma Acori Graminei.*

For cases with white tongue coating, loose stools, and absence of thirst, add 9 grams *Rhizoma Gastrodiae* and 9 grams *Rhizoma Atractylodis Macrocephalae.*

WIND SYMPTOM-COMPLEX DUE TO DEFICIENCY OF BLOOD. Manifestations: Protracted condition characterized by recurrent spells of vertigo or rotary vertigo, tinnitus and deafness, pale or sallow complexion, palpitation, lassitude, forgetfulness, insomnia, poor appetite, flat taste in the mouth, thin tongue coating, feeble and thready pulse.

Principle of treatment: Nourishing blood to subdue wind.

Prescription: Decoction of Schisandrae, with Modifications.

Fructus Schisandrae	9	grams
Semen Ziziphi Spinosae (stir-baked)	15	"
Rhizoma Dioscorea	9	"
Radix Angelicae Sinensis	9	"
Arillus Longan	15	"

Modifications include: For cases with severe deficiency of blood, administer Decoction of Eight Precious Ingredients to nourish *qi* and blood; and to subdue wind add 6 grams *Lumbricus,* 6 grams *Scorpio,* and 15 grams *Concha Magaritifera Usta* (decocted first).

For cases with intense heat in the liver, marked by insomnia, concentrated urine, constipation, red tongue with yellowish coating, and taut pulse, Decoction of Gentian for Purging the Liver may be given along with 6 grams *Lumbricus.*

Other Common Methods of Treating Meniere's Disease

PROVEN RECIPES

Decoction administered daily:

Rhizoma Gastrodiae	18	grams
Ramulus Uncariae cum Uncis	30	"

Preparation taken before meals: Meat of 3 walnuts and 1 water chestnut, crushed and cooked together.

ACUPUNCTURE TREATMENT

Main points: Fengchi (GB 20), Hegu (LI 4), Sanyinjiao (Sp 6), Zusanli (St 36), Neiguan (P 6), Taichong (Liv 3).

Uniform reinforcing-reducing method is applied. All points are used during each treatment.

EAR-ACUPUNCTURE THERAPY. Subcortex, Ear-Shenmen, Heart region.

One or two points are selected for each treatment. Needles are retained 20–30 minutes.

A FINAL NOTE

Throughout this book, the Chinese principle that the body is an integrated whole has been emphasized. The current volume has discussed how, on the basis of this principle, traditional Chinese medicine treats diseases. Other important principles reflected in this volume include the following: As a disease progresses through its various stages, treatment is modified according to the symptom-complex present at the time. Also, because each human body is in a unique dynamic equilibrium with its environment, each individual reacts differently during the course of a disease; therefore, each case must be analyzed and treated individually.

Traditional Chinese medicine has developed several kinds of therapy. Among them are acupuncture, *qi gong* (breathing exercises), and remedial massage. But by far, the primary mode of treatment in China today, as it has been since ancient times, is herbs. This, then, has been the main emphasis of this book. Indeed, in this volume, numerous herbs and herbal prescriptions have been presented. The existence of so many reflects, in part, both the principles mentioned in the previous paragraph and the long history of traditional Chinese medicine.

Names of Herbs

Actinolitum (actinolite, 陽起石)
Aloë (aloe, 蘆薈)
Alumen (alum, 明礬)
Ancistrodon Acutus (long-noded pit viper, 白花蛇)
Arillus Longan (longan aril, 龍眼肉)
Arisaemacum Bilis (arisaema with bile, 膽南星)
Aspongopus (stink-bug, 九香蟲)
Benzoinum (benzoin, 安息香)
Bombyx Batryticatus (batryticated silkworm, 僵蠶)
Borneolum (borneol, 冰片)
Bulbus Allii (garlic, 蒜瓣)
Bulbus Allii Macrostemi (onion bulb, 薤白)
Bulbus Cremastrae (edible tulip bulb, 山慈菇)
Bulbus Fritillariae (fritillary bulb, 貝母)
Bulbus Fritillariae Cirrhosae (tendril leaved fritillary bulb, 川貝母)
Bulbus Fritillariae Thunbergii (fritillary bulb, 浙貝母)
Bulbus Lilii (lily bulb, 百合)
Cacumen Biotae (oriental arbovitae twig, 側柏葉)
Calcitum (calcite, 方解石)
Calculus Bovis (ox-gallstone, 牛黃)
Calculus Pseudosciaena Encephalon (yellow croaker ear stone, 魚腦石)
Calomelas (calomel, 輕粉)
Calyx Kaki (persimmon calyx and receptacle, 柿蒂)

Carapax Trionycis (turtle shell, 鱉甲)
Caulis Akebiae (fiveleaf akebia stem, 木通)
Caulis Allii Fistulosum (green onion stalk, 生蔥)
Caulis Bambusae in Taenis (bamboo shavings, 竹茹)
Caulis Clematidis Armandii (Sichuan clematis stem, 川木通)
Caulis Phragmitis (common reed rhizome, 葦莖)
Caulis Polygoni Multiflori (vine of muliflower knotweed, 夜交藤)
Caulis Sargentodoxae (sargentgloryvine stem, 紅藤)
Caulis Spatholobi (spatholobus stem, 鷄血藤)
Caulis Trachelospermi (Chinese starjasmine stem, 絡石藤)
Chloriteschist (青礞石)
Cinnabaris (cinnabar, 朱砂)
Colla Corii Asini (donkey-hide gelatin, 阿膠)
Colla Cornus Cervi (deer horn glue, 鹿角膠)
Colla Plastri Testudinis (glue of tortoise plastron, 龜板膠)
Concha Haliotidis (sea-ear shell, 石決明)
Concha Margaritifera Usta (pearl shell, 珍珠母)
Concha Meretricis (clam shell, 海蛤殼)
Concha Ostreae (oyster shell, 牡犡)
Concretio Silicea Bambusae (tabasheer, 天竺黃)
Cordyceps (Chinese caterpillar fungus, 冬蟲夏草)
Cornu Antelopis (antelope horn, 羚羊角)
Cornu Bubali (buffalo horn, 水牛角)
Cornu Cervi Degelatinatum (deglued antler powder, 鹿角霜)
Cornu Cervi Pantotrichum (pilose antler, 鹿茸)
Cornu Rhinoceri (rhinoceros horn, 犀角)
Cortex Acanthopanacis Radicis (acanthopanax bark, 五加皮)
Cortex Ailanthi (heaven tree bark, 椿皮)
Cortex Albiziae (silktree bark, 合歡皮)
Cortex Cinnamomi (Chinese cassia tree bark, 肉桂)
Cortex Dictamni Radicis (ditlany root-bark, 白鮮皮)
Cortex Eucommiae (eucommia bark, 杜仲)
Cortex Fraxini (ash bark, 秦皮)
Cortex Lycii Radicis (wolfberry root-bark, 地骨皮)
Cortex Magnoliae Officinalis (official magnolia bark, 厚樸)
Cortex Meliae (Chinaberry bark, 苦楝皮)
Cortex Mori Radicis (mulberry root-bark, 桑白皮)
Cortex Moutan Radicis (peony root-bark, 牡丹皮)
Cortex Phellodendri (corktree bark, 黃柏)
Cortex Poria (tuckahoe bark, 茯苓皮)
Crinis Carbonisatus (burnt hair, 血餘炭)
Dens Draconis (dragon's teeth, 龍齒)

Dryobalanops Aromatica (common borneo camphor, 龍腦)

Endothelium Corneum Gigeriae Galli (chicken gizzard membrane, 鷄內金)

Eupolyphaga seu Steleophaga (ground beetle, 土鱉蟲)

Excrementum Bombycis (silkworm droppings, 蠶沙)

Exocarpium Benicasae (wax gourd peel, 冬瓜皮)

Exocarpium Citri Grandis (tangerine peel, 橘紅)

Exocarpium Citrulli (watermelon peel, 西瓜皮)

Exocarpium Zingiberis (ginger peel, 薑皮)

Faeces Trogopterorum (flying squirrel feces, 五靈脂)

Flos Albiziae (silktree flower, 合歡花)

Flos Buddleiae (pale butterflybush flower, 密蒙花)

Flos Carthami (safflower, 紅花)

Flos Caryophylli (clove flower, 丁香)

Flos Celosiae Cristatae (common cockscomb flower, 鷄冠花)

Flos Chrysanthemi (chrysanthemum flower, 菊花)

Flos Chrysanthemi Indici (mother chrysanthemum, 野菊花)

Flos Daturae Stramonii (jamestown weed flower, 蔓陀羅花)

Flos Dolichoris (flower of hyacinth dolichos, 扁豆花)

Flos Farfarae (common colsfoot flower, 欵冬花)

Flos Genkwa (lilac daphne flower, 芫花)

Flos Inulae (British inula flower, 旋復花)

Flos Lonicerae (honeysuckle flower, 金銀花)

Flos Magnoliae (magnolia flower, 辛夷花)

Flos Sophorae (Chinese scholartree flower, 槐花)

Flos Vinca (vinca rosea, 長春花)

Fluoritum (fluorite, 紫石英)

Folium Artemisiae Argyi (Chinese mugwort leaf, 艾葉)

Folium Clerodendri Trichotomi (harlequin glorybower leaf, 臭梧桐葉)

Folium Eriobotryae (loquat leaf, 枇杷葉)

Folium Ginkgo (gingko leaf, 白菓葉)

Folium Ilex (broad leaf holly, 苦丁茶)

Folium Isatidis (Dyer's Woad leaf, 大青葉)

Folium Kaki (persimmon leaf, 柿葉)

Folium Mori (white mulberry leaf, 桑葉)

Folium Nelumbinis (lotus leaf, 荷葉)

Folium Perillae (purple perilla leaf, 紫蘇葉)

Folium Pyrrosiae (pyrrosia leaf, 石葦)

Folium Sennae (senna leaf, 番瀉葉)

Folium seu Flos Hibisci (cottonrose hibiscus, 芙蓉葉或花)

Fructus Alpiniae Oxyphyllae (galangal fruit, 益智仁)

Fructus Amomi (amomum fruit, 砂仁)

Fructus Amomi Tsaoko (amomum tsaoko, 草果)
Fructus Arctii (great burdock achene, 牛蒡子)
Fructus Aristolochiae (birthwort fruit, 馬兜鈴)
Fructus Aurantii Immaturus (immature citron, 枳實)
Fructus Aurantii (bitter orange, 枳殼)
Fructus Bruceae (Java brucea fruit, 鴉膽子)
Fructus Cannabis (hemp seed, 火麻仁)
Fructus Capsici (hot pepper, 川椒)
Fructus Chaenomelis (Chinese flowering quince, 木瓜)
Fructus Chebulae (chebula fruit, 訶子)
Fructus Citri Sarcodactylis (citron, 佛手)
Fructus Cnidii (cnidium fruit, 蛇床子)
Fructus Corni (dogwood fruit, 山茱萸)
Fructus Crataegi (hawthorn fruit, 山楂)
Fructus Crotonis (croton fruit, 巴豆)
Fructus et Radix Camptotheca Acuminata (camptotheca acuminata, 喜樹)
Fructus Evodiae (evodia fruit, 吳茱萸)
Fructus Foeniculi (common fennel fruit, 小茴香)
Fructus Forsythiae (weeping forsythia fruit, 連翹)
Fructus Gardeniae (capejasmine fruit, 梔子)
Fructus Hordei Germinatus (malt, 麥芽)
Fructus Kochiae (broom cypress fruit, 地膚子)
Fructus Leonuri (motherwort fruit, 茺蔚子)
Fructus Ligustri Lucidi (glossy privet fruit, 女貞子)
Fructus Lycii (Chinese wolfberry fruit, 枸杞子)
Fructus Meliae Toosendan (Sichuan Chinaberry, 川楝子)
Fructus Mume (dark plum, 烏梅)
Fructus Oryzae Germinatus (rice sprout, 穀芽)
Fructus Perillae (purple perilla fruit, 紫蘇子)
Fructus Piperis Longi (long pepper fruit, 蓽拔)
Fructus Psoraleae (malaytea scurfpea fruit, 補骨脂)
Fructus Quisqualis (rangoon creeper fruit, 使君子)
Fructus Rosae Laevigatae (cherokee rose fruit, 金櫻子)
Fructus Rubi (red raspberry, 覆盆子)
Fructus Schisandrae (Chinese magnoliavine fruit, 五味子)
Fructus Tribuli (白蒺藜)
Fructus Trichosanthis (Mongolian snakegourd fruit, 瓜蔞)
Fructus Tritici (wheat, 小麥)
Fructus Tritici Levis (blighted wheat, 浮小麥)
Fructus Amomi Tsaoko (amomum tsao-ko fruit, 草菓)
Fructus Ulmus Macrocarpa (蕪荑)
Fructus Vitex (vitex fruit, 蔓荊子)

Fructus Ziziphi Jujubae (Chinese date, 大棗)
Galla Chinensis (Chinese gall, 五倍子)
Ganoderma Lucidum seu Japonicum (lucid ganoderma, 靈芝)
Gecko (gecko, 蛤蚧)
Glutinous Millei (cooked millet, 黃米飯)
Gypsum Fibrosum (gypsum, 石膏)
Halloysitum Rubrum (red kaoline, 赤石脂)
Herba Agastachis (wrinkled gianthyssop, 藿香)
Herba Agrimoniae (hairyvein agrimony, 仙鶴草)
Herba Ajugae Decumbens (bugle, 白毛夏枯草)
Herba Andrographitis (fresh creat, 穿心蓮)
Herba Apium Graveolens (celery, 旱芹菜)
Herba Artemisia Anomalas (劉寄奴)
Herba Artemisiae Chinghao (sweet wormwood, 青蒿)
Herba Artemisiae Scopariae (oriental wormwood, 茵陳)
Herba Asari (wildginger, 細辛)
Herba Cephalanoploris (field thistle, 小薊)
Herba Cistanchis (saline cistanche, 肉蓯蓉)
Herba Commelinae (dayflower herb, 鴨跖草)
Herba Crotalariae (crotalaria, 農吉利)
Herba Cynomorii (Chinese cynomorium, 鎖陽)
Herba Dendrobii (noble dendrobium, 石斛)
Herba Dianthi (fringed pink, 瞿麥)
Herba Ecliptae (eclipta, 旱蓮草)
Herba Elsholtziae seu Moslae (Chinese mosla, 香薷)
Herba Ephedrae (Chinese epedra, 麻黃)
Herba Epimedii (epimedium, 仙靈脾, 淫羊藿)
Herba Eupatorii (eupatorium, 佩蘭)
Herba Houttuyniae (cordate houttuynia, 魚腥草)
Herba Leonuri (motherwort, 益母草)
Herba Lophatheri (bamboo leaf, 淡竹葉)
Herba Lycopi (bugleweed, 澤蘭)
Herba Lysimachiae (loosestrife, 金錢草)
Herba Menthae (peppermint, 薄荷)
Herba Oldenlandiae (oldenlandia, 白花蛇舌草)
Herba Opuntia Dillenii (cactus, 仙人掌)
Herba Patriniae (patrinia, 敗醬草)
Herba Polygoni Avicularis (common knot-grass, 萹蓄)
Herba Portulacae (purslane, 馬齒莧)
Herba Schizonepetae (shizonepeta, 荊芥)
Herba Scutellariae Barbatae (sun-plant, 半枝蓮)
Herba seu Radix Cirsii Japonici (thistle, 大薊)

Herba Siegesbeckieae (common St. Paulswort, 豨薟草)

Herba Speranskiae (透骨草)

Herba Spirodelae (common duckweed, 浮萍)

Herba Taraxaci (dandelion herb, 蒲公英)

Herba Verbenae (European verbena, 馬鞭草)

Herba Violae (Chinese violet, 紫花地丁)

Herba Xanthii (cocklebur, 蒼耳草)

Hippocampus (sea horse, 海馬)

Hirudo (leech, 水蛭)

Indigo Naturalis (natural indigo, 青黛)

Lasiosphaera seu Calvatia (puff-ball, 馬勃)

Lignum Pini Poriaferum (the core of poria, 茯神)

Lignum Aquilariae Resinatum (eaglewood, 沉香)

Lignum Dalbergiae Odoriferae (dalbergia wood, 降香)

Lignum Santali (sandal wood, 檀香)

Lignum Sappan (sappan caesalpinia, 蘇木)

Limonitum (limonite, 禹餘糧)

Lithargyrum (litharge, 密陀僧)

Lumbricus (earthworm, 地龍)

Magnetitum (magnetite, 磁石)

Malt extract (飴糖)

Maltose (麥芽糖)

Margarita (pearl, 珍珠)

Massa Fermentata Medicinalis (medicated leaven, 神麴)

Medulla Tetrapanacis (stem pith of the rice-paper plant, 通草)

Mel (honey, 蜂蜜)

Moschus (musk, 麝香)

Mylabris (blister beetle, 斑蝥)

Natrii Sulfas (sodium sulfate, 芒硝)

Natrii Sulfas Exsiccatus (compound of Glauber's-salf and licorice, 玄明粉)

Nidus Vespae (cells in a honeycomb, 露蜂房)

Nodus Nelumbinis Rhizomatis (lotus rhizome, 藕節)

Ochra (red ochre, 代赭石)

Olium Stryrax (oil of styrax, 蘇合香油)

Omphalia lapidescens (stone-like omphalia, 雷丸)

Oötheca Mantidis (ovum of mantis, 桑螵蛸)

Os Draconis (dragon's bone, 龍骨)

Os Sepiae (cuttlefish bone, 烏賊骨, 海螵蛸)

Os Tigris (tiger bone, 虎骨)

Pericarpium Arecae (shell of areca nut, 大腹皮)

Pericarpium Citri Reticulatae (dried orange peel, 陳皮)

Pericarpium Citri Reticulatae Viride (dried green orange peel, 青皮)

Pericarpium Dolichoris Albae (hyacinth dolichos peel, 扁豆衣)

Pericarpium Granati (pomegranate bark, 石榴皮)

Pericarpium Papaveris (poppy shell, 罌粟殼)

Pericarpium Trichosanthis (peel of Mongolian snakegourd, 瓜蔞皮)

Pericarpium Zanthoxyli (peppertree pricklyash, 花椒)

Periostracum Cicadae (cicada slough, 蟬蛻)

Petiolus Nelumbinis (lotus petiole, 荷梗)

Petiolus Trachycarpi Carbonisatus (burnt petiole of windmill-palm, 棕櫚炭)

Placenta Hominis (dried human placenta, 紫河車)

Plastrum Testudinis (tortoise plastron, 龜板)

Plumula Nelumbinis (lotus plumule, 蓮子心)

Pollen Typhae (cattail pollen, 蒲黃)

Polyporus Umbellatus (umbellate pore fungus, 豬苓)

Poria (tuckahoe, 茯苓)

Pulvis Alumen (alum, 枯礬末)

Pulvis Bubali (buffalo horn powder, 水牛角粉)

Pulvis Cinnabaris (cinnabar powder, 朱砂粉)

Pulvis Concha Meretricis (concha powder, 海蛤粉)

Pulvis Corium Erinacei (hedgehog skin powder, 刺猬皮粉)

Pulvis Cornu Antelopis (antelope horn powder, 羚羊角粉)

Pulvis Cornu Cervi Pantotrichum (pilose antler, 鹿茸粉)

Pulvis Eupolyphaga seu Steleophage (土鱉蟲粉)

Pulvis Notoginseng (pseudo-ginseng powder, 三七粉)

Pulvis Placenta Hominis (human placenta powder, 胎盤粉)

Pulvis Receptaculum Nelumbinis Carbonisatus (burnt lotus seedpod, 蓮蓬炭粉)

Pulvis Rhinocori (rhinoceros horn powder, 犀角粉)

Pumex (pumice, 海浮石)

Radix Achyranthis Bidentatae (bidentate achyranthes root, 牛膝)

Radix Aconiti (Chinese monkshood root, 烏頭)

Radix Aconiti Kusnezoffii (kusnezoff monkshood root, 草烏)

Radix Aconiti Nigri Praeparata (black baked monkshood root, 黑附子)

Radix Aconiti Praeparata (monkshood root, 附子)

Radix Actinidiae (actinida, 藤梨根)

Radix Adenophorae Strictae (straight ladybell root, 南沙參)

Radix Ampelopsis (Japanese ampelopsis, 白蘞)

Radix Angelicae Dahuricae (dahurian angelica root, 白芷)

Radix Angelicae Pubescentis (pubescent angelica root, 獨活)

Radix Angelicae Sinensis (Chinese angelica root, 當歸)

Radix Aristolochiae (dutchmanspipe root, 青木香)

Radix Arnebiae seu Lithospermi (purple gromwell root, 紫草)

Radix Asparagi (lucid asparagus root, 天門冬)

Radix Asteris (tatarian aster root, 紫菀)

Radix Astragali (milk veteh root, 黃芪)

Radix Aucklandiae (costus root, 木香)

Radix Boehmeriae (ramie root, 苧蔴根)

Radix Bupleuri (Chinese thorowax root, 紫胡)

Radix Clematidis (Chinese clematis root, 威靈仙)

Radix Codonopsis Pilosulae (pilose asiabell root, 黨參)

Radix Curcumae (aromatic turmeric, 鬱金)

Radix Cyathulae (cyathula root, 川牛膝)

Radix Cynanchi Atrati (swallow wort root, 白薇)

Radix Dichroae (antipyretic dichroa root, 常山)

Radix Dipsaci (Himalaya teasel root, 續斷)

Radix Ephedrae (Chinese ephedra root, 麻黃根)

Radix et Rhizoma Rhei (rhubarb root, 大黃)

Radix Euphorbiae Ebracteolatae (ebracteolate euphorbia root, 狼毒)

Radix Euphorbiae Kansui (kansui root, 甘遂)

Radix Euphorbiae Pekinensis (Peking spurge, 大戟)

Radix Gentianae (Chinese gentian, 龍膽草)

Radix Gentianae Macrophyllae (largeleaf gentian root, 秦艽)

Radix Ginseng (ginseng root, 人參)

Radix Ginseng Rubra (ginseng prepared with honey, 紅參)

Radix Ginseng Americana (American ginseng, 西洋參)

Radix Glehniae (glehnia root, 北沙參)

Radix Glycyrrhizae (licorice root, 甘草)

Radix Ilicis Pubescentis (hairy holly root, 毛冬青)

Radix Isatidis (Dyer's Woad root, 板蘭根)

Radix Ledebouriellae (ledebouriella root, 防風)

Radix Linderae (three-nerved spicebush root, 烏藥)

Radix Morindae Officinalis (morinda root, 巴戟天)

Radix Notoginseng (pseudo-ginseng root, 三七)

Radix Ophiopogonis (tuber of dwarf lilyturf, 麥冬)

Radix Paeoniae Alba (white peony root, 白芍)

Radix Paeoniae Rubra (red peony root, 赤芍)

Radix Peucedani (purple-flowered peucedanum root, 前胡)

Radix Phytolaccae (India pokeberry, 商陸)

Radix Platycodi (balloonflower root, 桔梗)

Radix Polygalae (polygala root, 遠志)

Radix Polygoni Multiflori (multiflower knotweed tuber, 何首烏)

Radix Pseudostellariae (pseudostellaria root, 太子參)

Radix Puerariae (pueraria root, 葛根)

Radix Pulsatillae (Chinese pulsatilla root, 白頭翁)
Radix Rehmannia (rehmannia root, 生地黄)
Radix Rhapontici seu Echinopsis (globethistle root, 漏蘆)
Radix Rubiae (madder root, 茜草)
Radix Salviae Miltiorrhizae (red sage root, 丹參)
Radix Sanguisorbae (garden burned root, 地楡)
Radix Saussureae Laphae (costus root, 廣木香)
Radix Scrophulariae (figwort root, 玄參)
Radix Scutellariae (skullcap root, 黄芩)
Radix Semiaquilegiae (semiaquilegia root, 天葵子)
Radix Sophorae Flavescentis (flavescent sophora root, 苦參)
Radix Sophorae Subprostratae (subprostrate sophora root, 山豆根)
Radix Stellariae (starwort root, 銀柴胡)
Radix Stemonae (stemona root, 百部)
Radix Stephaniae Tetrandrae (tetrandra root, 防己)
Radix Trichosanthis (snakegourd root, 天花粉)
Radix Veratrum Nigum (藜蘆)
Ramulus Cinnamomi (cassia twigs, 桂枝)
Ramulus Loranthi (parasitic loranthus, 桑寄生)
Ramulus Mori (white mulberry branch, 桑枝)
Ramulus Sophorae (Chinese scholartree twig, 槐枝)
Ramulus Uncariae cum Uncis (uncaria stem with hooks, 鈎藤)
Realgar (red orpiment, 雄黄)
Resina Draconis (dragon's blood resin, 血竭)
Resina Myrrhae (myrrh, 沒藥)
Resina Olibani (olibanum, 乳香)
Retinervus Citri Fructus (tangerine pith, 橘絡)
Retinervus Luffae Fructus (pith loofah, 絲瓜絡)
Rhizoma Acori Graminei (grass-leaved sweetflag rhizome, 石菖蒲)
Rhizoma Alismatis (oriental water plantain rhizome, 澤瀉)
Rhizoma Alpiniae Officinarum (lesser galangal rhizome, 高良薑)
Rhizoma Anemarrhenae (wind-weed rhizome, 知母)
Rhizoma Arisaematis (jack-in-the-pulpit, 天南星)
Rhizoma Atractylodis (Chinese atractylodes, 蒼朮)
Rhizoma Atractylodis Macrocephalae (large-headed atractylodes rhizome, 白朮)
Rhizoma Belamcandae (blackberry lily rhizome, 射干)
Rhizoma Bletillae (hyacinth bletilla, 白芨)
Rhizoma Cibotii (chain fern rhizome, 狗脊)
Rhizoma Cimicifugae (skunk bugbane rhizome, 昇麻)
Rhizoma Coptidis (Chinese coptis root, 黄連)
Rhizoma Corydalis (corydalis tuber, 延胡索)

Rhizoma Curculiginis (curculigo rhizome, 仙茅)
Rhizoma Curcumae Longae (turmeric rhizome, 薑黃)
Rhizoma Cynanchi Stauntoni (white swallowwort, 白前)
Rhizoma Cyperi (nutgrass flatsedge rhizome, 香附)
Rhizoma Oyrtomii (cyrtomium rhizome, 貫眾)
Rhizoma Dioscoreae (Chinese yam rhizome, 山藥)
Rhizoma Dioscoreae Hypoglaucae (yam rhizome, 萆薢)
Rhizoma Drynariae (drynaria rhizome, 骨碎補)
Rhizoma et Radix Ligustici (ligusticum root, 藁本)
Rhizoma Gastrodiae (elevated gastrodia tuber, 天麻)
Rhizoma Imperatae (cogongrass rhizome, 白茅根)
Rhizoma Ligustici Chuanxiong (chuanxiong rhizome, 川芎)
Rhizoma Paridis (Paris rhizome, 蚤休)
Rhizoma Phragmitis (common reed rhizome, 蘆根)
Rhizoma Picrorrhizae (胡黃連)
Rhizoma Pinelliae (Pinellia tuber, 半夏)
Rhizoma Polygonati (siberian solomonseal rhizome, 黃精)
Rhizoma Polygonati Odorati (solomonseal rhizome, 玉竹, 葳蕤)
Rhizoma Polygoni Cuspidati (giant knotweed, 虎杖)
Rhizoma seu Radix Notopterygii (notopterygium root, 羌活)
Rhizoma Smilacis Glabrae (smilax glabra rhizome, 土茯苓)
Rhizoma Sparganii (burreed rhizome, 三棱)
Rhizoma Typhonii (typhonium tuber, 白附子)
Rhizoma Zedoariae (zedoary turmeric rhizome, 莪术)
Rhizoma Zingiberis (dried ginger rhizome, 乾薑)
Rhizoma Zingiberis Praeparata (baked ginger, 炮薑)
Rhizoma Zingiberis Recens (fresh ginger, 生薑)
Sargassum (kelp, 海藻)
Scolopendra (centipede, 蜈蚣)
Scorpio (scorpion, 全蝎)
Semen Allii Tuberosi (seed of fragrant flowered garlic, 韭菜子)
Semen Alpiniae Katsumadai (katsumadai seed, 草豆蔻)
Semen Arecae (betel nut, 檳榔)
Semen Armeniacae Amarum (apricot kernel, 杏仁)
Semen Astragali Complanati (milkvetch seed, 沙苑子)
Semen Benincasae (wax gourd seed, 冬瓜子)
Semen Biotae (oriental arborvitae seed, 柏子仁)
Semen Caesalpiniae (caesalpinia, 石蓮子)
Semen Cannabis (cannabis seed, 麻子仁)
Semen Cardamomi Rotundi (round cardamon seed, 白豆蔻)
Semen Cassiae (sickle senna seed, 決明子)
Semen Celosiae (feather cockscomb seed, 青葙子)

Semen Citri Reticulatae (tangerine seed, 橘核)
Semen Coicis (Job's tears seed, 薏苡仁)
Semen Cucurbitae Moschatae (pumpkin seed, 南瓜子)
Semen Cuscutae (Chinese dodder seed, 菟絲子)
Semen Dolichoris Album (bean of white hyacinth dolichos, 白扁豆)
Semen Euryales (euryale seed, 芡實)
Semen Ginkgo (gingko-nut, 白菓)
Semen Glycine Max (black soybean, 黑大豆)
Semen Juglandis Regiae (walnut meat, 胡桃仁)
Semen Lepidii seu Descurainiae (pepperweed or flixweed tansymustard
    seed, 葶藶子)
Semen Litchi (lychee-pit, 荔枝核)
Semen Myristicae (nutmeg, 肉豆蔻)
Semen Nelumbinis (Hindu lotus seed, 蓮子)
Semen Oryzae Nonglutinosae (nonglutinous rice, 粳米)
Semen Persicae (peach kernel, 桃仁)
Semen Pharbitidis (morning glory seed, 牽牛子)
Semen Phaseoli (adsuki bean, 赤小豆)
Semen Phaseoli Radiatus (mung bean, 綠豆)
Semen Plantaginis (asiatic plantain seed, 車前子)
Semen Pruni (bush cherry seed, 鬱李仁)
Semen Raphani (Chinese radish seed, 萊菔子)
Semen Ricini (castor bean, 蓖麻子)
Semen Sesami (black sesame, 黑芝蔴, 胡蔴仁)
Semen Sinapis Albae (white mustard seed, 白芥子)
Semen Sojae Germinatum (soya bean roll, 豆卷)
Semen Sojae Praeparatum (fermented soya beans, 豆豉)
Semen Strychni (nuxvomica poison nut, 馬錢子)
Semen Torreyae (Chinese torreya seed, 榧子)
Semen Trichosanthis (Mongolian snakegourd seed, 瓜蔞仁)
Semen Vaccariae (cowherb seed, 王不留行)
Semen Ziziphi Spinosae (wild jujube seed, 酸棗仁)
Spica Prunellae (selfhead spica, 夏枯草)
Spica Schizonepetae (schizonepeta spike, 荊芥穗)
Spine Gleditsiae (honeylocust thorn, 皂角刺)
Spora Lygodii (climbing fern, 海金沙)
Squama Manitis (pangolin scale, 穿山甲)
Stamen Nelumbinis (hindu lotus stamen, 蓮鬚)
Stigma Maydis (corn stamen, 玉米鬚)
Styrax Liquidus (storax, 蘇合香)
Succinum (amber, 琥珀)
Succum Bambusae (Bamboo juice 竹瀝)

Tabanus Bivittatus (gadfly, 虻蟲)
Talcum (talc, 滑石)
Thallus Laminariae seu Eckloniae (dried thallus, 昆布)
Zaocys (black snake, 烏梢蛇)

Names of Prescriptions

Angelicae Decoction 當歸飲子
Angelica Decoction for Acting on the Kidney 歸腎丸
Angelica Decoction for Treating Cold Limbs 當歸四逆湯
Antiasthmatic Decoction 定喘湯
Astiphlogistic Powder (Decoction) of Schizonepeta and Ledebouriella 荊防敗毒散(湯)
Antitussive Powder 止嗽散
Bezoar Bolus for Clearing Away Heart-Fire 牛黃清心丸
Bezoar Resurrection Bolus 安宮牛黃丸
Big Pearls for Stopping Wind 大定風珠
Biliary Lithagogue Decoction 膽道排石湯
Black Plum Bolus 烏梅丸
Blood Regulation Decoction of Semen Persicae 桃仁承氣湯
Blood Tonifying Decoction of Angelicae 當歸補血湯
Bolus for Calming the Mind 安神定志丸
Bolus for Invigorating the Function of the Gallbladder 利膽丸
Bolus for Reinforcing Deficiency of Vital Essence (*yin*) of the Kidney 左歸丸
Bolus for Reinforcing Deficiency of Vital Function (*yang*) of the Kidney 右歸丸
Bolus for Reinforcing the Spleen 健脾丸
Bolus for Seminal Consolidation 固精丸
Bolus for Supporting Impregnation 贊育丸

Bolus for Tonifying the Kidney 腎氣丸
Bolus of Cuscutae 菟絲子丸
Bolus of Four Magical Herbs 四神湯(丸)
Bolus of Six Ingredients with Rehmannia 六味地黃丸
Bolus to Regulate the Functioning of the Spleen and Stomach 理中丸
Bupleuri Decoction for Soothing the Liver 柴胡疏肝湯
Burn Extract 燙傷油
Burn Oleol 燙傷油劑
Calculus-Expelling Decoction 排石湯
Channel Warming Decoction 溫經湯
Compound Salviae Injection 複方丹參注射液
Coptidis and Mume Decoction for Tranquilizing Ascarids 連梅安蛔湯
Coptidis Decoction for Warming the Gallbladder 黃連溫膽湯
Coronary Heart Disease Pills 冠心丸
Coronary Heart Disease Prescription II 冠心二號方
Cough-Relieving Syrup 寧嗽露
Crushing Pain Relieving Pills 寬胸丸
Decoction (Pills) for Acting on the Spleen 歸脾(丸)湯
Decoction for Adjusting the Flow of Vital Energy by Nourishing the Liver
    and Kidney 一貫煎
Decoction for Arthralgia 宣痹湯
Decoction for Checking Hyperactivity of the Liver and Subduing Endo-
    genous Wind 鎮肝熄風湯
Decoction (Bolus) for Checking Menstruation 固經湯(丸)
Decoction for Constipation due to Hypofunction of the Kidney 濟川煎
Decoction for Controlling Water 眞武湯
Decoction (Pills) for Destroying Worms 化蟲湯(丸)
Decoction for Dispersing Pathogenic Wind 消風湯(散)
Decoction for Eliminating Blood Stasis 通瘀煎
Decoction for Eliminating Summer Heat and Invigorating Vital Energy
    清暑益氣湯
Decoction for Enriching the Body Fluid 增液湯
Decoction for Expelling Phlegm 導痰湯
Decoction for Expelling Stones from the Bile Ducts 膽道排石湯
Decoction (Powder) for Invigorating the Pulse-Beat 生脈湯(散)
Decoction for Longevity and Normal Speech Ability 資壽解語湯
Decoction for Nourishing the Kidney 大補元煎
Decoction for Preserving Vital Essence 保陰煎
Decoction for Prevention of Miscarriage 胎元飲
Decoction for Promoting Blood Circulation and Relieving Cold Limbs
    通脈四逆湯
Decoction for Prostration with Cold Limbs 四逆湯

Decoction for Recovery by Activating Blood Circulation 復元活血湯

Decoction for Recuperating from Hemiplegia by Reinforcing Vital Energy 補陽還五湯

Decoction for Reinforcing Vital Energy and Strengthening the Spleen and Stomach 補中益氣湯

Decoction for Reinforcing Vital Function of the Kidney 右歸飲

Decoction for Relieving Generalized Pain Due to Blood Stasis 身痛逐瘀湯

Decoction (Powder) for Removing Blood Stasis 失笑湯(散)

Decoction for Removing Blood Stasis from the Chest 血腑逐瘀湯

Decoction for Removing Blood Stasis under the Thoracic Diaphragm 膈下逐瘀湯

Decoction for Removing Dampness from the Kidney 腎着湯

Decoction (Powder) for Removing Heat from the Bones 清骨湯(散)

Decoction for Removing Obstruction from the Five Internal Organs 五磨飲

Decoction for Removing Stagnant Blood and Promoting Hemogenesis 生化湯

Decoction for Restoring Lung Function by Clearing Pathogenic Heat 清燥救肺湯

Decoction for Restoring the Ability to Walk 顧步湯

Decoction (Bolus) for Seminal Consolidation 固精湯(丸)

Decoction for Strengthening the Chong Channel 固冲湯

Decoction for Supporting Impregnation 贊育丹

Decoction for Treating Leukorrhea 完帶湯

Decoction of Adenophorae and Ophiopogonis 沙參麥冬湯

Decoction of Agastachis for Dispelling Turbidity 藿香正氣湯

Decoction of Angelicae Pubescentis and Loranthi 獨活寄生湯

Decoction of Angelica Sinensis and Six Other Yellow Ingredients 當歸六黃湯

Decoction of Antelopis and Uncariae 羚羊鉤藤湯

Decoction of Artemisiae 茵陳蒿湯

Decoction (Bolus) of Atractylodis and Cyperi for Removing Phlegm 蒼附導痰湯(丸)

Decoction (Powder) of Atractylodis Macrocephalae and Paeoniae 白术芍藥湯(散)（又名痛瀉要方）

Decoction of Aurantii and Atractylodis 枳术湯

Decoction of Bupleuri, Aurantii, and Pinelliae 柴枳半夏湯

Combination of Bupleuri Decoction for Soothing the Liver, Decoction of Orange Peel and Pinellia, and Decoction of Four Noble Ingredients 柴胡舒肝湯, 二陳湯, 四君子湯合方

Decoction of Caryophyllii and Calyx Kaki 丁香柿蒂湯

Decoction of Caulis Allii and Seven Other Herbs 葱白七味散

Decoction of Caulis Phragmitis 葦莖湯

Decoction of Cephalanoploris 小薊飲子

Decoction of Chinghao and Scutellariae for Gallbladder Clearing 蒿芩清
膽湯

Decoction of Chinghao et Carapax Trionycis 青蒿鱉甲湯

Decoction of Cimicifuga and Puerariae 昇麻葛根湯

Decoction of Codonopsis (or Ginseng) and Perillae 參蘇飲

Decoction (Powder) of Codonopsis, Poria, and Atractylodis 參芩白朮
飲(散)

Decoction of Cornu Antelopis and Uncariae 羚羊鈎藤湯

Decoction of Cyperi and Inulae 香附旋復湯

Decoction of Eight Precious Ingredients 八珍湯

Decoction of Ephedra 麻黃湯

Decoction of Ephedra, Armeniacae, Gypsum, and Glycyrrhizae 麻杏石
甘湯

Decoction of Ephedra, Forsythia, and Phaseoli 麻黃連翹赤小豆湯

Decoction of Evodiae 吳茱萸湯

Decoction of Fermentata Medicinalis and Atractylodis in Combination
with Stomach Beneficial Bolus 神朮湯(散)合保和湯(丸)

Decoction of Five Detoxicants 五味消毒飲

Decoction (Powder) of Five Ingredients Including Poria 五苓湯(散)

Decoction of Four Herbs 四物湯

Decoction of Four Herbs with Persicae and Carthami 桃紅四物湯

Decoction (Bolus) of Four Magical Herbs 四神湯(丸)

Decoction of Four Miraculous Herbs for Relief of Disorders 四妙勇安湯

Decoction of Four Noble Ingredients 四君子湯

Decoction (Bolus) of Four Wonderful Herbs 四妙湯(丸)

Decoction (Powder) of Fritillariae and Trichosanthis 貝母瓜蔞湯(散)

Decoction of Gastrodiae and Uncariae 天麻鈎藤飲

Decoction of Gentianae to Purge the Liver 龍膽瀉肝湯

Decoction of Ginseng 獨參湯

Decoction of Ginseng and Aconiti 參附湯

Decoction of Ginseng and Aconiti, Draconis, and Ostrear 參附龍牡湯

Decoction (Bolus) of Ginseng and Antler 參茸補湯(丸)

Decoction of Ginseng (or Codonopsis) and Perillae 參蘇飲

Decoction of Glycyrrhizae Praeparata 灸甘草湯(復脈湯)

Decoction of Glycyrrhizae, Wheat, and Jujube 甘麥大棗湯

Decoction (Powder) of Ledebouriella for Dispersing Superficial Wind
防風通聖湯(散)

Decoction of Lilii for Strengthening the Lung 百合固金湯

Decoction of Lophatheri and Gypsum 竹葉石膏湯

Decoction (Powder) of Lonicera and Forsythia 銀翹湯(散)

Decoction of Loranthi 桑寄生湯
Decoction of Magnoliae with Two Other Herbs 原樸三物湯
Decoction of Mori and Armeniacae 桑杏湯
Decoction of Mori and Chrysanthemi 桑菊飲
Decoction of Nine Herbs Including Notopterygium 九味羌活湯
Decoction of Ophiopogonis 麥門冬湯
Decoction of Orange Peel and Pinellia 二陳湯
Decoction of Peels of Five Herbs 五皮飲
Decoction of Pericarpium Citri and Caulis Bambusae in Taenis 橘皮竹茹湯
Decoction of Pinelliae and Magnoliae 半夏厚樸湯
Decoction of Pinelliae, Atractylodes, and Gastrodiae 半夏白朮天麻湯
Decoction of Pinelliae for Dispelling Pathogenic Heat from the Heart 半夏瀉心湯
Decoction of Perillae to Bring Down Vital Energy 蘇子降氣湯
Decoction of Polygonatum Odoratum 葳蕤湯
Decoction of Poria, Cinnamomi, Atractylodis, and Glycyrrhizae 苓桂朮甘湯
Decoction of Puerariae, Scutellariae, and Coptidis 葛根苓連湯
Decoction of Pulsatillae 白頭翁湯
Decoction of Ramulus Cinnamomi 桂枝湯
Decoction of Rehmannia 地黃飲子
Decoction of Rhei and Aconiti 大黃附子湯
Decoction of Rhei and Cortex Moutan 大黃牡丹皮湯
Decoction of Rhinoceros Cornu and Rehmannia 犀角地黃湯
Decoction of Salviae 丹參飲
Decoction of Sargentodoxae 紅藤煎
Decoction of Schisandrae 五味子飲
Decoction of Six Ingredients with Rehmannia 六味地黃湯
Decoction of Stephaniae and Astragali 防己黃芪湯
Decoction of Ten Jujubes 十棗湯
Decoction of Three Kinds of Seeds 三仁湯
Decoction of Three Kinds of Seeds for the Benefit of the Parents 三子養親湯
Decoction of Trichosanthis, Allium, and Pinelliae 瓜蔞薤白半夏湯
Decoction of Trichosanthis, Allium, and Spiritus 瓜蔞薤白白酒湯
Decoction of Trionycis, Ostrease, and Manitis for Removing Blood Stasis 三甲化瘀湯
Decoction (Powder) of Two Wonderful Herbs in Combination with Decoction of Diuretic Ingredients 二妙合八正湯(散)
Decoction of Ziziphi Spinosae 酸棗仁湯
Decoction to Replenish Vital Essence and Remove Pathogenic Factors from the Lung 養陰清肺湯

Detoxicant Decoction for Universal Relief 普濟消毒飲
Detoxicant Decoction of Coptidis 黃連解毒湯
Detoxicant Manna Decoction (Pills) 甘露消毒飲（丹）
Dioscoreae Decoction to Eliminate Damp-Turbidity 萆薢分清飲
Drastic Purgative Decoction 大承氣湯
Dysmenorrhea Powder 痛經散
Ease Decoction with Moutan and Gardeniae 丹梔消遙散
Ease Powder 消遙散
Fetus-Easing Decoction 聖愈湯
Fetus-Saving Decoction (Bolus) 壽胎湯（丸）
Gallbladder-Warming Decoction 溫膽湯
Ginseng Nutrition Decoction (Pills) 人參養營湯（丸）
Golden Bolus for Seminal Consolidation 金鎖固精丸
Green Moth Pills 青蛾丸
Jade Goddess Decoction 玉女煎
Jade Powder 碧玉散
Jade Screen Powder (Decoction) 玉屏風散（湯）
Magic Decoction for Rescuing Life 仙方活命飲
Magnolia Decoction to Warm the Spleen and Stomach 厚樸溫中湯
Magnolia Decoction with Seven Ingredients 厚樸七物湯
Major Bolus for Activating Blood Flow in Channels 大活絡丹
Major Decoction (Bolus) for Tonifying Vital Essence 大補陰湯（丸）
Major Decoction of Bupleurum 大柴胡湯
Mild Pills for Activating Blood Flow in Channels 小活絡丹
Mind-Easing Decoction (Pills) 補心湯（丹）
Minor Blue Dragon Decoction 小青龍湯
Minor Decoction for Functional Restoration of the Spleen and Stomach 小建中湯
Minor Decoction of Bupleurum 小柴胡湯
Minor Purgative Decoction 小承氣湯
Mixture of Chuanxiong with Tea 川芎茶調散
Notopterygium Decoction for Eliminating Dampness 羌活勝濕湯
Nourishing Kidney Bolus 濟生腎氣丸
Nutrient System Clearing Decoction 清營湯
Phlegm Eliminating Pills of Chloriteschist 礞石滾痰丸
Phragmitis Decoction Worth a Thousand Pieces of Gold 千金葦莖湯
Pills for Acting on the Spleen 歸脾丸
Pills for Clearing Away Heat and Phlegm 清氣化痰丸
Pills for Controlling Phlegm-Fluid 控涎丹
Pills for Consolidating semen with Three Herbs 三才封髓丹
Pills (Pulvis) of Alpiniae and Cyperus 艮附丸（散）
Pills of Aucklandiae and Arecae 木香檳榔丸

Pills of Coptis and Evodia 左金丸(萸連丸)
Pills of Four Fresh Herbs 四生丸
Pills of Rhei and Eupolyphuga 大黄䗪蟲丸
Pills of Rhinoceros Gallstone 犀黃丸
Pills of Scutellariae and Allii 芩蒜丸
Pills of Six Magic Ingredients 六神丸
Pills of Tangerine Seed 橘核丸
Pills of Three Herbs for Emergency 三物備急丸
Placenta Compound Restorative Pills 河車大造丸
Placenta Pills 胎盤丸
Powder for Clearing Away Stomach Heat 清胃散
Powder for Cold Limbs 四逆散
Powder for Correcting Facial Deviation 牽正散
Powder for Dispelling Heat from the Heart Channel 導赤散
Powder for Inducing Lactation 生乳散
Powder for Nourishing Viscera 眞人養臟散
Powder for Regulating the Function of the Stomach 平胃散
Powder for Removing Blood Stasis 失笑散
Powder for Removing Heat from the Bones 清骨散
Powder for the Welling Up of Lactation 下乳涌泉散
Powder of Agastachis for Dispelling Turbidity 藿香正氣散
Powder of Bitter Armeniacae and Perillae 杏蘇散
Powder of Five Ingredients Including Poria 五苓散
Powder of Lonicera and Forsythia 銀翹散
Powder of Ten Burnt Herbs 十灰散
Powder of Two Wonderful Ingredients 二妙散
Prescription for Extrauterine Gestation 宮外孕方
Priceless Treasure Pills 至寶丹
Pulse-Activating Decoction of Trionycis, Ostreae, and Manitis 三甲復
    脈湯
Pulvis Atractylodes and Paeonia 白朮芍藥散
Pulvis Elsholtzia 香薷散
Pulvis Ginseng for Antiphlogistic 人參敗毒散
Pulvis Mantis 桑螵蛸粉
Pulvis Meliae 金鈴子散
Pulvis Ostreae 牡蠣散
Pulvis Sophorae 槐花散
Purgative Decoction for Enriching the Body Fluid 增液承氣湯
Purple Snowy Powder 紫雪散
Recipe for Coughing Blood 咳血方
Rehabilitation Powder 再造散
Rehmannia Decoction (Bolus) of Anemarrhenae and Phellodendri 知柏地

黃湯(丸)
Rehmannia Decoction (Bolus) of Lycii and Chrysanthemum 杞菊地黃湯(丸)
Renewed Decoction of Elsholtzia 新加香薷飲
Restoring Kidney Decoction (Pills) Prescribed by the Golden Chamber 金匱腎氣湯(丹)
Royal Pills for Mind Easing 天王補心丹
Scrofula Bolus 清瘰丸
Sedative Cinnabar Bolus 朱砂安神丸
Semen Cannabis Bolus 麻子仁丸
Ship and Cart Pills 舟車丸
Six to One Powder 六一散
Siegesbeckiae and Clerodendri Pills 豨桐丸
Spleen Strengthening Decoction 實脾飲
Spleen-Warming Decoction 溫脾湯
Stomach Beneficial Bolus (Decoction) 保和丸(湯)
Stomachic Decoction of Poria 胃苓湯
Storax Bolus 蘇合香丸
Two Fairies Decoction 二仙湯
Universal Tonic Bolus (Decoction) with Ten Ingredients 十全大補丸(湯)
Vital Function Regulation Decoction 陽和湯
White-Tiger Decoction 白虎湯
Wind-Eliminating Powder 消風散
Yellow Dragon Decoction 黃龍湯
Yellow Golden Pulvis 如意金黃散

SELECTED BIBLIOGRAPHY

Annotated Collection of Prescriptions 醫方集解. Wang Ang 汪昂, 1682.

The Book of History 尚書. Confucius 孔子, 551–479 B.C.

Canon of Acupuncture 針經. (Also known as *Miraculous Pivot*, see below.)

A Classic of Acupuncture and Moxibustion 針灸甲乙經. Huangfu Mi 皇甫謐, 259.

Classic of Categories 類經. Zhang Jiebin 張介賓, 1624.

Classic of Internal Medicine 內經. Unknown author, c. 475–221 B.C.

Classic on Medical Problems 難經. Authorship ascribed to Qin Yueren 秦越人, c. 1st–2d century B.C.

    "The Sixty-First Problem" 六十一難.

    "The Sixty-Ninth Problem" 六十九難.

A Collection of Case Histories of Traditional Chinese Medicine 中醫醫話集錦. Pan Yangzhi 潘養之, Chen Jiayang 陳家揚, Pei Shenyi 裴慎醫, and Feng Jinming 馮金明. Gansu: Gansu People's Publishing House, 1981.

A Collection of Case Records by Dr. Yue Meizhong 岳美中醫案集. Academy of Traditional Chinese Medicine 中醫研究院. Beijing: People's Medical Publishing House, 1978.

Compendium of Materia Medica 本草綱目. Li Shizhen 李時珍, 1590.

Confucians' Duties to Their Parents 儒門事親. Zhang Congzheng 張從正, 1228.

Danxi's Experimental Therapy 丹溪心法. Zhu Danxi 朱丹溪, 1347.

Discussion of Cold-Induced Diseases 傷寒雜病論. (This book was originally a part of *Discussion of Cold-Induced and Miscellaneous Diseases*.)

Discussion of Cold-Induced and Miscellaneous Diseases 傷寒論. Zhang Zhongjing 張仲景, 219.

Disease Etiology According to Traditional Chinese Medicine 中醫病理研究. Kuang Tiaoyuan 匡調元, 1980.

Essentials of Correlation of Traditional Chinese and Western Medicines 中西滙通

醫經精義. Tang Zonghai 唐宗海, 1892.

Essentials of the Four Classics 四經心源. Huang Yuanyu 黃元御, 1753.

General Collection of Wise Healing 聖濟總錄. The Imperial Medical Institute, 1111–1117.

The General Treatise on Etiology and Symptoms 諸病源候論. Chao Yuanfang 巢元方, 610.

Illustrated Supplement to the Classic of Categories 類經圖翼. Zhang Jiebin 張介賓, 1624.

Insights into Traditional Chinese Surgery 中醫外科心得. Zhao Shanghua 趙尚華. Shanxi: Shanxi People's Publishing House, 1982.

Instructions to Coroners 洗冤錄. Song Ci 宋慈, 1247.

Jingyue's Complete Works 景岳全書.

"Treatise on the Common Cold" 傷風論. Zhang Jingyue 張景岳, 1624.

Journal of the Beijing College of Traditional Chinese Medicine 北京中醫學院學報 (1982), no. 4, "The Treatment of Nephrotic Syndrome" 腎病綜合症的治療. Liu Yanchi 劉燕池.

Journal of Traditional Chinese Medicine 中醫雜誌 (1964), no. 6. "The Treatment of Coronary Atherosclerotic Heart Disease" 冠心病的治療. Liu Yanchi 劉燕池.

Liu Fengwu's Experience in Gynecology 劉奉五婦科經驗. Beijing College of Traditional Chinese Medicine 北京中醫學院. Beijing: People's Medical Publishing House, 1977.

Medical Experiences of Dr. Pu Fuzhou 蒲輔周醫療經驗. Academy of Traditional Chinese Medicine 中醫研究院. Beijing: People's Medical Publishing House, 1976.

Miraculous Pivot 靈樞.

"Special Treatise on the Five Disorders of the Body Fluid" 五癃津液別篇.

"A Synopsis of Diagnostic Observations of Appearance and Color" 形色外診簡摩.

"Treatise on the Analysis of Yin-Yang in 25 Different Individuals" 陰陽二十五人.

"Treatise on the Channels and Collaterals" 經脈篇.

"Treatise on the Comparison of Channels to Rivers" 經水篇.

"Treatise on Defensive Energy" 衛氣論.

"Treatise on Exogenous Pathogenic Factors and Their Treatment" 邪客篇.

"Treatise on Fasting" 平人絕穀篇.

"Treatise on Functions" 官能篇.

"Treatise on the Intestines and Stomach" 腸胃篇.

"Treatise on the Length of Vessels" 脈度篇.

"Treatise on Longevity of the Firm or Gentle Disposition" 壽夭剛柔論.

"Treatise on Mental and Life Activity" 本神篇.

"Treatise on the Original Organs" 本臟篇.

"Treatise on the Pathology and Etiology of Visceral Diseases" 邪氣臟腑病形篇.

"Treatise on the Primary Occurrence of Diseases" 百病始生篇.

"Treatise on the Seas" 海論篇.

"Treatise on the Variations of *Qi* During the Day" 順氣一日爲四時篇.

Newly Revised Materia Medica 新修草本. Su Jing et al. 蘇敬等, 659.

Notes on Medicine 讀醫隨筆.

"Essay on the Ascending, Descending, Entering, and Exiting of *Qi*" 昇降出入論. Zhou Xuehai 周學海, 1891.

On the Origin and Source of Medicine 醫學源流論. Xu Lingtai 徐靈胎, 1764.

The Origin of Medicine 醫學原始. Wang Honghan 王宏翰, 1688.

Peaceful Holy Benevolent Prescriptions 太平聖惠方. Wang Huaiyin 王懷隱, 992.

Plain Questions 素問.

"Further Discussions of the Five *Zhang* Organs" 五臟別論.

"General Treatise on Essential Principles" 至眞要大論.

"Treatise on Abrupt Pains" 擧痛論.

"Treatise on Acupuncture" 刺法論. (In the Addendum to *Plain Questions* 素問遺篇.)

"Treatise on Communication of Vitality with Heaven" 生氣通天論.

"Treatise on the Correspondence Between Man and the Universe" 陰陽應象大論.

"Treatise on the Correspondence of the Skin to the Channels" 皮部論.

"Treatise on Deficiency and Excess" 通評虛實論.

"Treatise on the Division and Junction of *Yin* and *Yang*" 陰陽離合論.

"Treatise on Essential Laws of Disease Occurrence" 金匱眞言論.

"Treatise on the Feebleness of Limbs" 痿論.

"Treatise on Fevers" 評熱病論.

"Treatise on the Five Circuit Phase" 五運行大論.

"Treatise on How to Keep Healthy" 寶命全形篇.

"Treatise on the Matching of the Circuit Phases and Climatic Factors" 六元正紀大論.

"Treatise on Natural Essence in Ancient Times" 上古天眞論.

"Treatise on the Organ Picture" 六節臟象論.

"Treatise on the Regulation of Channels" 調經論.

"Treatise on the Relationship Between Outward Manifestations and the *Zang* Organs" 五臟生成論.

"Treatise on Seasonal Changes and Vitality" 八正神明論.

"Treatise on the Six Climatic Factors" 六微旨大論.

Practical Traditional Chinese Internal Medicine 實用中醫內科學. Luo Guojun

羅國鈞. Shanxi: Shanxi People's Publishing House, 1981.

Prescriptions Worth a Thousand Pieces of Gold 千金要方. Sun Simiao 孫思邈, 682.

The Pulse Classic 脈經. Wang Shuhe 王叔和, 265–317.

The Pulse Studies of Binhu 瀕湖脈學. Li Shizhen 李時珍, 1564.

Selected Case Records 醫案選編. Longhua Hospital (affiliated with Shanghai College of Traditional Chinese Medicine) 上海中醫學院附屬龍華醫院. Shanghai: Shanghai People's Publishing House, 1977.

Selected Successful Case Records of Traditional Doctors 中醫臨床驗案選編. Beijing Traditional Chinese Medical Hospital. Beijing: Beijing Institute of Traditional Chinese Medicine, 1965.

Shanghai Veteran Traditional Doctors' Experiences 上海老中醫經驗選編. Li Zunwu 李遵五. Shanghai Bureau of Health 上海衞生局. Shanghai: Scientific and Technical Publishing House of Shanghai, 1980.

Shen Nong's Herbal 神農本草經. Unknown author, c. 1st century B.C.

Shen's Work on the Importance of Life Preservation 沈氏尊生書. Shen Jinao 沈金鰲, 1773.

"The Causes of Miscellaneous Diseases" 染病源流犀燭.

Sub-Systematic Classic of Categories 類經附翼. Zhang Jiebin 張介賓, 1624.

A Supplement to the Compendium of Materia Medica 本草綱目拾遺. Zhao Xuemin 趙學敏, 1765.

Supplement to the Prescriptions Worth a Thousand Pieces of Gold 千金翼方. Sun Simiao 孫思邈, 682.

Synopsis of the Golden Chamber 金匱要略. Zhang Zhongjing 張仲景, 219.

The Treasured Classic 中藏經. Unknown author; attributed to Hua Tuo 華陀, during the Six Dynasties, c. 317–618.

A Treatise on Alchemy 抱樸子. Ge Hong 葛洪, 320.

Treatise on Spleen and Stomach 脾胃論. Li Dongyuan 李東垣, 1249.

Universal Prescriptions 普濟方. Zhu Su 朱橚, 1406.

Veteran Traditional Doctors' Experiences in Beijing 北京老中醫經驗選編. Guan Youbo 關幼波 and Wang Hongshi 王鴻士. Beijing: Beijing Publishing House, 1980.

INDEX

Entries followed by "t" denote tables. English common names of medicinal herbs are listed in appendix A.

liver and, 33
viral hepatitis and, 347
Encephalitis
acupuncture and, 364
case history, 365
children and, 356
collapse syndrome, 360
damp-heat and, 359
differentiation of symptom-complexes, 359
etiology, 356
extreme heat and, 360
Japanese B, 63t, 356-66
summer fever and, 356
treatment of, 357, 363-65
vital energy and, 362
vital essence and, 362
wind and, 361
Enteritis, acute, 62t; *see also* Gastroenteritis
Enuresis
infantile, 145t
kidney and, 132t, 147t
Environment, prescription composition and, 12-14, 153
Ephedrae, Herba, 152-53
asthma and, 49t
decoction of, 152, 159t, 163t
Ephedrae, Radix, spontaneous perspiration, 142t
Epidemic(s), 346; *see also* specific disease
Epidemic parotitis, *see* Mumps
Epilepsy
aromatic stimulants and, 91
resucitation and, 36
treatment of, 71t, 91t, 94-95t, 101t, 126t
Epimedii, Herba, arthalgia and, 131t
Epistaxis, 51t, 97t, 104t, 120t, 154
Equilibrium, 1-4
Eriobotriae, Folium, vomiting and, 74t
Erysipelas, 58t, 63t
Esophagus, cancer of, 122-24t
Eucommiae, Cortex, back pain and, 132t
Eupatorii, Herba, dampness resolving and, 78t
Euphorbiae Kan Sui, Radix
incompatibility, 129t
purgatives and, 88t
Euphorbiae Pekinensis, Radix
incompatibility, 129t
purgatives and, 89t
Euryales, Semen
chronic diarrhea and, 146t

urination and, 146t
Evacuants, indigestion and, 80; *see also* Purgatives
Evodiae, Fructus, 153
chronic diarrhea and, 93t
stomach warming and, 185t
Expectorants, 32, 70; *see also* Phlegm
Eyes
blurred vision, 134t, 147t
cataracts, 140t
improving of, 53t
infections of, 64t, 67-68t, 97t
night-blindness, 79t

Facial Deviation, powder for, 230t
Fallopian tubes, salpingitis and, 400-4
Farfarae, Flos, antitussives/antiasthmatics, 76t
Fatigue, viral hepatitis and, 347
Fear, hypertension and, 283
Febrifugal prescriptions, 25, 34, 176-84t, 219-20t
Febrile conditions, 10
bleeding with, 58-60t
Fetus
development of, 377
movement of, 396
Fever
acupuncture and, 253
blood and, 250, 253
case history of, 254
causes of, 248
diagnosis and treatment of, 248
internal injury and, 247, 253
prescriptions for, 183-84t
symptom-complexes of, 249
vital energy and, 250-53
vital essence and, 249, 251
Fire, hypertension and, 282
Flavors, of herbs, 45
Food
diarrhea and, 276
digestion of, 80t, 216-17t, 276
insomnia and, 331
overeating, 340
poisoning, 129t
retention of, 80t
stagnancy, 31
viral hepatitis, 347
see also Digestion
Forsythiae, Fructus
decoction of, 162t